The Fasting Fix

life

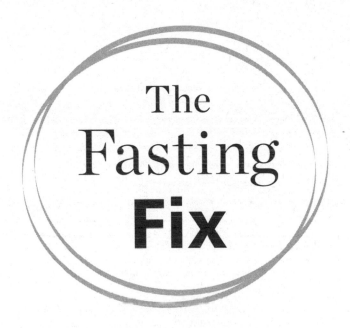

The Fasting Fix

Eat Smarter, Fast Better, Live Longer

Andreas Michalsen, MD, PHD

with Suzann Kirschner-Brouns

PENGUIN LIFE

VIKING
An imprint of Penguin Random House LLC
penguinrandomhouse.com

Originally published in German as *Mit Ernährung Heilen* by Insel Verlag Berlin, in 2019.
Copyright © 2019 by Insel Verlag Berlin. The German language
edition was edited by Friedrich-Karl Sandmann.

First English language edition published by Viking in 2020.

Translated from German by Laura Wagner.

English translation copyright © 2020 by Andreas Michalsen and Insel Verlag Berlin.

A Penguin Life Book

LIBRARY OF CONGRESS CATALOGING-IN-PUBLICATION DATA
Names: Michalsen, Andreas, author. | Kirschner-Brouns, Suzann, author.
Title: The fasting fix : eat smarter, fast better, live longer /
Andreas Michalsen, MD, PhD with Suzann Kirschner-Brouns.
Other titles: Mit Ernährung heilen. English
Description: First edition. | New York : Viking, [2020] |
This work was originally published in German as Mit Ernährung Heilen
by Insel Verlag Berlin, translated from German by Laura Wagner. |
Includes bibliographical references and index.
Identifiers: LCCN 2020027162 (print) | LCCN 2020027163 (ebook) |
ISBN 9781984880154 (hardcover) | ISBN 9781984880161 (ebook)
Subjects: LCSH: Fasting—Therapeutic use. | Diet therapy. |
Chronic diseases—Alternative treatment.
Classification: LCC RM226.5 .M5313 2020 (print) |
LCC RM226.5 (ebook) | DDC 615.8/54—dc23
LC record available at https://lccn.loc.gov/2020027162
LC ebook record available at https://lccn.loc.gov/2020027163

Printed in the United States of America
1 3 5 7 9 10 8 6 4 2

Book design by Daniel Lagin

Contents

Part Three

Fast Easier, Live Longer: The Healing
and Preventive Effect of Therapeutic Fasting
and Intermittent Fasting

Part Four

Healing Through Nutrition and Fasting:
My Therapeutic Program for a Healthy Life

Introduction

For ten years, I have been head of the department of internal and complementary medicine at Immanuel Hospital Berlin and a professor of clinical complementary medicine at Charité university medical center in Berlin—and right now, the health care practice I find most important, both personally and professionally, is nutrition. But I didn't always believe this. Growing up, I had learned that following a healthy diet should be considered a part of medicine. I absorbed this from my parents, particularly from my father, a doctor who focused on complementary medicine. In spite of this upbringing, I ate fast food and sweets, and even smoked during my time as a medical resident and during all those long nights working shifts in the intensive care unit and going out on emergency calls with ambulances. Vegetables and salads were rarely part of my diet; meals just had to be quick and filling. I got my comeuppance in my early thirties when an occupational medical exam showed that I had high blood pressure and significantly elevated blood lipid levels. My colleague advised me to change my lifestyle. Having witnessed many patients suffering from heart attacks and strokes, both of which are often consequences of an unhealthy diet or lifestyle, I took my colleague's advice to heart. I adopted a Mediterranean diet and quit smoking. Six months later, my blood pressure, cholesterol levels, and triglyceride levels were back to normal.

I began to consider how we should actually be researching and teaching patients how to use proper nutrition to protect ourselves from illnesses early on. In the department for internal medicine where I was working at the time, I shifted my clinical and scientific research to focus on developing specific lifestyle programs for patients, to prevent cardiovascular disease. Eventually, I turned to the field of complementary medicine. I was astonished to learn about the health benefits that could be achieved with a change in diet, especially when combined with therapeutic fasting. I examined the effects of fasting and healthy eating in clinical studies and wanted to understand the causes of these healthy effects. In 2008, researchers studying aging (and antiaging) arrived at the conclusion that there is no single drug or medical measure that can promise a long and healthy life. There is only one way: fasting![1] Inspired, I got in touch with scientists and fasting researchers all around the world. Together, we cultivated fruitful exchanges and nurtured an intense scientific occupation around the question: How is fasting able to prolong life in such a unique way?

When I considered my medical experience alongside new research, it became clear that fasting and eating fit together like lock and key. Through regular therapeutic fasting, intermittent fasting, and a mostly plant-based diet with few processed foods, we can prevent most chronic diseases. Fasting and eating complement each other perfectly. Research on fasting has revealed impressive findings and therapeutic success with thousands of patients, suggesting that combining regular fasting with healthy eating is the best thing we can do for our body.[2, 3]

The purpose of this book is to show you how you can eat better and fast easily and correctly, in order to improve your quality of life, achieve better health, and ultimately live longer.

I would like not only to convince you to engage with your diet and your health but also to give you the tools you need to actively take care of your health, because it is in your hands!

Do not rely on medications and procedures that only fight the symptoms. You have the power to address the root cause of illness. Seventy percent of the chronic diseases that we suffer from as we get older are partly caused by the wrong diet.[4] The long-term "Global Burden of Disease" study has shown that genes and medical care play only a small role in our health and, in fact, nutrition and lifestyle are the decisive factors in most chronic diseases.[5]

Hippocrates, the forefather of medicine, put nutrition and *díaita* (healing through lifestyle) at the center of all his therapies. Modern medicine recognizes the relationship between nutrition, lifestyle, and healing, yet even so, many doctors continue to push for medications and procedures that are expensive and come with numerous side effects: antihypertensive medications for high blood pressure, antidiabetic drugs for diabetes, anti-inflammatory drugs for inflammation, and statins for elevated levels of blood lipids. Obesity is more and more often treated with surgical procedures.

Counteracting and preventing diseases through nutrition and fasting, on the other hand, doesn't cost much—and it's highly effective for your health. Fasting should have a permanent place in our lives once more, as it did for our ancestors. After years of research, I decided to adopt a completely vegetarian diet—partly for health reasons, but also because I'm convinced that this is the diet that will ensure our planet's future.

Food is many things: a physical requirement for life, culture, enjoyment. But it's also a habit, and in some circumstances, it's an addiction. It can affect our body in so many ways. If we know how to engage with food correctly, it is pure medicine and pleasure together—and thus the best way to lead a long and healthy life.

ANDREAS MICHALSEN, MD, PHD

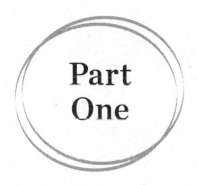

Part One

Our Evolution, Our Gut, Our Metabolism

Humanity's Evolutionary
Relationship with Food—
and How It Went Wrong

Chapter One

Rediscovering the Natural and Healthy Rhythm of Eating

Up until roughly ten thousand years ago, our ancestors roamed the earth as hunter-gatherers without a permanent home. They collected berries, seeds, roots, and mushrooms, hunted rabbits or buffalo. Gathering was more essential than hunting, because fruit, seeds, and insects covered most of their daily calorie needs and provided important vitamins and minerals. It is believed that meeting this daily caloric requirement took three to six hours of work.[1]

Once humans harnessed the power of fire, they were able to consume many parts of plants that had previously been inedible, broadening their diets considerably. Though scientists haven't been able to determine exactly when mankind learned to light fires, it's likely that even prehistoric humans such as *Homo erectus* were able to utilize natural fires caused by lightning as early as a million years ago. In any case, heating plants dissolved fibrous components and destroyed many toxins. It seems plausible, therefore, that many foods were made more digestible by being heated, and that this was beneficial to a person's health—which is still true today.

For a long time, it was undisputedly assumed that the consumption

Raw Foods

Nutrition experts and naturopaths have long been debating whether raw foods are healthy, and if so, in what quantity. The fact is that heating, chewing, and insalivating food relieves the gastrointestinal tract of a large share of its work. Heating food has likely protected people from infections in the past, and has therefore prevailed throughout evolution. But it is doubtful that, given the optimal storage and refrigeration options we have in our modern world, we still need to heat up everything we eat. Nevertheless, it's interesting to note that the bacteria required in our intestine to digest raw food are different than those needed to digest cooked food.[2] Where raw foods are concerned, my opinion is that everyone should decide for themselves, depending on their physical constitution, health, and tolerance. If, for example, your body is weakened due to an illness, your digestive tract is usually also affected. In that case, I would advise eating steamed or warmed-up meals rather than raw foods to relieve the stomach and the intestine.

of meat was of vital importance for the brain to increase in size, and therefore a crucial step in mankind's development. This was suggested by archaeological discoveries in Africa, which showed that the brain increased in weight just as early man left the African jungle behind and relocated to steppe-like regions. Where our ancestors had mainly been following a plant-based diet before, they now had to change their diet according to their new environment. In this new environment, they consumed desert hares and other animals, because these dry regions lacked fruit-bearing trees and bushes. This, at least, was the assumption for a long time. Since then researchers have come to the realization that this reasoning was faulty: Although nowadays we classify the regions to which early man migrated as steppe or even desert, at the time, these regions were in fact covered by forest.[3] As a result, the theory linking meat consumption and growth in brain size is no longer very convincing. It seems reasonable to say now that even if prehistoric man was an omnivore, meat was a rarity on his menu.

The diet of our ancestors was ideal from an evolutionary point of view: It was mainly plant based, and above all, it was highly diverse.[4] Excavations have shown that the hunter-gatherers of the Stone Age rarely suffered from malnutrition—they were larger in size and of better health than their descendants who had settled down.[5] Moreover, *Homo sapiens* of the time were very flexible. If there was a drought in one area, they simply moved on; if one food item became inedible due to a pest infestation, they just ate something else.[6] For this reason, the Stone Age hunter-gatherers were "the original affluent society," as they say, because they lived exceptionally well.[7] In addition to their balanced diets, they lived in communities without any major stress factors—at the very least, they never had to work to the point of burnout. They were in the fresh air all day and got plenty of exercise.

Of course, this doesn't mean that life wasn't hard, especially in regard to the lack of medical care. Nevertheless, I'd like to draw special attention to the dietary habits of the hunter-gatherers: largely plant based and diverse. This is similar to the traditional diets in the so-called Blue Zones—regions of the world where people live to an unusually old age while still remaining healthy.

It's also important to note the natural rhythm of food intake followed in the Stone Age. Nature dictated what and when people ate. If you found a bush laden with berries, you ate as many berries as you could; if you killed an animal, you ate it straightaway. Once an area had nothing more to give, you moved on. Sometimes you had to manage without food for days. Once the sun set, you went to bed. After sunrise, there was no breakfast waiting for you; you had to go out and procure it. The nearest source of food could be far away and hard to reach.

Allowing Your Digestive System to Rest

For tens of thousands of years, humans had to grapple with short and long periods of hunger. But this didn't seem to be a problem for our bodies. In fact, today we know that our cells recover and initiate repair mechanisms when our body is denied food for an extended period of time.[8]

When humans started to settle down—cultivating land, farming livestock, storing food for winter—they gained the ability to counter nature's unpredictability. Questions such as "What are we going to eat?" and "When are we going to eat?" became less of an issue. Even though people were plagued by famine due to occasional crop failures, and life became more exhausting because they had to toil in the fields and the stables from morning to night, there were now more regular meals than before. However, through the systematic cultivation of agricultural crops, food diversity was gradually lost. At the same time, people ate more animal protein (meat and dairy products).[9]

This process continued until the industrial revolution radically changed our dietary habits even more. Electricity, refrigerators, and fast transportation gave people almost unlimited access to food. Today, people in many areas of the world have the means to eat whatever they want, whenever they want. At first glance this seems like a victory over the unpredictability of nature; a second glance, however, reveals that this is a major problem for the biology of the human body.

Modern progress, particularly in the food industry, has actually had a negative effect on our genes and cells. The ancient program— eating, followed by periods of starvation, followed by eating—is still deeply rooted within them. There are a few recent genetic adaptations and changes in our body, but they are rare. Europeans, for example, have developed the ability to digest cow's milk over the past ten thousand years because of the advent of cattle farming. The enzyme lactase, which breaks down lactose, enables many people of European descent to consume cow's milk without getting stomach cramps.[10]

Disregarding the Needs of Our Metabolism

Other than a few adaptations, our digestive and metabolic systems have remained nearly unchanged for a hundred thousand years.[11] Change simply wasn't necessary. Over the course of evolution, the human organism has always been smart. It has continually tried to find the best path to remaining healthy in periods of both hunger and abundance.

But our bodies are completely overwhelmed by our twenty-first-century lifestyle. Modern methods of transportation and refrigeration allow for a permanent availability of food from around the world, at any time of the year. There has been a proliferation of industrially processed foods with numerous artificial additives, too much sugar, and too much salt. Moreover, consuming meat every day is another modern achievement our body's ancient metabolic system is unable to handle.

The problem is not just excess supply, but also how often we eat. Most of us are accustomed to eating even when we're not hungry, simply because we can. Food is always available in the affluent society in which we live: a little morning snack here, a coffee to go there, a piece of candy from the reception desk in the office, a slice of cake from the cafeteria in the afternoon, or a smoothie because it's "healthy."

What's perhaps most surprising is that in spite of the abundance of food available to us, what we're consuming is not only not healthy enough but also not diverse enough. In other words, we're eating too many carbohydrates, too much animal protein, and too many un-healthy fats and additives.

The Dramatic Increase of Chronic Diseases

We can all see and feel the consequences of our current way of eating. Cases of obesity- and diet-related diseases such as hypertension, arthrosis, diabetes, atherosclerosis, renal insufficiency, and back pain have been increasing dramatically for years.[12]

The most common chronic diseases throughout the Western world—and increasingly also in Asia and Africa—are arthrosis, rheumatism,

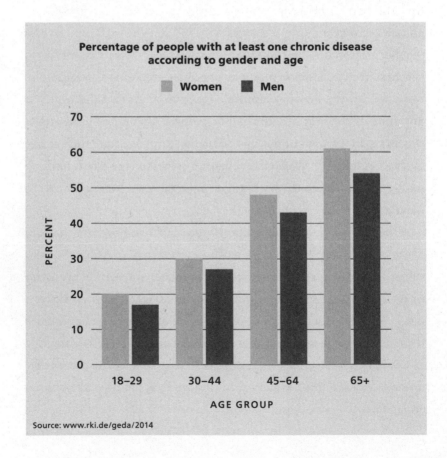

Percentage of people with at least one chronic disease according to gender and age

Source: www.rki.de/geda/2014

hypertension, diabetes, cardiovascular diseases such as coronary heart disease and stroke, respiratory disorders, and cancer. A study conducted by the Robert Koch Institute showed that 43 percent of women and 38 percent of men in Germany suffer from at least one chronic disease. With increasing age, the frequency of disease also increases. After the age of sixty-five, there is often the possibility of having multiple chronic diseases, regardless of gender.

Diet-related diseases, however, are not a biological fate. They've become an epidemic only because of our lifestyle and dietary habits.

Healing Chronic Diseases Through Nutrition

There have been enormous successes in the medical field over the past two hundred years. Through prevention, hygiene, vaccinations, and the effective treatment of infections and injuries we are now able to treat and cure many acute and severe diseases. Infant mortality has dropped drastically across the globe, and we're generally living longer and with better medical care. On the other hand, modern medicine lacks sustainable treatment plans for the epidemic of chronic diseases that are connected to the way we eat. Countless researchers are trying to develop innovative medications to try to fight these effects. But medications are never as perfectly tailored to our bodies as healthy eating and exercise.

Doctors and pharmacologists, for example, have found ways to use medication to lower high cholesterol levels caused by poor diet. But statins, the group of medications that block cholesterol synthesis, cause the body to search for alternatives to produce cholesterol, which leads to side effects. While for most people the benefits of using statins outweigh the risks, this is not true for all patients—especially when it comes to the elderly.[13]

An ideal therapy looks different. For example, by changing your

diet and exercising regularly, you can not only treat hypercholesterol-
emia but also prevent it.

The root of the problem, ironically, is that our bodies are very good
at utilizing food. In prehistoric times, the availability of food wasn't
always predictable. And so the body learned to build up fat reserves for
times of scarcity. Good utilizers of food—that is, *Homo sapiens* with
more fat reserves that could tide them over in times of need—were the
winners when it came to procreation. The ability to store sufficient fat
reserves was accordingly passed on to the following generations. But
since famines are now rare in Western civilization, our fat reserves make
little sense; external circumstances hardly require us to use them. And
so obesity, along with its related diseases, has long been on the rise.

Because evolution shaped our metabolism hundreds of thousands
of years ago, there is little we can do about the way our bodies utilize
food. What we can do is change how and what we eat. We must eat
less, lighter, and healthier food (and fast at regular intervals), because
we're no longer walking around outside for six hours a day. Instead,
most of us are sitting in offices for eight hours a day. Changing the way
we eat is the only sensible solution.

In Ancient Greece, Hippocrates, the forefather of medicine, put
díaita (dietary and lifestyle habits) at the center of all therapy. Interestingly, to treat obesity, he recommended physical exercise and only one
large meal within a twenty-four-hour period—which is essentially intermittent fasting!

Fasting Around the World

Fasting has been an established tradition across many cultures for centuries. Almost all world religions incorporate some sort of fasting,
which is considered a time of contemplation and self-examination; the
voluntary abstinence is an expression of faith and humility. The senses

become sharper, the body moves into an alert, clear, and euphoric state. The way hunger heightens our senses has been important in evolution, ensuring our ancestors wouldn't miss mushrooms concealed underneath the grass or the scent of an animal hidden behind a bush.

Every year during Lent, many Christians commit to fasting for forty days to replicate Jesus's forty-day fast in the desert. According to the Bible, Jesus was tempted toward the end of his fasting period, but he was undeterred. When the devil whispered to him, "If thou be the Son of God, command that these stones be made bread," he retorted, "Man shall not live by bread alone, but by every word that proceedeth out of the mouth of God" (Matthew 4:3–4, King James Version). In Judaism, two days of the year—Tishah-b'Ab and Yom Kippur—are observed with a twenty-five-hour fast. And within the Islamic tradition, the prophet Muḥammad was known to fast. For the purpose of fasting and meditation, he regularly retreated to the cave of Hira, where he is believed to have experienced his first revelation in 610 AD, in which the archangel Gabriel revealed to him the beginnings of what would become the Koran. This event is observed by Muslims every year during the month of Ramadan, the ninth month of the Islamic lunar calendar. During Ramadan, Muslims around the globe fast from sunrise to sunset.[14, 15] Within Hinduism, sadhus practice asceticism throughout their life, and in Buddhism many people fast during Wesak, the highest Buddhist holiday. In the Theravada tradition of Buddhism a form of intermittent fasting is commonly practiced, wherein people eat only once a day between late morning and noon.[16]

The effects of fasting were also used for purposes of war. In ancient times, Spartan and Persian soldiers fasted before battle. The Old Testament describes how the Maccabees, Jewish insurgents, fasted for three days before going into battle against King Antiochus. And the German emperor Otto I denied his army food before a crucial battle against the Hungarians.[17]

The Healing Effects of Fasting from Antiquity to Today

The ancient Greek writer and philosopher Plutarch was a firm believer in fasting. "Fast today instead of taking medicine," he said. Plato and his student Aristotle expressed similar views.

Later generations of writers had their own thoughts on fasting. Mark Twain wrote, "A little starvation can really do more for the average sick man than can the best medicines and the best doctors."[18] For Upton Sinclair, fasting was his personal salvation. He was in frail health after the stressful years of intensely researching and working on his novel *The Jungle*, which exposed the horrible conditions in Chicago's slaughterhouses. Medical treatments brought no improvement to his health, but long periods of fasting helped. In 1911, Sinclair dedicated an entire book to his positive experiences with fasting, *The Fasting Cure*. He remained a fan of fasting until his death at the age of ninety.[19] In Sinclair's time there already were a few physicians who specialized in fasting, pioneers who treated a large number of patients and publicized their impressive success. The British doctor Henry S. Tanner, who had immigrated to the United States, documented his first experiences with fasting in 1877 (he fasted for forty days), while Edward H. Dewey, an American physician, was almost simultaneously documenting successful treatments with fasting.[20, 21]

But only modern research and molecular biology have been able to scientifically prove the effects of fasting. In the following chapters, I am going to present the impressive therapeutic success that fasting can achieve in many chronic diseases. I am also going to teach you how to fast, and how to fight and prevent specific diseases through fasting.

Fasting has become increasingly popular in recent years. In 2018, gerontologist Valter Longo, from the University of Southern California, was named one of the fifty most influential people in the field of health care by *Time* magazine because of his research in the field of fasting.[22] His scientific work on fasting is groundbreaking, and I'm glad that we are currently working together on a few research projects.

Our modern dietary habits are, quite frankly, out of control. Studies show that most people eat up to ten times a day.[23] We rarely experience real hunger, since food is ingested constantly throughout the day. And it's not just about quantity. We are being inundated with sugar. Whereas hundreds of years ago the only sugar that was available was through fruit or, on very rare occasions, honey, now almost every processed food product contains sugar. And sugar, as we know, is hugely detrimental to health.

Never before has such an abundance of fresh fruit, vegetables, and spices been available to us. We can buy almost any food we want, any time of year. However, the transport of food across the globe has led to us no longer eating seasonally and locally. I believe that moving away from eating seasonally and locally is disadvantageous to our microbiome, our intestine, and our genes.

Most of us can instinctively feel how unnatural it is to find strawberries, tomatoes, and melons in supermarkets in December. The imported produce rarely tastes good, and the vitamin and nutrient content is questionable due to the ripening process being interrupted because the goods are often put into shipping containers when they are still green.

When you're shopping for fruit and vegetables, try to consider whether what you want to buy is local and in season. If something has traveled a long way to get to you, it's likely not the healthiest (or most environmentally friendly) choice!

Evolution's Clever Protective Mechanism

Morning sickness, or nausea during pregnancy, is a mechanism that developed over the course of evolution to protect the embryo from toxins. Pregnant women react strongly to smells, bitter tastes, and animal products, and thereby make healthy nutritional choices for their unborn baby. Or they "voluntarily" refrain from eating potentially harmful things.[24]

This explains why pregnant women are often repulsed by meat, fish, and eggs in particular, because animal products have long been a source of microbes and parasites. A survey of twenty-seven different communities around the world showed that in twenty of them morning sickness occurred; in the other seven it didn't. The members of those seven communities followed a predominantly vegetarian diet, living mainly off corn.[25] Nausea, therefore, is an evolutionary protective mechanism, even for people who aren't pregnant.

Modern food products often overpower this protective mechanism with additives such as sugar and salt. Without these smoke screens we would likely spare ourselves many modern diseases and subsequently a lot of suffering. No one would drink lemonade without sugar, eat candy without sugar, or buy ready-made sauces without flavor enhancers.

Interestingly, almost all fruit is naturally nontoxic. Most fruits have evolved to look beautifully bright and appealing so that they would be eaten by animals and humans alike, ensuring that their seeds are spread. It's only natural, therefore, that plants typically keep their fruit free of poisons.

Summary

- Long periods of hunger, punctuated by food intake, were frequent and common in the almost hundred-thousand-year-long history of *Homo sapiens*.[26] For a long time, the diet was diverse and plant based.[27]

- We adopted a regular but monotonous diet about twelve thousand years ago, with the advent of agriculture, animal husbandry, and food storage.[28] Now large quantities of animal protein have found their way into our modern diet.

- Since the mid-twentieth century in particular, people in industrial nations have enjoyed unlimited access to food. The emergence of food products that are rich in sugar, salt, and additives, along with the possibility of eating around the clock, has changed our eating habits in an unprecedented way.

- At the same time, obesity and chronic diseases are increasing dramatically. This is not surprising, since our genes and our metabolism have hardly changed in a hundred thousand years.[29] Our modern diet is essentially poisonous to our body, which has been accustomed to periods of hunger as well as a varied, mainly plant-based diet for centuries.

Our Bowels and Metabolism— How Nutrients Travel to Cells

Our organs and cells can exist only if they are regularly supplied with oxygen and energy. This is why we breathe and eat.

For food to benefit the body, it must first be broken down into smaller components: nutrients. This process of breaking down food into carbohydrates, fats, and proteins is called digestion. The resulting metabolized nutrients are released from the intestine into the blood and transported to the cells. With the aid of enzymes, these nutrients are chemically converted into energy in the cell's power stations, the mitochondria. This energy is then available to be used in the numerous processes happening in the body.

It may be surprising, but digestion doesn't start in the stomach. It starts in the kitchen. Cooking, frying, and boiling are the first, outsourced steps of digestion. When we cut and heat up food such as potatoes, broccoli, and carrots, their cell walls are broken open and minerals are released. This facilitates digestive processes in the gastrointestinal tract.

It's rather practical: Just looking at food and smelling the wonderful aromas of cooking stimulates our digestion. Our mouths literally water when we smell onions or garlic sautéed in olive oil. In this cephalic phase ("of or relating to the head"), thoughts about food and the smell of meals are released in the brain by corresponding signals—production of saliva begins, and messenger substances are sent to the organs involved in digestion.

The mouth is not just where food is broken down, it's also a critical early step in the digestive process, since food is mixed with the first digestive enzyme, salivary amylase. Carbohydrates are broken down 20 to 30 percent in the mouth. The more thoroughly this happens, the less work there is for the intestine later on. That's why I'm a big advocate of chewing food slowly and thoroughly.

The Journey of Food Through the Body

Once food is well mixed with saliva, it begins its extended journey through the body. Our brain has long since started to send signals and hormones to the lower digestive organs. The masticated food is swallowed and sent through the esophagus into the stomach, where it is already highly anticipated.

The very acidic pH of gastric acid—in an empty stomach it's between 1.5 and 2—eliminates practically all germs that enter the body through food. This, however, is a double-edged sword, because on one hand the gastric acid protects the body from bacteria; on the other hand, it's so aggressive that it can easily do harm outside the stomach. That's why the sphincter muscle between the stomach and esophagus is so important; it prevents the acidic food mass in the stomach from flowing back into the esophagus and thereby burning it. When this mechanism is faulty, we suffer from acid reflux. If this condition becomes chronic, it is called gastroesophageal reflux disease and causes more pain than heartburn, a sensation of pressure behind the sternum, and ructus (belching). Gastroesophageal reflux disease is the most common disease of the digestive tract, with about 20 percent of the population in the United States suffering from it.[30]

Gastric acid, enzymes, and muscular contractions of the stomach break down most of the food we eat very effectively. This is called the gastric digestive phase (*gaster* is Greek and means "stomach"). The amount of food ingested determines how much the stomach wall stretches; the ingredients in the food—proteins and spices in particular—determine the intensity of the stomach's movements. Peristalsis, wavelike muscle contractions, mix the food with acid and enzymes.

The stomach is also active when it's empty. After a short period of rest, when the food mass has slid farther down into the small intestine, the stomach begins to contract. These contractions can flow through the entire digestive tract like a wave and can be very pronounced. As a result of the turbulence, a noise can occur when air is pressed through the pyloric orifice. This is called a stomach rumble. Physicians call these contractions without a digestive purpose "housekeeper waves."

The stomach controls the entire digestive process. If food was insufficiently chewed or is very fatty, the stomach nerves slow down the ensuing digestive process. Then the intestine and the digestive juices from the pancreas and gallbladder have to wait a bit because the stomach is occupied with its digestive work for a longer period of time. Carbohydrates are processed in the stomach in about two hours; meat and fat take up to six hours.

Our Intestines and Liver— The Center of Our Metabolism

Once the food mass has passed from the stomach into the small intestine, the intestinal phase of digestion begins. The small intestine is five to six meters long and consists of three segments: the duodenum, the jejunum, and the ileum. Digestive juices from the pancreas are fed into the duodenum; they neutralize the acidity of the stomach and break down proteins, sugar, and fat. The sufficiently broken-down food components required by the body are absorbed into the lymphatic and the blood systems via the mucous membrane of the small intestine. Because of its villi, crypts, and microvilli, this membrane has a surface of almost four hundred square meters and thus provides an optimal surface for absorption. The small intestine, therefore, is highly equipped for digestion to take place.

Blood enriched with nutrients flows directly to the liver, the hub of the metabolism. The liver is where sugar is stored; this stored sugar is called glycogen. A certain amount of glycogen provides energy reserves for twelve to twenty-four hours. This is of vital importance for the metabolism during fasting. Only when glycogen stored in the liver is used up does the liver send signals to initiate fat loss.

The liver is also responsible for the synthesis of cholesterol, fat, and protein, as well as blood purification. Endogenous substances (internal substances such as hormones and red blood cells) and exogenous substances (external substances such as alcohol and medications, etc.) are broken down in the liver and prepared for excretion. This way, blood is cleansed of toxins before reaching the heart and eventually the cells, muscles, organs, and connective tissues.

While proteins and carbohydrates are absorbed into the blood vessels of the small intestine, fat metabolism is a little more complicated. Dietary fats have to be made fit for transport first because they aren't water-soluble. Part of this process starts in the mouth and the stomach. In the small intestine, certain enzymes (lipases) break down dietary fats into smaller components such as free fatty acids, glycerin, and mono- and diglycerides. These are then absorbed by the cells of the small intestine. Short-chain fatty acids and medium-chain fatty acids pass through the portal vein into the liver, while long-chain fatty acids are passed through the lymph into the venous bloodstream and then to the liver.

The mucous membrane of the small intestine absorbs water, and it is where the body decides which substances are urgently needed and which substances can or must be excreted.

From the small intestine, everything that remains at this stage is transported into the large intestine (colon), which is about one to one-and-a-half meters long. Just as there's a valve between the passage from the esophagus to the stomach, here too is a valve, between the small and large intestines, that prevents the food residue from sliding back into the small intestine. If this valve, the Bauhin's valve, is affected by intestinal inflammation, then flatulence, pain, and a feeling of pressure can occur.

In the large intestine, the last bit of food residue is utilized. Minerals such as calcium are absorbed here, and liquids are extracted once more. When someone is suffering from diarrhea, their stool is liquid because the large intestine is stinted by inflammation and little or no water can be extracted. Under normal circumstances, however, the concentrated stool is lubricated with mucus so that it can be excreted with desquamated intestinal cells. On a side note, mucus and intestinal cells are the reason why bowel movements can still be regular even after multiple days of fasting.

A Newly Discovered Organ—The Microbiome

The large intestine is home to the microbiome or microbiota (also known as the intestinal flora). It consists of roughly 100 trillion bacteria and microbes and is now considered an autonomous organ. This aggregate of microorganisms weighs between 3.3 and 4.4 pounds.

For a long time, very few germs or bacteria could be grown or detected using stool samples in the laboratory. New methods of analysis—specifically, genetic sequencing—have made it possible to examine all the germs on human skin and in the body. In 2012, scientists sequenced the entirety of human germs for the first time and found that 99 percent of the 100 trillion germs can be assigned to roughly 1,000 species of bacteria.[31] Since it does, in fact, consist almost exclusively of bacteria, the entirety of the genes of all germs in the human body is called the microbiome (which is Greek for "small lives"). These settle almost exclusively in the intestine, which is why today the word *microbiome* is used synonymously with *intestinal flora*.

Thousands of studies are currently being conducted around the world to research the microbiome. This is not an exaggeration: It's *the* hot topic in scientific research, and it has already revolutionized our understanding of health and the development of diseases.

It is not surprising that intestinal diseases are linked to the microbiome, but it's hard to believe that rheumatism, stroke, Parkinson's disease, and depression are also affected by the microbiome. Yet we now know that the microbiome seems to play a part in the development or prevention of almost all diseases. It plays a crucial role in our immune system, and as our "stomach brain" it also has a greater influence on our psyche than we might want to believe.

Our relationship with our small bacterial roommates is quite simple: They receive free room and board from us and in return they help retrieve benefits from food. The intestinal bacteria break down sugar molecules, produce healthy short-chain fatty acids for the intestine, and even produce some vitamins and amino acids that in turn are the building blocks for important proteins. Our small intestinal helpers also remove toxins that occur, for example, when bile acid is broken down. Moreover, they ensure an acidic pH value in the intestine to protect us from diarrheal pathogens and other harmful germs. But first and foremost, they have an essential influence on the immune system.

A newborn baby has practically no microbiome; it receives only a few germs from the mother's vagina when it passes through the birth canal. The infant gets exposed to other bacteria from the skin of the mother's breast during breastfeeding. Over time, the infant is also exposed to microbes from its environment. At about two years old, a child's microbiome resembles that of an adult.[32] But our intestinal flora remains a dynamic place that will change and adapt throughout our lives, due to environmental factors, climate, place of residence, diet, and the use of medication. Today, it is possible to roughly classify which species of bacteria are beneficial to a healthy metabolism and which are rather undesirable. A healthy intestinal flora functions, metaphorically speaking, like a vacuum cleaner, keeping the bad germs at bay or destroying them so they can't cause any harm.

The composition of the microbiome varies not only over the course of one's life but also from person to person. For example, identical twins who have the exact same genes will have different intestinal floras.[33] Interestingly, however, many of the bacteria living in the rectum are the same in most people. This indicates a shared genetic origin.[34] The microbiomes of indigenous peoples in the Amazon region and members of other indigenous tribes contain twice as many "good" species of bacteria as the intestinal floras of people living in Western industrial nations.[35, 36] But whether this is due to genetics or diet remains to be seen.

A diversity of species is an important factor for any ecosystem to be healthy. When animals, plants, insects, and microbes cohabitate, they complement and benefit from one another. Some live off the waste or excretions of others and vice versa. The symbiosis—the mutually beneficial cooperation—of microbiomes and humans functions the same way. The more diverse the species in the microbiome, the more stable our health and the better protected we are from diseases. In other words, the healthier we eat, the more biodiverse our microbiome is and the more it works to our benefit. One thing is clear: Nothing works in our body without a balanced microbiome. A healthy diet is essential here too, because the bacteria need the right food. The right food will facilitate the reproduction of good bacteria, which is always why I recommend whole-grain products, fresh vegetables, and other prebiotics that are high in fiber (more on this in the chapter on nutrition).

Many medications (including antibiotics and antacids), food additives, sweeteners, and alcohol can disturb the balance of the intestinal flora. However, some medications, such as the antidiabetic drug metformin, can have positive effects. The best food for intestinal bacteria, however, is not a drug; it's dietary fiber.

THIS DIET SUPPORTS YOUR MICROBIOME

- Unprocessed foods and whole-grain products (such as whole-grain rice and whole-grain pasta).
- Bread made from whole-grain rye meal or whole-grain rye flour, whole-grain wheat meal or whole-grain wheat flour, spelt, green spelt, or oats.
- High-fiber vegetables such as broccoli, sunchoke, spinach, green cabbage, asparagus, artichoke, savoy cabbage, fennel, sweet potato, rutabaga, beets, pumpkin, garlic, and many others.

- Potatoes, which are healthy when cooked, cooled down, and then eaten cold or reheated. When you allow potatoes to cool down, you create a "resistant" starch that is good for the microbiome.
- Legumes such as peas, chickpeas, beans, soybeans, and lentils.
- Use little salt.
- Fruit such as berries (blueberries, currants, blackberries), cherries, pineapple, kumquat, avocado, and citrus.
- Probiotic, fermented foods such as sauerkraut, kimchi, yogurt, kefir, kombucha, tempeh, miso, and tofu.
- Omega-3 fatty acids (especially in flaxseed oil, leafy green vegetables, and walnuts).
- Almonds, walnuts, hazelnuts, pistachios, and sesame seeds.

A change in diet affects the composition of the microbiome quickly, as scientists at Harvard University have shown. If you switch from a diet that is rich in meat to a vegetarian diet, you can observe a change in the composition of the microbiome after just twenty-four hours. There's an increase in anti-inflammatory bacteria that produce short-chain fatty acids.[37] And more and more studies are showing that fasting increases the diversity of bacteria in the intestine and the microbiome.[38]

Sensational Findings in Microbiome Research

One particularly stunning experiment was able to show that when mice ate unhealthy diets (leading to a reduction in their diversity of intestinal bacteria), their offspring became overweight and suffered from health problems.[39] With an unhealthy diet we're harming not just ourselves, but possibly even our children!

Research on microbiomes has also nullified a long-standing assumption in the world of nutritional science. Before, there was a simple formula to determine whether a person would become overweight: A calorie is a calorie, and if people consume more calories than they use, then they will become overweight. For years, the importance of the microbiome was ignored in this thinking. We now know that people who are overweight have a different microbiome. Their bacteria process food better, extracting and storing more calories from food than those of people who are not obese.

Researchers at the Weizmann Institute of Science in Rehovot, Israel, were able to prove that the microbiome even possesses its own biorhythm. Its circadian rhythm is determined by the time of food intake.[40] Which means that irregular meals, due to shift work or jet lag, for instance, confuse not only us but our little roommates too. This can have a negative effect on our weight. But intermittent fasting (fasting over a certain number of hours) can help. I believe its positive effect on our weight can in part be traced back to the stabilization of our circadian clock.

The microbiome also plays a role in certain types of food intolerances. If the small intestine is unable to sufficiently digest nutrients, such as lactose in the case of lactose intolerance or fructose in the case of fructose intolerance, the incompletely digested sugars reach the large intestine. There, bacterial decomposition and putrefaction bacteria cause stomach cramps, flatulence, and diarrhea.

Worse than unpleasant intestinal complaints are the hugely detrimental effects on the body's immune system if the ecological balance of the intestinal bacteria is significantly disturbed. It is now believed that rheumatoid arthritis, Bekhterev's disease, Parkinson's disease, multiple sclerosis, and other chronic diseases are "triggered" by an unbalanced intestinal flora.[41, 42] It will take some time for us to find out how targeted bacterial treatments may be able to effectively treat and even prevent diseases. There are already a number of live intestinal bacteria cultures (probiotics) available in stores and pharmacies, and they do show certain effects in some diseases. But so far, the effects are usually weak and short-lived. The same is true for stool transplants, in which the stool of a healthy person is transferred to the intestine of a sick person (these transplants are used only in very severe cases of acute intestinal infections or chronic inflammatory bowel diseases).

For now, we should concentrate on fasting and nutrition as the best way to promote a balanced, diverse microbiome.

Where Our Energy Comes From

Our body derives energy from three sources: fat, protein, and carbohydrates. Our energy is stored for both short-term and long-term use. The storage sugar glycogen in the liver is the short-term option; body fat is the long-term reserve. Protein cannot be stored by our body. That is one reason it's bad to eat too much protein. Since we cannot store protein, having too much of it in the body can cause (negative) growth and inflammation.

The Canadian nephrologist Jason Fung compares the storage facilities in our body to the refrigerators in our homes.[43] Glycogen is like the refrigerator in our kitchen; the fat reserves are like the deep freezers in our basement. Glycogen is readily available to us—the fridge is in close proximity—but we have to go to the basement for the fat reserves. We usually only head down to the basement when there is nothing left in the fridge. If you visualize this concept, it's easy to understand why it is so hard to get rid of fat in our fat reserves.

Insulin—The "Key" Hormone

The hormone insulin plays an important role in carbohydrate and fat metabolism. In order for fat to be broken down, two conditions must be met: The majority of the glycogen in the liver must be used up, and the insulin level in the blood has to be low enough to release the fat reserves. Neither of these conditions is easy to meet. If the glycogen reserves in the liver are running low, the body sends out hunger signals. If we then eat, new sugar is stored again as glycogen in the liver, so no fat is burned. Instead, excess carbohydrates are converted into fat and stored at high insulin levels.

This is because insulin is produced in the pancreatic cells and released into the blood with the meal. The sugar metabolized from the food must somehow get into the cells. This is where insulin takes center stage: It unlocks the cells, so to speak; without this insulin "key" that fits in the lock, sugar cannot enter the cell.

If we continually eat too much food, too much sugar, and too much animal protein, the pancreas must release increasing amounts of insulin to unlock the cells. But the cells are already full. What now? Since they don't need any more sugar and energy, they revert to a protective mechanism. They block the receptors at their cell walls for the insulin key—this is called insulin resistance.

As a result, blood sugar levels rise, because the insulin is powerless and unable to clear away sugar in the blood. The pancreas misunderstands the situation, believing it needs to create more insulin to unlock the cells. So the pancreas runs at full speed and releases more of the hormone; over time the disease diabetes sets in, and insulin levels rise and rise. At some point the pancreas is exhausted and surrenders—and from that moment onward, diabetes is very hard to cure.

Obesity and diabetes go hand in hand. High insulin levels prevent fat loss, because the cells believe enough sugar, or energy, is in circulation. Remember the image of the refrigerator and the freezer: The fridge is full, and so the freezer—the fat reserves—don't need to be accessed. That's why it becomes extremely difficult for someone suffering from advanced diabetes to lose weight in the long term through dieting. Obesity, high insulin levels, and diabetes are a vicious cycle.

Most conventional weight-loss diets only make the situation worse.

Conventional diets cause the glycogen reserves to be emptied first, but because of the chronically high insulin levels, the body hardly breaks down any fat and if it does, it does so with great difficulty. Now the body does what it always does when it thinks energy is running low: It slows down the basal metabolism so that it burns less energy. And voilà: There is further weight gain, creating a yo-yo effect. This is why I'm a staunch opponent of conventional diets.

With type 1 diabetes, the situation is essentially reversed. The patients—who are often young—are usually underweight. Their pancreas is no longer able to produce insulin, and without insulin the body cannot create fat stores.

In addition to insulin, our metabolism is regulated by many other control molecules and control systems. I'll explore this further later in the book, but the basic principle of all these controls and control systems is simple. When we eat too much sugar or animal protein, the body signals: "Attention, clear away the excess!" In order to clear away this excess, our body initiates fat storage, inflammation, and cell growth. But too much growth ultimately means an increased risk of cancer.[44] That's another reason I keep advocating therapeutic and intermittent fasting!

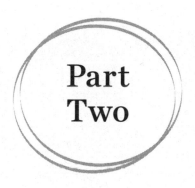

Part Two

Eat Better, Live Healthier

New Awareness of Nutrition

Chapter Two

The Healthiest Places in the World

A huge range of diet and nutrition trends have emerged over the past few years: Atkins, raw food, juicing, Paleo, keto, the list goes on and on. With new trends constantly emerging, what is actually healthy?

In the following chapter, I will introduce you to the latest research on healthy diet and nutrition and point out the correlations between these findings and my own observations from decades of clinical experience. My focus is on what diet can do for your health. To begin, I will take you on a short trip around the world.

Gianni Pes, an Italian physician and age researcher, and Michel Poulain, a Belgian astrophysicist and demographer, had the brilliant idea to examine diet and health from a rather unusual angle. Instead of feeding lab mice a diet that would *potentially* lead to longevity and waiting to see where this might lead, Pes and Poulain conducted a demographic survey in which they identified the regions on our planet where the oldest, healthiest people live. They marked these locations on a map with a blue pen, which is why these areas are now known as Blue Zones.[1] American journalist Dan Buettner heard about Pes and

Poulain's work and, together with the National Institute on Aging in Bethesda, Maryland, expanded on the concept. With Pes and Poulain on board, Buettner and his team identified six zones where the most one-hundred-year-olds (centenarians) and the most 110-year-olds (supercentenarians) lived. They wanted to find out why the people in these Blue Zones reach such a high age—looking into factors such as how they live, their diet, whether they smoke, family life and social involvement, and physical exercise. The result: Diet proved to be a decisive factor for a long and healthy life. More precisely, following a "traditional diet" is a decisive factor for a long and healthy life. Many of the people in these Blue Zones ate foods that had traditionally been eaten in those respective regions for many decades. Globalization has allowed us to access almost any kind of food, anytime we want. But perhaps this has actually been a disadvantage when it comes to our health and nutrition. Let's dive deeper into this by taking a look at these regions where people live healthily into old age.

Okinawa

Okinawa is also known as the Island of Immortality because a three-digit age is, statistically speaking, much more common here than anywhere else. Why is that? What is so special about the people who live there? Okinawa is situated in the East China Sea, about nine hundred miles from Tokyo. And even though the people on this Japanese island experienced a great deal of suffering during World War II, more than nine hundred of the 1.3 million people who live there are a hundred years old or older. Most of them live independently and are still very physically active. Perhaps that's why they don't have a word for *retirement*.

Almost all families in Okinawa, particularly those who live in the countryside, grow their own food. Everything else they buy in local markets—regional products, therefore—and not in big supermarket chains, so no imported foods. For decades, the sweet potato (imo) has been a staple food in Okinawa. For breakfast, people usually eat miso soup with vegetables. Seaweed, tofu, natto (fermented soybeans), and rice seasoned with onions, pepper, and turmeric are added to the other meals. A common addition to meals is bitter melon (goya) and mugwort. People drink green tea throughout the day. Animal protein such as fish is rarely eaten, and meat, usually pork, is eaten only on holidays.

> There is another striking factor when you observe the dietary habits on Okinawa: People practice "hara hachi bun me," a Confucian teaching that translates to mean "eat until you are only 80 percent full." No diet could be simpler. Caloric restriction is an integral part of the food culture on this Japanese island.

Unfortunately, centenarians are becoming increasingly rare on Okinawa. This is connected to the fact that the standard of living in Okinawa has become Westernized, including a preference for fast food. As a result, the very low percentage of dietary fat rose from 10 percent in the 1960s to roughly 30 percent today—that is, to the level of the Western world. Nowadays, almost every second islander between the ages of 20 and 69 is overweight.[2]

The low fat content in the food was once maintained by the sweet potato—it is considered the true secret for the longevity in this region.[3] Studies show its excellent effect on the blood circulation in the vessels.[4] Unfortunately, the sweet potato isn't as much of a staple food in Japan as it once was.

> **Try sweet potato!** Cut a thick sweet potato into half-inch slices and put them in an oven dish. Toss with olive oil, salt, and pepper and bake in the oven for thirty minutes at 400°F (flip the slices halfway through to ensure they don't burn).

The diet in Okinawa is very rich in seaweed, and I believe that seaweed is another major reason for longevity due to its high content of unsaturated omega-3 fatty acids and other phytochemicals.

The third factor in ensuring a long and healthy life is most likely the leafy greens that are consumed often in Asia: garland chrysanthemum, Osaka Shirona, and nozawana. Their high nitrate content protects the vessels and the metabolism—they're what we refer to as superfoods.

Beyond Okinawa, Japan in general is the country with the highest average life expectancy (83.9 years), according to the latest findings of an Organisation for Economic Co-operation and Development (OECD) study.[5] Currently, there are almost seventy thousand people in Japan who are over one hundred years old—this is unrivaled across the world.[6]

We can achieve the health benefits of Japanese cuisine by consuming local leafy greens such as spinach, arugula, Swiss chard, and beet

> ### Fennel Seeds
>
> Most Indian restaurants serve colorful candied fennel seeds after dinner to freshen your breath. The sugar in the candy coating isn't very healthy, but the fennel seeds themselves are great for you. You can stir-fry them with vegetables or cook them with rice. The nutrients (among them essential oils) pack a punch; they are small but powerful.

greens. The high levels of nitrate they contain protect our blood vessels and heart. Fennel seeds also protect us from atherosclerosis and keep our vessels supple.

Ikaria and Sardinia

It's not only in Asia that people live to a healthy old age; they do so in Europe as well. Specifically, on the Greek island of Ikaria in the Aegean Sea, and on the Italian island of Sardinia in the Mediterranean Sea.

Roughly eighty-five hundred people live on Ikaria, which is quite barren in places. The percentage of ninety-year-olds living here is ten times higher than the European average. Here, the islanders eat a lot of legumes, wild vegetables, herbs, and olives. They consume roughly eight ounces of vegetables a day—this is much more than Germans or Americans do.

Most of the centenarians on Sardinia live in small villages in the mountain region of Barbagia. In addition to a diet rich in vegetables and fruit, people also eat generous amounts of goat's and sheep's milk and cheese. Interestingly, the life expectancy of men and women in this mountainous region is almost the same.[7] This is surprising because women around the world usually live two to five years longer than men. Monks and nuns are an exception to this.[8] One possibility is that the men in monastic communities are exposed to less stress and have a healthier diet.

On Sardinia, in any case, physical labor and exercise also foster longevity.[9] And people there take siestas, which observational studies have proved are beneficial.[10] The siesta has many benefits: You avoid the exhausting midday heat, and this period of rest de-stresses you.

Both Italy and Greece follow the Mediterranean diet, and I consider it so important that I would like to elaborate on it.

The Mediterranean Diet

What is the Mediterranean diet? Is it the traditional diet of Morocco, Turkey, Greece, Italy, Portugal, or Croatia? Anyone who has traveled to a few of these countries knows that there are considerable differences here when it comes to food. The success of the diet undoubtedly owes a lot to the positive image of the Mediterranean Sea and memories of fantastic vacations. A Mediterranean diet certainly sounds more appealing than a North German diet, for example. But the traditional Mediterranean diet has less in common with what is mainly served in the tourist regions, such as souvlaki, gyros, Serrano ham, mozzarella, and overflowing red wine. Instead, it's centered on vegetables, fruit, nuts, legumes, spices, whole grains, and healthy oils.

When it comes to the Mediterranean diet, both physicians and demographers agree (which is rare) that it is very healthy. Anyone who has ever visited a Mediterranean country knows the culinary diversity. I too remember it well. I first encountered it at nineteen. I had finally arrived in warm, sunny northern Spain after a long train ride with my girlfriend at the time. We were lucky to find a room in a small boardinghouse at the edge of the city, since all the larger hotels were booked. A few older Spanish people were having dinner at the boardinghouse, and my girlfriend and I decided to eat there as well. There was only one dish on the menu—the house special. I was excited, picturing calamari, Manchego cheese, and paella—this was what I imagined Mediterranean food in Spain to be. But to my surprise there was none of that. Instead there were the following four courses: a vegetable soup, salad, two plates filled with vegetables—eggplant, zucchini, artichoke, white beans, green asparagus, fried bell pepper, and spinach with generous amounts of onions and garlic—as well as a sweet dessert made from pistachios, honey, and almonds. The food was served with freshly baked bread and olives. At the time, I was rather disappointed with this "simple" meal. But today I know that I was served an authentic, traditionally Mediterranean, incredibly healthy meal.

This is what traditional Mediterranean food is all about: vegetables, fruit, nuts, legumes, spices, whole grains, and healthy oils.

Ancel Keys Discovers the Phenomenal Effects of the Mediterranean Diet

One of the most notable people to draw the world's attention to the health benefits of the Mediterranean diet was the American scientist Ancel Benjamin Keys. Keys was a biologist and physiologist. At the time of World War II, he was researching how people react to unusual living conditions, hunger, and the physiological effects of dietary fats. He wanted to find out how a person could survive in extremely cold, high-altitude mountainous areas.[11] His work caught the attention of the US Department of Defense. On the basis of his research, Keys developed food rations for soldiers called K rations. Each of his waterproof K ration cartons contained 3,200 kcal of food consisting of cheese, chocolate, hard biscuits, powdered lemon, as well as chewing gum and cigarettes—the latter of which served to boost morale among the troops.[12]

But what made Keys truly famous was his Minnesota Starvation Experiment, a study on hunger and starvation. To motivate healthy men to participate voluntarily, he designed a poster to arouse curiosity: "Will You Starve That They Be Better Fed?"

The 32 participants received only 1,000 kcal a day for several months, but despite the sparse meals, they had to walk 12 to 18 miles every day. Through this extreme study, Keys was able to prove the enormous negative effects that great hunger has on the mind and body. He also showed how important it is to eat carefully and slowly following such prolonged deprivation, in order to avoid organ damage.[13] Keys's research results have since often been wrongfully used as evidence of the dangerous consequences of fasting. Yet his study had nothing to do with medical fasting. Its aim was to develop effective countermeasures against the effects of hunger.

After 1945, Keys had access to a lot of data on Europe's population. He observed that the malnutrition in the postwar period was accompanied by a very low rate of heart disease in some countries, but that strokes and heart attacks, on the other hand, surged with emerging prosperity. He also noted that mortality from heart attacks remained negligibly small in southern Italy.[14]

So he traveled to Italy and built a lab in Naples to measure blood lipid levels on-site. As a result, he wanted to investigate the connection between animal fat in food, cholesterol levels in the blood, and risk of heart attack. In 1958, he started the first systematic multicountry epidemiological study, the famous Seven Countries Study. Despite modest financial resources, he succeeded in exhaustively examining twelve thousand people from seven countries including Japan, Finland, Greece, and the United States. Laboratory and EKG data were documented and people were asked about their lifestyle habits. Any illnesses that had been suffered were recorded at the five- and ten-year marks.[15]

The results were astonishing: Heart attacks and coronary heart disease occurred in only 0.1 percent of the population of Crete and in only 1 percent of the population of Japan, but in 5.7 percent of the people in the United States and a whopping 9.5 percent in Finland. Heightened blood cholesterol levels were found in 77 percent of the Fins examined for the study but in only 3 percent of the Japanese.[16] Given how different dietary habits were between these two countries, these results probably shouldn't be that surprising to us now.

Keys was the first to recognize that not every type of fat is harmful to health. On Crete, people traditionally use substantial amounts of olive oil, which doesn't initially sound like a low-fat diet. Nevertheless, the heart attack rate was very low in comparison to places where people consumed a lot of animal fat. It was Keys's achievement to recognize the protective mechanism of olive oil for blood vessels and to differentiate the effects of different kinds of fat. He was also the first to classify the Mediterranean diet as wholly healthy. Moreover, he concluded that the secret to the health of the inhabitants of Crete and southern Italy was that they ate plenty of vegetables, fruit, and "complex" carbohydrates.

Keys's scientific research shaped his own personal life. He implemented his dietary recommendations in his own day-to-day living and died at age 101 in his adoptive home of Naples.

All data from elaborate clinical studies that possess medical validity are clear. They show that after switching to a Mediterranean diet, people suffer fewer heart attacks and strokes and are less likely to develop diabetes and hypertension. There is improvement in rheumatic pains, as well as in the early stages of dementia in elderly people.[17]

> The Mediterranean diet appears to have a preventive effect even for breast cancer and colon cancer.[18]

Without question, the Mediterranean diet in its traditional, plant-based form is one of the world's healthiest diets!

The Mediterranean Diet in Practice

In 2016, the leading researchers on the Mediterranean diet (nutritionists and cardiologists from Spain, Greece, France, the United States, and Great Britain) were interviewed by the renowned professional journal

BMC Medicine about their assessment of the Mediterranean diet.[19] According to the interview, these are the ten guidelines for following this diet:

CONSUME THESE FOODS GENEROUSLY:

- Olive oil as the main cooking fat (at least four teaspoons a day)
- Nuts (at least three times a week, ideally 30 grams a day, which is about a handful)
- Plenty of fresh fruit (ideally three times a day, preferably berries or grapes)
- Plenty of fresh vegetables (ideally two to three times a day)
- Legumes (several times a week, ideally every day)
- Spices, onions, garlic (as often as possible)
- Whole-grain foods with a lot of dietary fiber (bread, pasta, rice)

CONSUME THESE FOODS EXTREMELY SPARINGLY OR NOT AT ALL:

- Sweets and sugary drinks
- Meat and sausage
- Dairy products

Milk in the Mediterranean Diet

If you consume dairy products, avoid industrially, mass-produced products and opt for sheep or goat cheese. And aim to use cheese as the Southern Europeans do—sprinkle small amounts of feta, pecorino, and parmesan on food for taste, not a thick slice on bread. Yogurt and fermented drinks such as ayran and kefir are regularly consumed in Mediterranean countries and contain healthy probiotic bacteria. But there the overall consumption of dairy products is very low.

Fish in the Mediterranean Diet

I'm not an advocate of eating fish, for health reasons and for ecological reasons. But of course, fish embodies the Mediterranean diet like no other food, especially in coastal regions. Beyond the seaside towns, however, things are different and it's not necessarily on the menu. If you're choosing between fish and meat, you should choose fish; it's the lesser of two evils, so to speak. But the Mediterranean diet should not be defined by consumption of fish. The diet is characterized, first and foremost, by the consumption of a lot of vegetables as well as plant-based oils—and not by eating fish.

Fats in the Mediterranean Diet

Antonia Trichopoulou of the University of Athens and president of the Hellenic Health Foundation, who got major modern population studies on the Mediterranean diet off the ground, describes the diet as an essentially plant-based, vegan diet that, surprisingly, is not low fat. On the subject of olive oil, she likes to point out that this oil is actually a fruit juice.

Time and again we hear that you shouldn't heat up olive oil, that it's not suitable for frying and cooking—but that's not true. On the contrary, recent studies show that the chemical composition of olive oil remains stable even at high temperatures and that it is therefore suited to be heated up for long periods of time without developing harmful substances.[20]

I'll discuss this more in depth later on, but I would like to mention one thing at this point: Keys was slightly wrong on the topic of cholesterol. (He regarded high blood cholesterol levels as bad for health, which is true, but then he concluded that any dietary fat intake was harmful—which is not true, because fats cannot be generalized. There are "bad," saturated fats and "good," plant-based, monounsaturated and polyunsaturated fats.) The Mediterranean diet protects against heart attack and stroke without lowering cholesterol levels. Most recent data shows that the more good fats from healthy oils and nuts we eat instead of bad fats from animal products, the healthier it is for our heart, no matter how high or low our cholesterol levels are.[21]

Alcohol in the Mediterranean Diet

A warm summer night on a terrace by the sea, a slice of bread with olive oil, sea salt, and pimentos—what more could you need? Maybe a glass of red wine? Wine is undoubtedly part of meals in the southern European countries. However—and most people fail to recognize this—in modest amounts.

Nowadays, many scientists and doctors recommend restricting the consumption of wine and alcohol. I agree. For a long time, a sip of red wine was considered healthy, but this concept was retired in 2018. The data published up until that point usually focused on examining cardiovascular diseases.[22] Most recent surveys, however, suggest that even small amounts of alcohol are more harmful than we assumed.[23, 24] Even though there still is evidence of a small advantage in terms of cardiovascular diseases with regular, moderate consumption, we know now that alcohol promotes the development of cancer.[25]

If you don't want to give up having wine with your meals, you should keep the Mediterranean tradition in mind: Wine is drunk during meals, not as an end in itself.

The "MediterrAsian" Diet

As healthy as the Mediterranean diet is, this doesn't mean that other diets are not. There is increasing scientific evidence for the health effects of Asian cuisine.[26] Some nutritional scientists are claiming that the "MediterrAsian" diet is the ideal form of nutrition.[27]

The foundation of Japanese cuisine—according to the Japanese Food Guide Spinning Top model—consists of carbohydrates such as grain, noodles, pasta, and rice. This is followed by a slightly smaller portion of vegetable-based dishes. The third portion—fish, eggs, soy, and meat—is eaten even less often by the Japanese. The fourth section—dairy products and fruit—is rarely consumed.[28] A study published in *The BMJ* in 2016 showed a connection between this form of nutrition, life expectancy, and cardiovascular diseases. The more people eat according to the traditional Japanese style of cooking, the healthier they are and the longer they live.[29]

The China Study, conducted by the British biochemist T. Colin Campbell on behalf of the Chinese government, investigated the health of the inhabitants of central China. The diet in China's rural areas consisted mainly of grain and vegetables, with little meat or freshwater fish. As a result, the amount of animal protein in the diet was a mere 10 percent. The fat content of the food was also low and the percentage of dietary fiber high. Obesity, hypertension, elevated cholesterol levels, and cardiovascular disease rarely occurred in the people who were examined across 130 villages in central China. Cases of breast and intestinal cancer and autoimmune diseases such as multiple sclerosis and type 1 diabetes were also rare. In comparison, American men died of a heart attack sixteen times more often than Chinese men.[30]

Loma Linda and Nicoya

Let's continue on our journey to the healthiest places on earth, from Japan across Europe to the West Coast of the United States. We are now heading to Loma Linda, an area not far from Los Angeles. Within this California city is a community of people called Seventh-day Adventists who enjoy long, healthy life spans. The members of this Protestant church believe that the human body is a house of God.[31] Because of their religious beliefs, they follow a healthy, plant-based diet—most of them are vegetarian or vegan—and place great value on a healthy lifestyle. This includes avoiding nicotine, alcohol, and meat. Instead, their diet consists of mainly nuts, vegetables, legumes, and fruit; some eat fish and only a few eat meat. Scientists at Loma Linda University had an ideal research situation here—they were able to identify a large group of people who followed a very uniform diet with few differences in everyday routine and lifestyle due to their shared religion. As a result, there was only a small possibility of falsified data, something many studies have to contend with. The Adventist Health Study started more than two decades ago; extensive long-term analyses were compiled for sixty thousand and ninety-seven thousand participants. What I found most impressive was that the Adventists tended to live about ten years longer than the average American citizen; "Ten Years of Life" was the title of the study.[32] Five factors were essential for this longer life span: abstaining from nicotine use, following a vegetarian diet, consumption of nuts, regular exercise, and close social relationships.

Other interesting findings of this study, in addition to the protective effect of a vegetarian diet, included the discoveries that the consumption of tomatoes protects against ovarian cancer and prostate cancer, and drinking five glasses of water every day protects the heart.[33, 34]

There is yet another Blue Zone with a higher-than-average number of energetic one-hundred-year-olds. They can be found on the Nicoya Peninsula in Costa Rica in Central America. Here too, traditional lifestyle and dietary habits have been preserved due to the isolated location, just as they were on Sardinia, Crete, and Ikaria. The dietary pattern is the same as in the other Blue Zones: a lot of vegetables (mainly beans here) and plenty of fruit. Carbohydrates are provided by the area's staple food, corn. An additional factor for the longevity of the Nicoyans is a kind of daily intermittent fasting. Traditionally, very little is eaten in the evenings.[35]

More Discoveries from Traditional Forms of Nutrition

Beyond the Blue Zones project, other population groups who live exceedingly healthy lives while reaching a very old age are being examined around the world. A closer look at medical databases reveals interesting data from studies that investigated traditional forms of nutrition in Africa. In 1959, epidemiologists reported astonishing findings from Uganda. The scientists compared the results of autopsies of the hearts of more than six hundred people of the same age from the United States and Uganda. Among the Americans, 136 heart attacks were identified as the cause of death. Among the Ugandans, there was only one.[36, 37] This discovery was confirmed in further studies.[38] While searching for the reason behind this, scientists came across the dietary habits of Ugandans. Compared to Americans, Ugandans ate a lot of vegetables, legumes, whole grains, very little meat, and no industrially processed products.

Similar observations were made in Kenya earlier. In the 1920s, scientists recorded blood pressure values of about a thousand Kenyans who followed a predominantly plant-based and whole-food diet. In contrast to Americans and Europeans, they did not present with heightened blood pressure levels as they got older. In the group of Kenyans who were sixty and older, scientists were even able to measure lower blood pressure levels (110/70 mmHg on average), while these were heightened in people from the West (over 140/90 mmHg).[39] Another study examined the causes of diseases in eighteen hundred Kenyans who received inpatient treatment in hospitals. There was not a single case of hypertension or heart attack![40]

A very remote area in the Amazon region of Bolivia also reinforces the findings of the research conducted in Blue Zones. In this region, roughly ten thousand Tsimane—members of an indigenous tribe— live in about eighty villages. In 2001, anthropologists began to examine the lifestyle of the Tsimane more closely as part of the Tsimane Health and Life History Project. Life in the jungle has its challenges; there is no electricity or running water. The inhabitants spend many hours of the day on their feet collecting fruit and roots, growing grain and cassava, a starchy tuber. Because of the many insects and parasites, infections that lead to inflammation in the body and on the skin are common. Medical care is lacking. Nevertheless, the average life expectancy of seventy-two is relatively high.

The Tsimane research project focused on this inflammation and its effects on cardiovascular diseases (such as heart attacks and strokes). It has long been known that atherosclerosis is also a result of inflammatory processes. For that reason, the researchers wanted to look into the state of cardiovascular health among the Tsimane. They carried out cardiological examinations on 705 members of this tribe between the ages of forty and ninety-four.

The results of the study were such a sensation that when they were published in 2017, the Tsimane were declared the heart-healthiest people in the world. The average atherosclerosis of an eighty-year-old Tsimane corresponded to that of an American in his or her early fifties. Even though the Tsimane had high levels of inflammation in their blood, this seemed to be insignificant for heart health. Instead, researchers found that there was no increase in weight, cholesterol, blood sugar levels, or blood pressure, even through old age—all seemingly inevitable signs of aging in the United States and Europe.

In 85 percent of the Tsimane examined, the risk of a heart attack was zero, even in old age!

So how do the Tsimane eat? Definitely high-carb: 72 percent of calories come from carbohydrates, mainly corn, rice, cassava, and plantains. They consume very little fat (14 percent of calories) and little protein (14 percent; mainly from legumes, seeds, and a little fish). Of course, everything they eat is fresh and hasn't been industrially processed.

In recent years, the Tsimane have had more and more contact with the outside world. Through the construction of roads and the use of motorboats, Western products have reached previously remote areas. This has changed the dietary habits in these parts as well. Unfortunately, refined sugar has found its way into the villages, as well as industrially produced fats. On the other hand, medical care has improved. It remains to be seen whether one will outweigh the other.[41]

Conclusions from Our Around-the-World Trip to the Blue Zones

It seems clear that people who stick to traditional eating habits and consume local products can enjoy great health. Dan Buettner observed how people in the Blue Zones not only were healthy, but appeared quite satisfied with their lives.[42]

THE OLDEST AND HEALTHIEST PEOPLE IN THE WORLD EAT:

- Predominantly whole foods, no industrially processed foods
- A lot of vegetables and/or fruit

- Nuts
- Little or no meat, little fish
- Little or no dairy products
- A lot of grain and complex carbohydrates
- Little or no sugar
- Mostly low-fat foods
- In Mediterranean regions: a lot of plant-based fats (nuts, olive oil)
- Lots of fiber (vegetables, fruit, whole grains)

FURTHERMORE, THE MOST LONG-LIVED PEOPLE:

- Usually eat smaller portions, i.e., restrict calories
- Are active
- Usually have strong social connections

Chapter Three

Essential Nutrients
and Where They Are Found

The major essential nutrients—fat, protein, and carbohydrates—are technically called macronutrients. I've thought long and hard about whether I should stick with this classification. Basically, I consider it one of the greatest sins of modern nutritional science to focus too much on individual nutrients. If we only ever talk about fat instead of the foods that contain them—that is, if we talk about saturated fats and not about pork chops or butter—we lose touch with real foods, and we get the wrong idea.

For years, people were advised to avoid fat completely. But plant-based fats actually protect the heart. In addition, health risks increase if we use sugar instead of fat. So the right foods (low sugar or sugar-free) must be put on the table so that giving up fat can make sense. Even "healthy" low-fat products are not a solution, because they're not really filling. It's hard to resist cravings when you're not eating foods that fill you up. In the following pages, I would like to consider the most essential nutrients and corresponding foods in a more nuanced way.

Fats

By now it's a fact widely known: Fat isn't as bad as we used to think, and fat in and of itself doesn't make us fat. Nevertheless, this nutrient still has a negative reputation, even though as a macronutrient fat actually has quite a few positive qualities.

We love fat, because it's a wonderful flavor carrier. Think of how much more delicious toast is when butter is spread across it, or how much more flavorful a piece of bread is when dipped in olive oil. Moreover, nothing is as filling as fat. When we're hungry, the smell of fried food draws us in like magic. Fat is also essential for the absorption of vitamins A, D, E, and K. Vitamin A precursors (beta-carotene, contained, for example, in carrots) can sufficiently be metabolized in the body only if we add fat.[1]

The unique capacity for fat to be stored can be both good and bad. The body, as I have already mentioned, is unable to store any protein and only a small amount of carbohydrates, but to the chagrin of many people, it has no problem storing fat. In past centuries, it was a clear evolutionary advantage to possess fat reserves. They were biological life insurance for bad times, so to say. Even today, being able to rely on fat reserves is still an advantage when facing serious, protracted, and debilitating diseases, such as cancer.

As great as it is for when times are tough, fat is fatal for our health in times of abundance. The important biological ability of the body to survive even without regular intake of food is rooted in our genes and cells. Today, it has become a global problem as the world's population becomes increasingly overweight.

My scientific stance on fat can be summarized in one sentence: It is absolutely not necessary to eat less fat overall (although you can, especially when suffering from heart disease and diabetes), but we should eat more of the good fats and less of the unhealthy, bad fats. The fat in a pepperoni pizza is not healthy, whereas a salad of avocado with chopped tomatoes, onions, walnuts, and plenty of olive oil is bursting with healthy fats.

Reduce Saturated Fat as Much as Possible

Meat and dairy products (butter, milk, cheese) contain large amounts of saturated fatty acids. Even some plant-based fats such as palm oil and coconut oil belong in this category. According to the current studies, saturated fatty acids are associated with an increased risk of heart attack or stroke.[2]

Nutrition experts are always trying to mitigate or reduce warnings about saturated fats. But even if saturated fatty acids aren't as unhealthy as was assumed for decades, they are still far from being healthy! The overwhelming majority of studies show that cardiovascular diseases in particular increase as a result of eating large amounts of saturated fats.[3] In my medical work I see the adverse effects every day. If patients change their diet so that they eat fewer saturated animal fats and more plant-based ones, an impressive effect can be seen after just a few weeks: Elevated blood pressure lowers, the skin calms down, inflammation in the body (including in the joints) decreases, digestion normalizes. In short, people are healthier, and they look it—younger, more relaxed, refreshed!

There are studies that paint saturated fats in a good light. A famous recent—and quite frankly annoying—example of this is the international PURE (Prospective Urban Rural Epidemiology) study, which caused quite a stir. The dietary habits of 135,000 participants from eighteen countries and five continents were documented and the subjects' state of health was observed over a period of seven years. The result: People who ate large amounts of saturated fatty acids every day died a little less frequently than those who ate more carbohydrates. Upon examination, however, it became clear that most participants came from Asia, especially China and Bangladesh. In those countries, the question of whether a person eats saturated fats or carbohydrates often isn't a matter of preference or choice, but one of wealth. Essentially, groups of people who could afford to buy meat and dairy products were being compared with those who could afford only white rice and less expensive processed foods. Inexplicably, the study also did not differentiate between the types of carbohydrate intake: It did not matter whether whole grains or junk food made up the majority of daily diet. Thus, an unhealthy lifestyle (eating carbohydrates from junk food, sweets, and white rice) due to existential poverty was being compared with the lifestyle of wealthy people who ate high-quality fiber from grains and vegetables in addition to a lot of animal fat.[4] An imprecise and negligent method, in my opinion.

Unsurprisingly, a large number of lab experiments painted a completely different picture: The adverse effect of saturated fatty acids on blood vessels, the heart, and the brain was clearly confirmed. Clinical studies with random group selection showed even more clearly that diets with very little saturated fatty acids protect against heart attack, stroke, diabetes, breast cancer, and a few other types of cancer.[5, 6] And if we look at the long-lived people in the Blue Zones, none of them ingest large quantities of saturated fats. Very few studies come to a different conclusion. Those that do are often funded by the American meat industry.

It is healthy to reduce saturated fats as much as possible—I generally advise against eating meat. There is nothing wrong with small amounts of organic butter and organic dairy products, ideally from grazing livestock. They are also part of many traditional diets.

You don't need to avoid saturated fatty acids altogether, but they don't do us any good. Anytime saturated fatty acids are replaced with plant-based fats or whole-grain carbohydrates, there are proven health-promoting effects.

Plant-Based Saturated Fats

In addition to animal fats, there are also plant-based saturated fats. These include coconut and palm oil.

You should avoid palm oil altogether; it is not healthy and its production is responsible for deforestation in the rain forest. Palm oil is often added to many processed foods, even to organic products that might seem healthy. Read ingredient labels carefully. You don't want these products to end up in your shopping cart.

Coconut oil contains plenty of saturated fats and is the subject of almost absurd scientific disputes: Some glorify it as a universal remedy, others consider it a poison. Here too, it pays to take a closer look. Coconut oil undoubtedly contains a large amount of saturated fats (up to 90 percent), but it also contains medium-chain fatty acids. According to most recent findings, these are said to be very good for gut health.[7] However, a recent meta-analysis of all clinical studies that tested coconut oil found no beneficial metabolic effects, and in fact saw an increase in "bad," LDL-cholesterol blood levels. Thus, coconut oil cannot be regarded as a healthy oil.

Monounsaturated Fatty Acids Are Very Healthy

The most famous source of monounsaturated fatty acids is olive oil, *the* embodiment of the Mediterranean diet. In antiquity it was called "liquid gold."[8] The largest study on the Mediterranean diet was the PREDIMED study, which was conducted in Spain. Its results are famous within the field of medicine. It compared one group of participants who followed a Mediterranean diet—which included consuming either a lot of olive oil or a lot of nuts—with another group that ate normally. After five

A Short Course on Olive Oil

The quality of olive oil is often hard to gauge at first glance. Ultimately, the choice is a matter of taste. Make sure to buy organic. And if possible, try the olive oil before buying it. Does it taste fruity or does it have a spicy, bitter note? Is the liquid clear or cloudy? Also keep in mind, you're probably not going to be able to buy oil of excellent quality for three dollars in the supermarket.

To me, olive oil is delicious when it's spicy and bitter. This is the case when it contains plenty of phytochemicals—that is, polyphenols and oleocanthal. At home we have one kind of olive oil for the grown-ups and a milder kind for the children, who don't like the bitter kind. The spiciness and the bitterness of olive oil can be so strong that it triggers a cough reflex. That is nothing to worry about—in fact it's a sign of quality. Olive oil that is virtually tasteless is usually not particularly good or healthy.

Contrary to popular belief, olive oil can be heated up to high temperatures for a long time without developing unhealthy substances. This is even true for extra virgin olive oil, which is rich in polyphenols. Surprisingly, polyphenols appear to stabilize the oil when heated. But don't use particularly expensive oil for cooking—that's a waste of money; the taste suffers from the heating. Pay attention to the smoke point: If you fry with olive oil (or any other oil) and smoke develops in the pan, lower the temperature. The smoke point is usually reached at 356°F, but sometimes up to 446°F. Unfiltered bottled olive oils, the Flor de Aceite, are the exception here; their smoke point is 266°F. These precious oils shouldn't be used for frying and should only be enjoyed cold. It's best to buy two types of olive oil, one for roasting and baking, and one for salads and antipasti. All edible oils should be stored in a cool, dark, dry place.

years, there were considerable health benefits for both the olive oil and the nut groups—fewer heart attacks, strokes, and incidences of diabetes, and fewer cases of breast cancer in the participating women. Those in the olive oil group, who showed very good health results, ate fifty grams (five tablespoons) of olive oil every day.[9] This is a rather significant amount—over ten days it amounts to more than two cups. This amount isn't obligatory, but I recommend using olive oil generously in salads, with raw foods, or to cook vegetables. I like to prepare an appetizer consisting of a plate of olive oil, the Arabic spice mixture za'atar (which contains wild thyme), finely chopped tomatoes, red onions, and olives. Served with a fresh whole wheat baguette, it's delicious!

Other good sources of monounsaturated fatty acids are canola oil, peanut butter, and avocado. The healthiest source is nut butter, made from almonds, hazelnuts, cashews, Brazil nuts, or pecans. And I always have a nut mix on the dining table or in a drawer—unsalted, of course.

Polyunsaturated Fatty Acids

Polyunsaturated fatty acids protect the heart and blood vessels particularly well. The most famous representatives are omega-3 fatty acids and omega-6 fatty acids. Their name and number refer to the position of their double bond in the chemical structure.

OMEGA-3 FATTY ACIDS

Medium-chain omega-3 fatty acids such as alpha-linolenic acid are found in flaxseed and flaxseed oil, canola oil, walnuts, soybean oil, wheat germ oil, leafy greens, and grasses. Long-chain omega-3 fatty acids such as eicosapentaenoic acid (EPA) and docosahexaenoic acid (DHA) are also known as marine omega fatty acids or fish oil. Fatty fish such as mackerel and herring contain a particularly large amount of omega-3 fatty acids; the original source of the fatty acids is the algae these fish eat.

What most people don't know: When grazing livestock are kept in their natural environment and able to consume mainly grass and hay, their milk and meat end up being rich in omega-3 fatty acids.

EPA lowers the risk of heart attack and hypertension and has an anti-inflammatory effect (e.g., for rheumatism), and there is evidence that DHA has a protective effect on the brain, such as from diseases like dementia. DHA is also said to support optimal brain performance in infantile and adolescent growth periods. Pregnant women in the United States often take omega-3 fatty acids as dietary supplements.

I often see claims that an exclusively plant-based diet doesn't allow us to meet our body's requirement for long-chain omega-3 fatty acids. That is not true. Our body has the ability to produce EPA from plant-based alpha-linolenic acid, but not in a ratio of one to one. We need a significantly larger amount of alpha-linolenic acid to produce the corresponding amount of EPA. This was demonstrated in an experiment called the Muffin Study, by Delfin Rodriguez-Leyva of the Lenin Hospital in Holguin, Cuba. Thirty grams of flaxseed was "hidden" in muffin batter. One group of participants ate one flaxseed muffin a day, while the other group ate a "generic" muffin, without flaxseed. Neither group of participants knew what ingredients the muffins contained (this is called a blind study design). After several weeks, the participants in the flaxseed group had significantly lower blood pressure compared to the other group—by almost 10 mmHg systolic. Moreover, there was a second surprise: A significant increase in EPA was measured in the blood of the flaxseed eaters. The alpha-linolenic acid contained in the flaxseed had been converted into marine omega-3 fatty acid (fish oil). This proved that EPA can be obtained through a purely plant-based diet.[10]

Two other studies have shown that our body can produce DHA from alpha-linolenic acid if we add a little turmeric to our food.[11]

You can also get omega-3 fatty acids by eating seaweed—which is, after all, one of the reasons why the inhabitants of Okinawa and the Japanese in general are so healthy. In the mornings they often have hot miso soup with wakame seaweed, or rice wrapped in sheets of nori. I believe that seaweed, or "salad of the sea," is going to become an important part of our diets in the future.

Is Fish Healthy?

Fish has a reputation for being healthy. Is this true? The first major studies on fish oil extracts showed positive results for its possibility of reducing the risk of heart attack and cardiac arrhythmias.[12] And in lab tests, all fish oils were able to curb the production of pro-inflammatory substances in the body, so-called eicosanoids, in an impressive way.[13] Yet after many studies were grouped together in extensive meta-analyses, there wasn't much evidence for the beneficial effect of fish oils.[14]

Only a few years ago, researchers at Harvard University were able to show that the proteins contained in fish are healthier than those in meat, but still less healthy than plant-based proteins.[15] If around 3 percent of the total protein calorie intake from fish is replaced by plant-based proteins, the risk of heart disease is reduced by 12 percent. Therefore, fish protein is not as harmful as meat protein (which causes a 39 percent risk increase!), but it's not a protection, either.

The origins of the idea that fish is healthy might be traced to the "Eskimo legend." In the 1970s, Danish scientists Hans Olaf Bang and Jørn Dyerberg traveled to Greenland to study the Inuit and their seemingly impressive heart health. The studies they published surprised other nutritional researchers, because the Inuit ate almost no vegetables or fruits—the opposite of what we've long believed is healthy for the heart. But the heart health of the Inuit was theorized to be the result of all the omega-3 fatty acids they consumed. The fact was, however, that the researchers didn't actually examine heart health and athero- sclerosis of the Inuit, but merely analyzed the fatty acid levels in their blood. Then, from data pulled from public death registries, they assumed that relatively few Inuit died of heart attacks. On closer inspection, this low rate of heart attack was due to the fact that the life expectancy of Inuit at fifty years was so low that the typical age for heart attacks wasn't even reached.[16] Later studies showed that the age-related rate of heart attacks in the Inuit people wasn't lower than that of mainland Danes or Americans.[17, 18] Interestingly enough, the life expectancy of the Inuit is rising now, since they have adopted a typical Western diet.[19] They are probably the only people in the world who have improved their health through a Western diet!

As a result of Bang and Dyerberg's work, there were more research projects conducted in Denmark examining the health benefits of con- suming fish. In the DART-1 (Diet and Reinfarction Trial) study, half of 2,033 patients who had suffered from a heart attack were advised to eat fatty saltwater fish at least twice a week or, alternatively, to take fish oil capsules. The initial results were promising: There was a 30 percent reduction in mortality risk after several months of following this ad- vice. But three years later, the result changed to the contrary. The mor- tality risk of the fish eaters had suddenly increased by 30 percent.[20] The result for the fish eaters in a follow-up study, the DART-2 study, was even worse. This study was conducted with 3,314 patients who suffered from heart disease and heart trouble (angina pectoris). There was no positive effect whatsoever for the fish eaters; the risk of mortality actu- ally increased in some of the patients who took fish oil capsules.[21] On the other hand, some observational studies (which provide little evi- dence) have described a slightly reduced risk of heart attack, diabetes, and cardiovascular disease with two to three servings of fatty saltwater fish per week.[22] However, we have to take into account what was being compared. It's very possible that participants in these studies ate fish when they would have normally eaten meat. Compared to meat, fish is the healthier alternative. But it is not inherently healthy. I hold fast to the belief that fish offers no advantage when it comes to omega-3 fatty acids—plant-based sources are sufficient.

And we must not forget that the problems within our oceans are also reducing the quality of the fish we eat. The oceans have been swallowing a lot of waste for centuries, but garbage—specifically plastic—is becoming a bigger and bigger ecological problem. The exposure of edible fish to toxic substances is high, resulting in biomagnification—the accumulation of substances such as dioxin, PCB (toxic and carcinogenic chlorine compounds), DDT (insecticide) and other pesticides, and heavy metals such as mercury, cadmium, and lead. The often-recommended fatty cold-water fish such as salmon and mackerel are affected by biomagnification. Elevated concentrations of these heavy metals can be detected in people who eat fish often.[23, 24] In addition, microplastics are increasingly being detected in fish. In the North Sea it is found in five out of seven animals.[25] Moreover, microplastics are a magnet for other harmful substances, including dioxin and PCB. What seems even more relevant to me is that fishing is no longer sustainable.[26] The Food and Agriculture Organization of the United Nations has already determined that only 13 percent of fish populations are large enough to regenerate without any problems.[27] Almost all calculations show that by the end of this century there will be no fish swimming in the sea unless fishing regulations are changed drastically.[28] Therefore, fish is not the best prospect for us as a food source. I don't think aquaculture is a good solution, either. Up to two hundred thousand salmon are kept in coarse-meshed enclosures in Norwegian aquacultures. As with any type of factory farming, the problem is that these fish live in spaces that are far too restricted. Parasites spread, which in turn are controlled with pesticides. The pesticides end up in the salmon and in the Norwegian fjords.[29] Conditions are even worse in the farms for animals such as scampi and prawns in Thailand and Vietnam. That's where most of the frozen shellfish sold in supermarkets comes from. If you would like to consume omega-3 fatty acids, I recommend that you eat mainly plant-based sources.

Eating fish is not sustainable, and with the increasing pollution of the oceans, the risk of fish being harmful to your health is increasing. If you don't want to give up fish, make sure to buy organic, even if it may unfortunately be expensive. I would advise against eating salmon, mackerel, cod, pollock, and tuna. Ecologically speaking, things are not looking good for these species of fish. Above all, I'd advise staying far away from shellfish.

OMEGA-6 FATTY ACIDS

These fatty acids are found mainly in vegetable oils, such as sunflower oil and corn oil. These oils lower blood cholesterol levels and are better than animal-derived fat, coconut oil, and palm oil with their high amounts of saturated fatty acids. However, due to their given inflammatory side effect, sunflower oil and corn oil should not be the primary oils you use in the kitchen. Sesame oil, however, is rich in omega-6 fatty acids and contains many antioxidants; studies show that it lowers blood lipid levels. I prepare almost all Asian dishes with sesame oil and garnish with toasted sesame seeds before serving.

Trans Fats or Trans-fatty Acids

Trans fats can occur naturally or through food processing. They can be created when liquid oils are turned into solid, spreadable, harder fats such as margarine—that's why they are also called hardened fats. Trans fats are the bad boys among the fats. They massively increase LDL-cholesterol and triglyceride levels. They intensify inflammatory processes in the body, lead to insulin resistance, and are linked to an increased risk of heart and vascular diseases as well as certain types of cancer.[30] In 2015, the FDA banned the use of trans fats; manufacturers were given three years to eliminate any artificial trans fats from their food products.[31] Trans fats are often found in potato chips, doughnuts, and the kinds of deep-fried treats we often see at fairs—give these foods a wide berth.

The Ornish Diet

One of the pioneers of plant-based nutrition is the American cardiologist Dean Ornish. In several studies, he worked with patients whose heart diseases were so severe that they were no longer treatable with modern cardiology. Ornish would ask them to follow a plant-based (vegan), strictly low-fat diet—and the results showed astonishing success.[32] Other cardiologists have been able to corroborate his success.[33] The Ornish diet requires strong willpower, since the diet's low fat restriction makes it easy to get hungry. Most patients I know who follow this diet often keep containers filled with vegetables on hand to satiate their hunger.

But the Ornish diet is, without a doubt, a cure for coronary arteriosclerosis. This has been confirmed time and again in my consultations. Not only does it lead to weight loss and a drop in LDL-cholesterol levels, it also leads to stabilization of heart disease and causes coronary artery disease to diminish. It seems important to me that the Ornish diet causes LDL-cholesterol values to drop to levels that are otherwise achieved only with high doses of statins or other modern cholesterol medications. LDL levels are generally below 100 mg/dl, but they're often even lower in patients on the Ornish diet (50–70 mg/dl). We usually see these levels only in newborns or indigenous peoples who are barely affected by heart disease.[34]

Choosing such a drastic diet is always a personal decision. If the Ornish diet is too extreme for you, you might try the vegetarian PRED-IMED diet—that is, a Mediterranean diet rich in vegetables and fruit, olive oil, and nuts.

My Conclusion on Fats

- You should largely avoid saturated fats, ideally by not eating meat. If you eat animal fat in the form of butter and dairy products, then you should have only small amounts and pay attention to organic quality.
- Polyunsaturated fatty acids are better than saturated fatty acids, but some studies have shown slight inflammatory effects,[35] so I recommend avoiding sunflower oil and corn oil, especially if you suffer from inflammatory or rheumatic illnesses.
- Monounsaturated fatty acids are healthy: olive oil, canola oil, and nut butter made from almonds, hazelnuts, cashews, or pecans.
- Omega-3 fatty acids should be eaten in large quantities, but not in the form of fish oil. A recent study showed that heart patients with high blood-lipid levels can benefit from high doses of eicosapentaenoic acid (EPA). As I mentioned earlier, EPA can also be metabolized from plant-based alpha-linolenic acid.[36] The main source of omega-3 fatty acids should be flaxseed, flaxseed oil, walnuts, and leafy greens.

Protein

Proteins have long maintained a good reputation in the world of nutrition. They are undoubtedly important for our somatic cells, and they

A Different Way of Using Fat: Oil Pulling

Oil pulling, the practice of washing one's mouth with cooking oil, comes from Ayurvedic medicine. Although it doesn't make the body discharge toxins, as is often claimed, oil pulling can activate digestion via saliva early in the day. Studies have shown that oil pulling is an effective therapy for periodontitis, fights germs in the mouth, and prevents bad breath. And it has fewer side effects than chemical mouthwashes.

How to practice oil pulling:

- Every morning put a teaspoon of cooking oil, such as organic sunflower oil, in your mouth.
- Swish the oil around your mouth for three to five minutes—make sure to get it in between your teeth by pressing it through the gaps.
- Spit the oil out (in the trash, so your sink won't clog) and rinse your mouth with water. Do not swallow the oil!
- Brush your teeth.

are the most critical building blocks for organ systems such as the heart, brain, muscles, skin, and hair. Furthermore, enzymes, hormones, and antibodies are ultimately proteins. This macronutrient is much more complex than carbohydrates or fats. To put it simply, carbohydrates and fats serve mainly as energy sources, while proteins fulfill more complicated tasks.

Proteins are made up of small building blocks called amino acids. There are twenty standard amino acids that make up all of life's proteins. These twenty amino acids can be assembled in different combinations into more complex chains. A protein can consist of more than one thousand amino acids. Eight amino acids (valine, isoleucine, leucine, lysine, methionine, phenylalanine, threonine, and tryptophan) are considered essential, and it was long believed we could only get them through food. However, recent studies suggest that the body is able to produce these amino acids on its own, after all.[37, 38]

Unlike fat and carbohydrates, protein can't be stored by humans. In emergencies, such as during prolonged periods of hunger, proteins are released by the muscles as reserve energy. These muscle proteins are then used to create sugar for our brain. But muscle loss is never sensible or healthy. That's why for long periods of therapeutic fasting, a minimum amount of calories is consumed in the form of juice or vegetable broth to avoid protein breakdown from the muscles. Protein deficiency is rare in the developed world; we might see it in cases of extreme malnutrition or some serious illnesses.

Just as deficiency is unhealthy, an excess of nutritional proteins is also unhealthy. The consequences include kidney problems, digestive disorders, and above all, the promotion of inflammatory processes in the body. That's why I advise staying away from those protein shakes you sometimes see sold at gyms. You should also beware of high-protein powders; they are an unhealthy waste of money. Instead, it's best to eat plenty of vegetable proteins, ideally pure—that is, not canned, frozen, or ready-made, but as natural as possible (nuts, legumes, whole grains, leafy greens, and seeds).

Protein Has Three Important Qualities

PROTEIN MAKES YOU FEEL FULL

Protein satiates much better than carbohydrates and fat. Even if it initially seems like fat is more filling because it has more calories (1 gram of protein has 4 kcal; 1 gram of fat, a little over 9 kcal), studies show that this is not true. If you ingest the same number of calories in protein and fat, the protein will keep you feeling full for longer. In terms of evolutionary biology, this makes sense, since protein can't be stored but is exceedingly important for many processes in our body (more important than fat). When given the choice, we're always going to opt for the nutrient that satiates us for longer.

PROTEIN FACILITATES WEIGHT LOSS—BUT ONLY IN THE SHORT TERM

Protein doesn't raise the blood sugar level, and for that reason, insulin doesn't need to be released for protein alone. When insulin levels are low, fat is burned, even overnight. So if you make your evening meal high in protein rather than in fat or carbohydrates, protein can actually help you lose weight.

Time and again, we read that eating a diet that is protein heavy (30 percent or more) works wonders for weight loss.[39] This can indeed help reduce weight quickly in the short term. And for the treatment of a fatty liver, a temporary protein diet can be helpful. But in the long run, a protein-rich diet is not the healthiest option, for reasons I'll explain in the next section.

PROTEIN FACILITATES GROWTH—BUT ALSO AGING

The renowned Italian American age researcher Valter Longo said in an interview for *Spiegel* magazine in 2018, "I don't know any demographic group with a long life expectancy that has relied on a high intake of protein and fat."[40] His criticism of protein is based on the results of many years of research in which he investigated the secrets of cell aging. Working with other researchers, he realized that there was nothing to gain from antiaging medications and vitamins. Instead, they discovered that aging can be delayed by 20 to 40 percent through a reduction of caloric intake and repeated fasting in all organisms, from yeast to mice.

Longo then systematically pursued the question of whether this antiaging effect could be achieved only by reducing the overall energy intake, or if it could also be achieved by omitting individual nutritional components. And indeed, it was primarily the amino acids, particularly those of animal origin, that accelerated the aging process. The result was astonishing: Protein, which is so essential for our growth, is also what makes us age faster.

Two protein actors that control somatic cell growth and cause aging are essential to this paradox of growth but aging: the protein mTOR and the peptide hormone IGF-1. The first, mTOR, is a kind of control center for growth: It regulates the proliferation, differentiation, and reproduction of cells. Bodybuilders drink protein shakes to stimulate their muscle growth. IGF-1 is a (muscle) growth factor that is primarily triggered (in other words, released) by animal protein and for the most part produced in the liver. It's not surprising that this insulin-like growth factor is used as an illegal doping substance.

Growth is desirable in childhood, but eventually we become fully grown. If adults ingest proteins in concentrated amounts and in substances such as fitness drinks or doping drugs, they also facilitate the growth of cancer cells. In lab experiments this connection between mTOR, IGF-1, and the growth of cancer cells is clear.[41] When test animals with cancer are fed a high-protein diet, they die much more often than animals who are fed a low-protein diet.[42] Interestingly, taller people generally have a slightly higher risk of cancer.

As important as growth is when we are young, exceedingly strong growth signals are dangerous for older organisms. Cancer, after all, is characterized by uncontrolled growth.

Therefore, a protein-rich, high-calorie diet becomes a breeding ground for cancer growth. But calcification of the vessels and inflammation such as atherosclerosis are also fueled by too much animal protein. Inflammation at the cellular level is probably one of the main causes of premature aging.

So How Much Protein Should We Consume?

How much protein is just healthy enough to satisfy our hunger and supply the body with sufficient amounts of all the essential amino acids, and how much of it is harmful? The answer is relatively simple: The body should be nourished with plenty of plant-based proteins but never with large amounts of animal protein.

In the Blue Zones, proteins make up about 14 to 17 percent of the total energy intake through food. In 1950, when researchers noted the impressive longevity of the people in Okinawa, it was at a mere 9 percent![43]

Stay Away from a High-Protein Diet

Animal protein is still the main source of protein in the Western world—we eat a lot of meat, milk, cheese, butter, and fish. I think this is a catastrophe. We've been able to observe alarming health effects when people eat too much protein—the high-fat Atkins diet, for example.

Robert Atkins was an American cardiologist and nutritionist who, in the past century, promoted a high-fat, high-protein diet. He started to market it aggressively after achieving very good weight loss results in obese patients with his diet. What he didn't know or didn't want to know: Despite the weight loss, his diet usually led to a significant deterioration of the metabolism and circulation as well as hypertension after only a few months. A clinical study by Shane A. Phillips, a professor at the University of Illinois at Chicago, showed severe impairment of the blood vessel walls after only six weeks of following the Atkins diet.

Robert Atkins himself died at age seventy-two and suffered from coronary artery calcification, severe heart failure, and obesity—which his followers tried to hide for a long time.[44]

Glycoproteins

Glycoproteins, the so-called AGEs (advanced glycation end products), are glycated or caramelized proteins. They are formed when proteins are heated up at high temperatures in combination with sugar or carbohydrates—for example, when breaded chicken is deep-fried. They seem to play a role in age-related chronic diseases such as type 2 diabetes, kidney damage, and atherosclerosis.[45] They are also said to have a negative effect on bone density.[46]

Microscopically speaking, AGEs are indeed toxins. It is believed that during fasting, AGEs are activated and broken down, which is one of the reasons fasting is so healthy for the body.

Protein Requirements in Old Age

Around the age of forty, we start to lose muscle mass. That's why as we get older, we have to work harder to prevent this muscle loss (also known as sarcopenia in medical jargon). I recommend targeted strength training from the age of fifty at the latest. It is the best way to prevent muscle loss. After the age of sixty-five, the muscles also need more protein than they did before.

We therefore have to adapt our protein intake to the different phases of our life. Children and adolescents need more protein during phases of growth, and adults need less protein. Protein becomes important again with advancing age. In one observational study, to which Valter Longo also contributed, more than six thousand Americans over the age of fifty were examined and observed over the course of eighteen years. Participants who ate a lot of animal protein between the ages of fifty and sixty-five had major detrimental health effects. Not only were they at higher risk for diabetes, they were four times more likely to develop cancer and had a 75 percent higher risk of death. Meanwhile, the study participants who ate exclusively plant-based proteins showed no adverse effects on cancer risk and mortality rate.

However, after age sixty-five, a distinct change would occur. Now the participants who ate a high-protein diet, no matter whether the protein was animal- or plant-based, had an advantage. Higher protein intake, whether animal- or plant-based, was now associated with reduced mortality and cancer risk. Diabetes risk, though, remained increased with higher protein intake.[47]

Only when it came to participants with diabetes did animal protein remain an unfavorable factor in all age groups. This is likely because the alkaline quality of vegetables, which buffers acids, is believed to protect us from muscle loss. Normally, the kidneys ensure most of the buffering of acids in the body. With increasing age, however, kidney function deteriorates. Animal protein means more acid load for the body; plant-based meals, on the other hand, counteract this.

When the Acid-Base Balance Is Unsettled

In order for our metabolic processes to run optimally, our blood should have a pH value of 7.4. The pH value is the measure of the acidity of a solution. Depending on what we eat, our acid-base balance can be unsettled. Bases can buffer acids, but when the body's buffer systems are overwhelmed—for example, by an intake of too much acid—the body mobilizes minerals such as calcium from the bones to restore balance. But this process facilitates osteoporosis. This in turn affects the connective tissues, which become more pain-sensitive when exposed to too much acid. Furthermore, an acid-rich diet promotes kidney stones and muscle loss in old age. Patients with kidney disease are more likely to be affected by this, since the acid load affects the kidneys directly. When we eat foods that are rich in acid, the kidneys produce ammonia, a base, which neutralizes the acid. In the long run, however, ammonia damages the kidneys because it is a cytotoxin. It's a vicious cycle. And with increasing age, kidney function generally declines, and with it the ability to buffer acids.

A Healthy Acid-Base Balance

Alkaline	Acidic
• Fruit and vegetables	• Meat and fish
• Fruit and vegetable juices	• Dairy products and eggs
• Mineral water with a high bicarbonate content	• Bread and grain products
• Exercise and relaxation	• A stressful lifestyle

A modern diet with a lot of animal protein often leads to an insidious overacidification of the body. Foods with an alkaline effect, along with a healthy lifestyle, bring the acid-base ratio back into balance.

Animal proteins—meat, fish, eggs, and dairy products such as cheese (particularly processed cheese)—have an especially negative effect on our acid-base balance. Canned tuna is very acidic, while soft drinks such as cola, grain products, and bread are slightly acidic (fortunately, pasta isn't). It's the phosphorus in the grain that has a chemically acidic effect.

Which foods produce what amount of acid can't be determined precisely. But there are the so-called PRAL values (potential renal acid load), which tell us the estimated potential acid load on the body for every 100 grams of food. You can find lists of PRAL values for differ-ent foods online. Foods that have an acidifying effect on the body have a high positive value, while foods that have an alkalizing effect on the body have a negative value. Canned tuna, for example, has a PRAL value of around +12, while orange juice has a PRAL value of around -3. This evaluation was developed by Thomas Remer and Friedrich Manz, a nutritionist and a nephrologist, and provides helpful guiding principles. If acid production is high due to the consumption of a lot of meat or fish, for example, it helps to drink a glass of orange or veg-etable juice. This buffers the acid and creates a balance. Drinking min-eral water rich in bicarbonate helps with chronic kidney diseases. Detox clinics often recommend an alkaline powder; in our clinic we occasionally use it in therapeutic fasting. In everyday life, however, it makes more sense to follow a diet rich in bases rather than relying on an alkaline powder or pill. And almost all vegetables and fruits are rich in bases.

Milk Is Not Healthy

Milk is the source of life for all newborns in the world; all mammals are reared with it. In fact, breast milk contains all the ingredients the offspring needs to thrive in the first few months of life. It is not for nothing that milk has been a particularly valuable food source for thousands of years. However, human and animal breast milk differ. Human breast milk contains only a third of the amount of protein in cow's milk. Human milk is very low in protein, whereas cow's milk works almost like a growth cocktail.[48] This is because calves need to start putting on weight extremely fast right after birth (about a pound and a half a day), while a human newborn grows much more slowly.[49] And that's why for adult humans, the hormones contained in cow's milk trigger inflammation and premature aging.[50]

It's fair to assume that thousands of years ago, adult humans could not drink milk. Their bodies could not tolerate it, because only infants and toddlers were able to produce the increased amounts of the lactase enzyme that is essential for the digestion of milk sugar (lactose) contained in milk. It makes sense for children to be able to produce lactase while they are being breastfed. But the body produces large quantities of lactase only in infancy. From an evolutionary standpoint, humans no longer needed lactase once they stopped being breastfed. But scientists have calculated that a gene variant that occurred about eight thousand years ago allowed humans to continue producing lactase into adulthood.[51] The ability to drink cow's milk became an evolutionary advantage, so it's not surprising that this gene has prevailed, particu-

---

Lactose Intolerance

Suffering from lactose intolerance is not the same as having an allergy. With an allergy, even the tiniest amount can trigger a severe, sometimes life-threatening reaction. With lactose intolerance, on the other hand, a little milk can usually be tolerated. It is only after a certain amount that the stomach might start to grumble, because lactose cannot be broken down and digested in the upper intestinal tract. The undigested lactose moves on to the large intestine, where bacteria break it down, causing flatulence and diarrhea, about fifteen to thirty minutes after the milk is first ingested.

Lactose intolerance can be diagnosed with a breath test. If you are suffering from lactose intolerance but don't want to live a dairy-free lifestyle, then you should continue to eat small amounts of dairy products so that your body doesn't completely shut down the production of lactase. Well-aged, grainy cheese (parmesan) or kefir are generally well tolerated. Lactase powder as an enzyme replacement is available commercially, but studies on these powders have only been able to demonstrate a placebo effect.

larly in the northern hemisphere, with its long winters. Today, the lactase enzyme can be detected in 80 to 90 percent of the population in Northern Europe but only in 30 percent of people worldwide.[52]

Up until a few years ago, nutritionists agreed that milk was generally beneficial for health. It has many indisputably valuable ingredients—vitamins, minerals, and proteins. But age researchers saw things a little differently. As important as the growth factors and proteins contained in breast milk are for infants, they are unnecessary and can be harmful for adults.[53, 54] Research on animals has shown that milk and its proteins can promote premature aging and cancer growth.[55] However clear these results in animal studies are, they are not easily transferrable to humans. However, milk and dairy products are suspected to contribute to autoimmune diseases such as multiple sclerosis, rheumatoid arthritis, and inflammatory bowel diseases.[56] What has been scientifically proven beyond a doubt is that milk promotes acne.[57]

For a long time, women going through menopause were advised to drink milk to aid in the prevention of osteoporosis (because of milk's high calcium content). But a study from Scandinavia showed the opposite: Excessive milk consumption causes bones to become more brittle.[58] Apparently, the benefit of calcium is negated by phosphoproteins and the sulfurous amino acids methionine and cysteine, which are also contained in milk. These proteins have an inflammatory and chemical effect like an acid. The body tries to buffer this acid load with calcium, which is mobilized from the bones. By the way, osteoporosis occurs much less often in menopausal women in Japan and China, where milk is drunk only very rarely.[59]

Another argument against consuming milk is milk fat, which consists mainly of saturated fatty acids. A Harvard study with more than two hundred thousand participants showed that the risk of heart attack and stroke was reduced by 24 percent if only 5 percent of dietary energy from milk fat was replaced with plant-based fat.[60] Researchers from

Sweden confirmed this: They put participants in a study on a diet rich in milk fat (butter, cream, and cheese) for three weeks, and the control group on a diet rich in canola oil (canola oil and margarine made from canola oil). In the canola oil group, blood lipid levels improved significantly.[61] In the Scandinavian study I mentioned in the previous paragraph, researchers noted that in addition to higher bone fragility, they also noticed an increased mortality rate if participants drank a lot of milk.[62]

Things are a little better with cheese and yogurt than with milk, because these contain less lactose and therefore less galactose, a component of lactose that fosters inflammation and cell aging. Scientists have used galactose specifically to provoke premature aging and geriatric diseases in lab animals. Dementia and low fertility were observed in these experiments.[63] Cheese and yogurt contain bacteria that feed on milk sugar, which is why the lactose and galactose content in these dairy products is lower. Lactose-free milk contains pre-broken-down lactose but just as much galactose.

Reduce Milk and Dairy Products in Your Diet

In order to keep producing milk, dairy cows are constantly artificially inseminated. They are milked even during pregnancy. Because of this, significant amounts of sex hormones (which are produced in large quantities during pregnancy) are present in the milk we drink. This also applies to organic milk. These excess hormones that we ingest through milk are partially, but not completely, deactivated in the liver. Acne is then triggered hormonally by milk, and in men the consumption of milk also leads to reduced fertility.

What is more worrisome are the growth hormones insulin, IGF-1, and mTOR, whose concentration increases in the blood with the consumption of milk, to detrimental effect. These growth hormones are associated with an increased risk of cancer. In various experiments, milk was directly dripped onto prostate cancer cells. In each of these experiments, the growth of the cancer cells was stimulated by this process. Almond milk, on the other hand, reduced growth. Even though lab experiments can't be transferred to humans one-to-one, these results are worth paying attention to.

There are, ultimately, few convincing arguments for considering milk healthy. A glass of milk here and there is fine, but constant consumption is a problem. Moreover, milk is a true "killjoy" even in small amounts: Coffee has clear health-promoting effects, but if you add milk, this effect is canceled. The Graz, Austria–based researcher Frank Madeo found that coffee promotes autophagy, the self-cleaning of the cells. Within up to four hours after having coffee, cellular autophagy is boosted immensely. These effects occur both in coffee containing caffeine as well as decaffeinated coffee. Adding milk, however, almost completely negates this effect. These findings have also occurred in connection with black tea. Verena Stangl, a cardiologist at the Charité hospital, and her team researched the effect of tea on blood vessels. One group of subjects drank about two cups of black tea every day, while the other group drank black tea with low-fat milk. The group that drank unadulterated black tea showed improved vessel reaction, while the group that drank tea with milk showed no beneficial effects whatsoever. In further experiments, scientists were able to show that milk protein slows down the beneficial effect tea has on the vessels. The milk protein casein neutralizes the effective catechin of the tea.

> **Tip:** If you like drinking coffee with milk, try adding a plant-based milk such as almond, oat, or soy milk. They don't destroy the healthy effects of the coffee and have plenty of health-promoting, plant-based proteins.

The detrimental effect of milk is also why dark chocolate is healthier than milk chocolate. In milk chocolate, the percentage of cocoa is low and the milk proteins block the healthy effect of the cocoa.

Some studies have shown that milk and dairy products have a slightly antihypertensive property. On the other hand, countless clinical studies have proven that diabetes and hypertension can be avoided or treated very effectively with a vegan diet. Researchers from Toronto have summarized studies in which diabetics replaced animal protein with plant-based protein, concluding that consuming plant-based protein revealed a significant advantage: Blood pressure and sugar levels improved, and insulin and other hormone levels stayed within the normal range.

Yogurt, however, keeps getting very good results in many studies, particularly in terms of weight loss. It's likely that the bacteria contained in yogurt are responsible for this effect. But now there are plant-based yogurt products with similar bacteria available. Plant-based foods that are fermented in particular contain healthy bacteria. These include sauerkraut, kimchi, bread drink, fermented juices, and soy sauce.

If you don't want to skip dairy products altogether, then try to do the following:

- Use only small amounts.
- Use organic products made from the milk of free-range, grass-fed cows.
- Try to consume only unsweetened organic yogurt or kefir.
- Use cheese as a seasoning, such as pasta sprinkled with parmesan or pecorino.

Eggs

Having eggs for breakfast is a modern habit; our ancestors didn't eat them regularly or in large quantities. In addition, eggs are added to countless foods, usually to create a yellow color. Or they serve as a kind of glue so that cakes, pasta, and dough do not crumble.

When Ancel Keys discovered that high cholesterol levels significantly increase the risk of fatal heart attacks, the reputation of eggs was severely damaged, since egg yolks contain a lot of cholesterol. Later, however, it became clear that cholesterol itself isn't necessarily dangerous—rather, what's dangerous are saturated fats in food that are converted into cholesterol in the liver. There have since been numerous observational studies giving chicken eggs a more or less neutral status.

But there's a case to be made against the consumption of eggs. Like milk, eggs aren't meant to be a staple food. They're designed to support the development of a newborn chick. The high protein and cholesterol content of eggs may seem valuable at first, but it can be detrimental to adults. Just like milk, eggs have been shown to foster inflammation in the body in lab experiments. New studies strongly indicate that eggs increase the risk of atherosclerosis and heart attacks after all. Cholesterol doesn't appear to be the causal agent as much as choline and phosphatidylcholine (better known as lecithin), substances that occur in meat and cheese as well, but their concentration is especially high in eggs. Choline and phosphatidylcholine are converted into TMAO (trimethylamine N-oxide) by intestinal bacteria. High levels of TMAO in the blood have been linked to a higher risk for heart attack, stroke, other cardiovascular problems, and chronic kidney disease. So, should we eat eggs or not? I recommend limiting your consumption of eggs, or, ideally, not eating them at all. In a study by researchers at Cleveland State University, two hard-boiled eggs were enough to produce higher levels of TMAO in the blood. Another reason I advise against eating eggs is that the egg industry is the epitome of the terrible factory farm industry. Foodborne infections and food poisoning are most commonly caused by eggs. There are new scandals almost every year, and only recently the pesticide Fipronil was found in eggs.

You might be able to give up eggs for breakfast if you have other delicious options: fresh bread with savory vegetable spreads or oatmeal with berries and nuts. Instead of scrambled eggs, you could try scrambled tofu. And there are numerous plant-based alternatives to eggs when it comes to cooking and baking.

Meat

"The best meat is the flesh of fruit." I often refer to this quote by the nutritionist Claus Leitzmann in lectures to lightheartedly make the case for a meatless diet. I know this isn't an easy message for many people to hear. But the data doesn't lie!

A wealth of nutritional studies has revealed that a whole-food, plant-based, meatless or at least low-meat diet is the healthiest possible diet.[64] Two decades ago, Leitzmann recommended two options for an optimal diet: a vegetarian—ideally vegan—whole-food diet, or a diet in which meat and fish are eaten only on special occasions.[65, 66]

But Leitzmann was a pioneer in another way as well. He pointed out that when it comes to the consumption of meat and fish, the question isn't just which diet is the healthiest for us—ecology should be a central question too. All ecological, social, and animal welfare arguments convincingly point in one direction: A world without the consumption of meat would definitely have fewer problems!

Meat has a high carbon footprint: 70 percent of arable land is used to breed animals worldwide.[67] Four thousand gallons of water are needed to produce about two pounds of beef.[68] And let's not forget, the livestock industry is responsible for 15 to 20 percent of greenhouse gases.[69]

Quitting meat is probably the only way to feed everyone on earth without destroying our planet's ecology. But despite the rising number of vegetarians and vegans around the world, it is still hard for many people to imagine giving up meat. A juicy burger or steak still embodies, for many, the height of pleasure. Nevertheless, there's a lot to be said for issues that could be improved by avoiding meat: animal welfare, the climate, environmental resources (such as water), and the global fight against hunger. Every day when talking to my patients, I witness how dietary habits can change even though our tastes have been shaped by our culture and our upbringing for centuries.

It's become much easier to give up meat now than it was even a decade earlier. There are fresh vegetables, legumes, and plant-based sources of protein available in every supermarket. You can order vegetarian or vegan dishes in almost every restaurant nowadays without being scrutinized. It wasn't always this easy. When I decided to stop eating meat thirteen years ago, ordering meals in restaurants would often lead to an intense interrogation from the waiter: "No meat? But a little bacon in the sauce is fine, isn't it? It's not? How about fish? No?"

In Germany, Austria, and Switzerland, meat is a central component of almost every meal. In my hometown of Upper Swabia, Germany, almost all traditional dishes contain meat, sausage, or bacon in some form. Yet these days the local cuisine has changed as well; there is at least one vegetarian alternative on the menu of almost every restaurant.

Of course, eating meat doesn't make you sick right away; nobody drops dead out of their chair if they eat a single hamburger. But consuming meat regularly and in large quantities is responsible for many diseases in the Western world, including heart attacks, strokes, diabetes, hypertension, as well as arthrosis, arthritis, even dementia and some types of cancer (colon cancer, breast cancer, prostate cancer).[70, 71, 72] Substantial consumption of meat is unhealthy; there's no argument about it.

Processed meat, such as sausage, is the most harmful. With sausage, the problem lies within the many substances that are added. Sausage often includes curing salt, nitrates, and a lot of saturated fat. Over the past two decades, the majority of studies indicate that the consumption of sausage products—as little as two ounces a day (this is the equivalent of one sausage or a slice of ham)—increases the risk of intestinal cancer by 15 to 20 percent, of cardiovascular diseases by up to 40 percent, and of diabetes by 20 to 51 percent.[73] Even unprocessed meat is harmful to health. Eating 3.5 ounces of beef, pork, lamb, or venison a day increases your risk of developing diabetes by 19 percent and your risk of getting colon cancer by 17 percent.

Paleo, the "Stone Age Diet"

The word *Paleo* is short for *Paleolithic*, referring to the Paleolithic age that lasted from 2,500,000 to 8,000 BCE. Followers of the Paleo diet believe that our digestive system is still wired the way it was back then, when humans were hunter-gatherers. And so eating like our Stone Age ancestors is the principle of the Paleo diet, which promotes eating food that is as unprocessed as possible: lots of meat, lots of fish, root vegetables, and herbs. It rejects modern foods such as bread and other wheat products, dairy products, pressed oils, refined sugar, and alcohol. I'm rather critical of Paleo because many people—especially men—see it as a free ticket to unlimited meat consumption.

What Happens If You Stop Eating Meat and Fish?

Every one-sided diet has disadvantages. This is true for the vegan diet as well as for the Paleo diet—even if the former is mostly healthy and the latter mostly unhealthy. The most important thing is to eat a balanced, whole-food diet! I recommend a vegan diet for everyone (including children and pregnant women)—alongside other healthy forms of nutrition, such as the Mediterranean diet. A vegan who eats sugary cereal or toast with jam for breakfast, white wheat pasta with tomato sauce for lunch, and a tofu sausage with French fries for dinner is not healthy, of course.

If you follow a vegan diet, you need to be aware of your vitamin B12 levels. This vitamin plays an essential role in important metabolic processes and supports hematopoiesis. Meat, fish, eggs, milk, and dairy products are good sources of vitamin B12. If you avoid those, I recommend taking a supplement or using a toothpaste enriched with vitamin B12. The vitamin can also be administered by injection.

Vegetarians or vegans may suffer from Iron deficiency. The iron contained in meat and animal products is indeed better absorbed by the small intestine in the form of divalent iron than the plant-based trivalent iron. However, for the majority of people in the developed world it's not iron deficiency that's the problem but an excess of iron. Due to our high meat consumption, iron levels tend to be high rather than low—which increases the risk of diabetes, hypertension, fatty liver, and cardiovascular diseases, potentially even of some types of cancer. This can be counteracted with a vegetarian or vegan diet, or even by donating blood on a regular basis. Vegan women who have heavy periods need to pay special attention to their iron levels. Whole grains, legumes, seeds, nuts, and vegetables contain iron. If you ingest vitamin C or acidic foods at the same time, trivalent iron is converted into divalent iron and absorption is increased. So if you suffer from iron deficiency, you should eat a slice of bell pepper or drink a glass of orange juice along with your whole-grain bread.

Red and White Meat

So-called red meat includes beef, pork, and lamb. People who want to reduce their meat consumption usually start by giving up pork first, since they suspect that it is particularly bad for their health. Beef and lamb, however, aren't any healthier.

White meat—that is, poultry—performs slightly better in health risk calculations, at least in the case of heart diseases.[74] But due to factory farming, poultry is linked to infections and measurable drug residues in the meat.

Unfortunately, factory farming has contributed to a decline in the quality of meat. Meat was once a privilege of the aristocracy; today it is a health risk. But the past is still present in people's minds—many continue to measure the idea of being privileged and wealthy by the ability to afford meat every day. This brings us to the next myth: that eating meat is "masculine" and helps men boost libido. Statistics show that women eat less meat and adopt a vegetarian diet more often than men.[75] In fact, however, men who follow a vegetarian diet or one that doesn't include a lot of meat have higher testosterone levels and suffer less from erectile dysfunction than men who eat meat.[76, 77] So there you have it, gentlemen—there are no more excuses!

Stop Eating Meat and Live Healthier

Perhaps you are someone who wants to switch to a meat-free diet but are finding it more challenging than you anticipated. You might be wondering if there are tips or tricks to make it easy to stop eating meat completely.

I want to be honest, there is ultimately only one way: You must grit your teeth and do it. We humans are heavily fixated on our habits, and the reward and happiness centers in our brain have been programmed accordingly over many years. Eating a steak is almost as great as having sex, it seems to suggest to us. When we anticipate or expect a craving to be fulfilled, the brain is flooded by neurotransmitters or hormones that create a sense of joy.[78] If we want to change a habit, there's no way to do it without experiencing withdrawal symptoms.[79] This may not be physiological, but it is at least psychological. It's important to know this so that you won't stumble into this feeling of withdrawal without warning. Know that this feeling that something is missing doesn't last and will recede over time.

I was in my early forties when I decided to become a vegetarian. I still remember how difficult it was for me to stop eating meat completely. Most patients who stop eating meat and fish for health reasons have an easier time of it, since they see the health benefits rather quickly. After one year at the most, giving up meat is no longer a problem for them. During this transitional phase I don't object to meat substitutes such as veggie burger patties or sausages made from tofu or seitan. Having something on the plate that at least looks familiar is comforting. Eventually, people who have been vegetarian for a long time often develop a big collection of delicious recipes and no longer turn to meat substitutes.

Reducing your consumption of meat little by little, for example to once a week or once a fortnight, is a practical method. In any case, make sure to buy meat of free-range, organic quality.

If you can't (yet) imagine giving up meat completely, I recommend a challenge. Be a vegetarian for three months! During this time, observe your energy levels and overall health. Also note if and when you are actually missing meat.

Umami

As a vegetarian you don't have to miss out on umami, the savory flavor that can be found in fried or grilled meat. The term for this fifth sense of taste—next to sweet, sour, salty, and bitter—is Japanese and means "flavorful," "aromatic," "the essence." The umami taste is mainly caused by glutamic acid, which is an amino acid found in proteins.

If you're overcome with "umami greed," try cooking with foods such as tomatoes, celery, mushrooms, garlic, vegetable broth, and fermented foods such as miso and soy sauce—they all provide a lot of the umami taste. Aged cheese such as parmesan also has umami.

The pleasure of food is not dependent on meat. Vegetarian cuisine is incredibly delicious and imaginative, and you can enjoy the additional pleasure of knowing that your dietary choices are good for our planet.

Patient History: Hypertension, Renal Infarction

Martin H., a fifty-six-year-old recruitment consultant and coach from Berlin, almost died because of a tear in his aorta. He subsequently discovered how therapeutic fasting and vegetable juice can act as natural antihypertensive medicine.

"It was almost too late when I realized that I needed to change ..."

I was taken to the emergency room after a renal infarction struck me down. I was very lucky that the attending doctor had previously worked in cardiology and recognized the rare cause: renal infarction—a large tear in my aorta caused by hypertension.

I had known for years that my blood pressure tended to be high—190/100 instead of the healthy 120/80. I was taking medication for it, but the medication wasn't always able to keep my blood pressure under control. My lifestyle exacerbated the problem. I took frequent business trips, always quickly eating on the go. I didn't care about what I ate, as long as it was filling. Now, I have an eight-inch-long metal stent that supports my aorta. It's quite the reminder.

My doctor said that I should try to make some changes in my life. I decided to try a fasting cure, and went to see Dr. Michalsen at his clinic. With the right reasons and motivation, I can follow through on things that may seem hard, like not eating for days. I quickly understood why giving up food could give my body the chance to reset and free my taste buds of their addiction to salt and sugar, which had become normal to me.

In addition to fasting, I took nutritional courses in the hospital. After those courses, I decided to seize the moment and mostly stop eating meat, white-flour grain products, dairy products, salt, and sugar. This doesn't mean that I won't prepare a special dish once or twice a month and enjoy goose breast with red cabbage and dumplings with my wife, but it does mean that I now consider this a special pleasure and not the norm! My everyday diet is now more purposeful, and I'm doing well with it: In the morning I drink freshly squeezed orange juice blended with carrots. For my days at the office I prepare salads or vegetable soups. Every now and again I'll eat a sandwich, but I won't put any meat or cheese on it; instead I'll add vegetables and eggs instead. Fruit or vegetable smoothies are handy for when I'm on the go. If I have a meeting at a restaurant, I order fish. I don't eat anything after five p.m. Intermittent fasting—in which you don't eat anything for a period of sixteen hours—works well for my schedule, and I don't feel like I'm hungry or missing anything.

My weight has dropped from 220 to 207 pounds (I'm 6'1"); I practice endurance sports such as swimming; and I've rearranged my work commitments so I don't travel quite as much. This combination, together with the healthy diet, ensures that my blood pressure is now permanently at 140/80 or 130/80, without medication. Almost perfect. It was almost too late when I realized that I needed to change—and that change could be so easy.

Artificial Lab Meat Is the Future

The philosopher Richard David Precht once said in an interview, "We won't need factory farming for much longer, because soon we'll be able to produce meat in cell cultures."[80] Since many people enjoy eating meat, we must assume that not everyone is going to want to stop eating it in the foreseeable future. And so artificial or lab-grown meat is an important topic to consider.

Mark Post, a pharmacologist at Maastricht University in the Netherlands, has been working on creating artificial meat. The first artificial burger created by Post after years of work in the lab cost $250,000 because of the immense molecular and equipment-based expenses. But the price is dropping dramatically. It's possible that we will be able to buy a burger made with artificial meat for five to nine dollars in two or three years.[81] To produce cultured meat—also called in vitro meat or clean meat—muscle stem cells are taken from a living cow via biopsy and grown into muscle tissue on a culture medium in a lab.

Lab meat is being seriously discussed as an alternative source of meat. Post estimates that instead of 1.5 billion cattle, only thirty thousand animals would be needed to meet the global demand for cultured meat.[82] At first glance, eating artificial meat seems to contradict my recommendation for eating "natural" food. But the idea intrigues me. If people can't succeed in giving up meat completely, this would be the only way for us to eat meat without killing animals. In addition, the ecological burden associated with meat production could be avoided. And last but not least, this meat would be free from substances such as antibiotics, growth hormones, viruses, bacteria, and pesticides that accompany every piece of meat produced in factory-farming conditions.

In the near future, there are probably only going to be two options for meat lovers or lovers of animal protein: cultured meat and insects. Between these two options, artificial meat is likely the more appealing choice. But people might ultimately prefer a delicious vegetarian dish over an artificial steak.

My Conclusion on Protein

There is one factor in the discussion of proteins that I find especially important: We always eat protein as part of a food. In other words, the combination is what makes the poison. Plant-based proteins are ingested almost exclusively with healthy dietary fiber, such as in legumes (like beans, lentils, and peas), whole-grain products, leafy greens, tofu, seeds, and nuts. The sources of plant-based protein are inexhaustible, which is why vegans rarely suffer from protein deficiency.

On the other hand, the animal proteins we consume come with a lot of saturated fats, unless the meat is organic. I think this is the secret behind why plant-based protein is so much healthier.

Protein requirements depend on what stage of life we're in. Children and adolescents as well as people over the age of sixty-five need more protein; adults up to age sixty-five generally need less. Avoid high-protein diets and protein shakes for muscle growth—you might lose a few pounds or gain muscle faster, but it'll come at the expense of your health.

Carbohydrates

Many nutritionists recommend cutting carbohydrates out of your diet altogether. To them, carbohydrates are the main cause of obesity and diseases such as diabetes, heart disease, and fatty liver. But if you look at the dietary recommendations of the most well-respected medical societies around the world, you'll see that they recommend making sure that at least half of our daily caloric intake comes from carbohydrates. When we traveled to the healthiest places in the world, the Blue Zones, we saw that ultimately all healthy diets contain surprisingly large amounts of carbohydrates. The rule is: A diet is healthy if the grain and carbohydrates are whole and if the overall diet is balanced.

Simplified terms such as "low carb" and "high carb" don't help us assess the benefit or harm of carbohydrates as a large nutrient group. Neither does the general demonization of carbs—because whole-grain bread, whole-grain pasta, parsnips, carrots, amaranth, buckwheat, apples, and berries are healthy! The risk of stroke and heart attack is generally reduced by 20 percent with a whole-grain-based diet. For diabetes, the risk is lowered by 50 percent.[83] Potatoes don't perform quite as well—they are not harmful, but they aren't very beneficial either.[84, 85] The most extensive study summary on this topic to date has shown that the risk of cancer and circulatory diseases is significantly reduced if you eat at least three servings of whole grain (three ounces) a day; for example, two slices of whole-grain bread and a small amount of oatmeal.[86, 87]

But foods that contain simple, "useless" carbohydrates—such as lemonade, soft drinks, frozen yogurt, ice cream, white flour, bread rolls with jam, sugary cereal, and milk chocolate bars—aren't healthy. Whole-grain bread and oatmeal are not to blame for the carbohydrates' bad image; it's the monosaccharides, also known as simple sugars, that are to blame. This primarily means household sugar or granulated sugar, also called sucrose, which consists of glucose (dextrose) and fructose (fruit sugar). In the years when fat and cholesterol were seen as particularly harmful, nutritional medicine didn't really take sugar into consideration. While it was known that sugar only provides "empty" calories, overweight patients and diabetics were advised to stir artificial sweeteners instead of sugar into their coffee. But we now know that this recommendation was wrong.

There are also complex carbohydrates such as starch, which is composed of thousands of sugar molecules.

In the following sections, we'll take a closer look at these "good" and "bad" carbohydrates.

Sugar

Our ancestors were no strangers to sugar, because fruit has always been a part of human nutrition. Fruit is sweet because fruit-bearing plants evolved over time to entice animals, especially birds, to eat their fruit. Once eaten, the fruit's seeds are excreted—guaranteeing the survival of the plant species.

Our brain requires sugar in order to function. The reward and happiness centers in our brain are strongly activated by anything sweet—something that has enabled the food industry to drive the consumption of sugar to incredible heights. Sugar, which was once a rare delicacy that was previously available only in the form of honey, ripe fruit in summer, and preserved fruit in winter, is now in almost every processed food. This escalation in our consumption of sugar is worrisome. Sweets can be addictive, as brain researchers found out years ago; children get hooked especially easily.[88]

Sugar makes it possible to sell even qualitatively bad foods well, just as salt and fat are able to do. And sugar is one thing above all: cheap. These days, there's no question that high sugar consumption increases the risk of fatal cardiovascular diseases. Depending on the study, the risk is between 10 and 40 percent; with an extremely high consumption of sugar the risk can even double or triple.[89, 90]

Our overconsumption of sugar usually starts with breakfast. Breakfast cereals were developed by John Harvey Kellogg, an American doctor and naturopath. He created them with the intention of giving people a healthier option for breakfast (at the time, the meal usually consisted of bacon and eggs). But these cereals have mutated into an unhealthy combination of white flour and a lot of sugar. Even in organic supermarkets, you'll usually find a limited variety of oats and a wide variety of sugary cereals.

If you enjoy having cereal for breakfast, I recommend creating your own mixture of oats, flaxseed, nuts, and berries. Whenever I'm staying at a hotel, I try to find out whether they offer traditional Bircher muesli. This muesli was created by the Swiss doctor and naturopath Max Bircher-Benner. Essentially, it contains rolled oats, grated apple, and nuts. It tastes delicious. But you should pay attention to the quantity: If you eat too much of it, flatulence may occur.

What Happens When We Eat Sugar?

The purer a sugar is—pure fructose, dextrose, or sucrose in the worst-case scenario—the faster the sugar molecules reach our bloodstream. The body reacts to this with something akin to panic, because it worries that the sugar molecules can't be converted into energy for the cells quickly enough. This is why large amounts of insulin ("insult peaks"), which is responsible for the transport of sugar into the cells, are released from the pancreas. A consistently high level of sugar in the bloodstream has serious consequences. In the long run, it exhausts the pancreas. The somatic cells, into which sugar is meant to be transported, can't handle the constant supply either. They develop insulin resistance, resulting in high levels of sugar remaining in the bloodstream, which can cause damage to vessels and cells.

Finally, excessive sugar consumption shortens telomeres—an essential part of the human cell—and thereby accelerates cell aging.[91] Soft drinks are the most unhealthy, and should be taxed the way we tax alcohol.[92]

Use Sugar like a Spice

In the past, sugar was used like a spice, sparingly and purposefully—in desserts, for example. For centuries, only 3 to 4 percent of nutritional energy came from sugar—today it's 15 to 20 percent.[93] Sugar damages not only the teeth but also the heart and the brain.[94, 95] If blood sugar levels are high, cognitive performance and concentration diminish.[96] Researchers such as American biochemist Lewis C. Cantley even believe that cancer can be triggered by high sugar consumption, because people who suffer from obesity and diabetes show a higher risk of cancer.[97] Robert Lustig, a pediatric endocrinologist researching metabolic syndrome, condemns sugar. He was able to prove that lab animals, once they have become accustomed to sugar, show the same symptoms that occur in heroin withdrawal when they undergo sugar withdrawal.[98]

If you have ever tried to avoid sugar for a couple of days, you know how hard it is. It really does resemble withdrawal, a feeling that does not occur when you go without other foods such as potatoes or tomatoes. This explains why more than 200 million chocolate Easter bunnies and 150 million chocolate Santa Clauses are sold every year in German supermarkets. On average, every German consumes sixty-six pounds of white sugar a year, plus fructose, lactose, and galactose.

> Our body is not genetically prepared to deal with the dramatically high levels of sugar we currently consume. So it's not surprising that insulin, which regulates the utilization of carbohydrates in the body, is out of balance in more and more people. More than 34 million Americans now suffer from diabetes.

What can we do to wean ourselves off sugar? Try to reserve sugar for special occasions. A piece of dark chocolate can be an indulgent treat. In fact, chocolate supports health through the polyphenols it contains. The benefit of milk chocolate is small and disappears if you eat more than two ounces a week. On the other hand, one study showed that eating 3.5 ounces of dark chocolate a day can have beneficial effects on blood lipid levels, the heart, the circulatory system, and hypertension.[99] Do you like dark chocolate? I love it, but I can't eat 3.5 ounces a day. But perhaps that is the advantage of dark chocolate—you're usually satisfied after just three or four pieces of it. The combination of dark chocolate and almonds is especially healthy; chocolate with hazelnuts is also a good choice.

I don't believe in total abstinence when it comes to sugar. A piece of chocolate or a slice of cake every now and again are what make life worth living. The problem is that sugar is now everywhere, particularly in foods where you wouldn't expect them. This includes chips, ham, pizza, ketchup, tomato sauce, instant soups, and so on. When you're out shopping, make an effort to study ingredient labels. I do this regularly, and I'm constantly surprised. Above all, I'm continually stunned by how much sugar and other artificial substances are added to things like a simple cup of fruit yogurt.

What Types of Sugar Are There?

- **Fruit sugar (fructose):** A component of sugar composites, also contained in fruits and berries. Fructose is healthy when consumed in the form of fruit, since its negative effects are counterbalanced by healthy fiber and other plant substances in the fruit. But fructose on its own, such as in the form of agave syrup, can cause fatty liver disease and digestive problems. Consume in moderate amounts.

- **Table sugar (sucrose):** Consists of a combination of glucose and fructose; comes from sugarcane and sugar beets. Table sugar is not healthy but can be eaten in reasonable amounts.
- **Dextrose (glucose):** Is mostly manufactured industrially; also contained in sweet fruits. Recommended in (rare) cases of hypoglycemia; for example, during exercise.
- **Milk sugar (lactose):** Consists of glucose and galactose and is contained in milk and non-fermented dairy products; hardly found in yogurt and aged cheese. Should be avoided in cases of lactose intolerance, which tends to become more severe as we age. Otherwise, it can be consumed in moderation.
- **Malt sugar (maltose):** Contained in beer, barley malt, breakfast cereals. Not recommended.
- **Galactose:** This sugar is found in milk and is assumed to promote inflammation, aging, and osteoporosis. Not recommended.
- **Sorbitol:** Occurs naturally in apples, pears, plums, and dried fruit, but can also be manufactured industrially and used as sugar substitute. In the body, sorbitol is converted into fructose and glucose and can cause diarrhea and flatulence. Not recommended.
- **Xylitol:** Small amounts can be found in vegetables, berries, and fruit. The body can't absorb xylitol well; it has marginally fewer calories than other types of sugar and is not cariogenic, which is why it is found in many chewing gums. Can cause flatulence and diarrhea; not recommended.
- **Corn syrup:** Is industrially produced from corn starch; intensely sweet; promotes fatty liver and belly fat. Not recommended.
- **Brown sugar:** If sugar from beets or sugarcane is not well purified, it will retain molasses, which contains small amounts of vitamins and minerals. This sugar is not really healthier than table sugar—in order to gain a benefit from the micronutrients, you would have to eat it by the pound. I love its caramel-like

taste, especially in coffee. The disadvantage: It tends to clump together.

- **Sucralose:** Until recently, sucralose was thought to be neutral, but it's since been shown that this sweetener can contribute to the development of diabetes.[100] Therefore, not recommended.

Artificial Sweeteners
Are Not a Healthy Substitute for Sugar

Even though artificial sweeteners such as saccharin, cyclamate, aspartame, and sucralose have no calories, it is believed that their sweet taste stimulates hormonal release in the small intestine and therefore promotes insulin release. Insulin, in turn, makes us hungry, so that the actual aim of artificial sweeteners, which is to save calories, is negated. Additionally, artificial sweeteners confuse the brain. Your brain registers that it's tasting something sweet and thus expects an increase in blood glucose. When that increase in blood glucose doesn't happen, the brain isn't satiated, setting in motion a vicious cycle that requires larger and larger amounts of sweet things. Studies have demonstrated that the increased use of artificial sweeteners could not reduce the disease rate for type 2 diabetes or obesity. On the contrary: Artificial sweeteners have fostered the obesity and diabetes epidemic.[101]

It's now believed that this is due to the unhealthy effect of these sweeteners on the microbiome. Their consumption upsets the balance of the gut bacteria as those bacteria strains that have a negative effect on the metabolism multiply. Therefore, it's best to just not use artificial sweeteners. If you can't manage without them, use stevia or erythritol, sugar substitutes that have little or at least fewer undesired side effects.

Is Fructose the Best Sugar?

For a long time, fructose (fruit sugar) was recommended to diabetics, because it does not cause an increase in insulin. It reaches the liver directly from the gastrointestinal tract. But a few years ago, the German Federal Institute for Risk Assessment started advising diabetics to stop consuming foods sweetened with fructose, because if your fructose consumption exceeds a certain level, the sugar is immediately converted into fat in the liver.[102] And we now know that fatty liver disease, which millions of people in Germany suffer from, is caused not so much by fat but by fructose overload. Unfortunately, fructose in concentrated form—for example, glucose-fructose syrup—is being added to more and more foods, ready-made products, and soft drinks. Because it does sweeten things wonderfully, after all.

Many people these days also suffer from fructose intolerance. Like lactose intolerance, this is not a real allergy. The body can digest fructose to a certain degree, usually 30 to 50 grams. However, this amount is often exceeded today due to the many fructose-containing foods. The result: Undigested fruit sugar travels down to the large intestine, where bacteria ferment it and putrefaction gasses develop. This causes diarrhea, flatulence, and pain. This is why patients often stop eating fresh fruit altogether. But I don't recommend cutting fresh fruit out of your diet. If you suffer from fructose intolerance, first try to avoid all foods to which this sugar is added artificially. Afterward, try eating fresh fruit (whole with the peel, not as a smoothie) and see whether you can tolerate it.

Fructose contained in fruit isn't dangerous, because the fiber, nutrients, vitamins, and phytochemicals it also contains create a healthy balance. Observational studies show that fruit juices increase the risk of diabetes, while eating whole fruits lowers the risk. Natural sweetness in fruit can be delicious; I particularly enjoy fresh figs or dates. But you should be careful with dried fruit. A raisin, for example, contains the same amount of fructose as a fresh grape. Since dried fruit is smaller in volume, it's easier to eat more than the fresh alternative—meaning a much higher fructose intake. You should always opt for fresh fruit.

A particularly unhealthy fructose-based artificial sweetener is high-fructose corn syrup (HFCS), made from corn. High-fructose corn syrup is used often and generously in the food industry because it's durable and cheap. Unfortunately, this syrup is suspected of increasing the risk of many diseases, from hypertension to cancer.[103]

Agave syrup isn't a healthy alternative either, since it contains mainly fructose and is therefore ultimately less healthy than conventional table sugar.

Finally, because fructose reaches the liver directly from the gastrointestinal tract, the brain receives the message "You haven't eaten that much sugar yet," and activates feelings of hunger. That's why soft drinks or high-calorie meals sweetened with fructose don't really satiate this feeling of hunger.

Sugar in Fruit Juice

In some studies, fruit and vegetable juices were shown to be unhealthy because they contain large amounts of fructose and therefore a lot of calories.[104, 105] During the production process, much of the good fiber is lost, so that the juice no longer has the same healthy effect that the whole fruit has. That's why I recommend that you always eat fruit in its natural form. If you love juice, buy a juicer that leaves the natural components of the fruit in the juice. A masticating juicer is better for this than a centrifugal juicer. Juice made by squeezing contains a lot of vitamins and phytochemicals, even if some of the fiber is still lost. This is always a pity, because fiber binds sugar molecules, which are released into the blood bit by bit as a result. This way, the body isn't flooded with fructose, glucose, or insulin. If you like to drink smoothies, I recommend mixing fruit with vegetables or leafy greens (such as spinach or arugula) and herbs so that the sweetness won't be too overpowering.

The Glycemic Index

The glycemic index (GI) is a system of ranking carbohydrates in foods based on how much they affect blood glucose levels. Carbohydrates with a low GI cause a lower, slower rise in blood glucose, whereas those with a high GI quickly raise blood glucose levels. So foods with a low GI value are said to be healthy, while foods with a high GI are said to be unhealthy. Dextrose has the highest GI value (100; it goes straight into the blood), white bread has a GI of 75, and peanuts have a GI of 14.

But this value says relatively little about the actual increase of glucose and insulin in the body, because our blood glucose levels are also determined by the density of carbohydrates and the degree of processing of the food: How was the food heated up or cooked? How long was the cooking time? Were the vegetables cut? How were they prepared? How long food stays in the stomach as well as fiber and vitamin content also play a role. It stands to reason, therefore, that a single numeric value isn't a good standard of measurement here.

I prefer the term "glycemic load." It is calculated by multiplying the GI by the amount of carbohydrates in the food. At least this way the number of carbohydrates actually contained in the respective foods is taken into account. This approach changes a lot (less than 10 is low and therefore healthy, 11 to 19 is moderate, and 20 is high, or unhealthy). Let's use an example to illustrate this: Raw carrots and white bread have approximately the same GI (around 70). However, the glycemic load for carrots is 4. For white bread, the glycemic load is 20 (since carrots contain fewer carbohydrates than white bread).

That's why you should try to mainly eat carbohydrates with a glycemic load of less than 10 (which is the case for almost all types of fruits and vegetables).

Having said this, glycemic load can be changed by many factors.

If grain is ground up or if vegetables are cut into small pieces, the load increases; if pasta, potatoes, or rice are eaten cold, the load is reduced. This fluctuating value brings us to the topic of fiber and resistant starch.

Dietary Fiber

In the past, fiber was believed to be largely insignificant. But in fact it is extremely important for our gut health; it is the fodder for our 100 trillion intestinal bacteria.[106] These bacteria, in turn, are an essential factor for a healthy immune system. Gut bacteria—the microbiome—protect us from metabolic disorders, autoimmune diseases, and bowel diseases including intestinal cancer.[107]

I recommend a daily fiber intake of about 30 grams. This amount is easy to achieve if you follow a whole-food, plant-based diet. The main source of fiber is all types of whole grains, as well as vegetables and fruit. Surprisingly, fiber is also found in coffee.

Resistant starch is a special type of fiber that cannot be broken down by the small intestine and therefore is able to reach the large intestine, where it feeds bacteria, along with other fibers and a few complex carbohydrates. If you are avoiding carbohydrates such as potatoes, pasta, or rice to maintain your weight, resistant starch can be an interesting option for you.

Starch is a polysaccharide, consisting of amylose and amylopectin. The starch grains in potatoes, rice, and pasta swell when heated in liquid and become water-soluble. If starch is boiled, the grains burst open. They are then broken down into small units of sugar by the intestine and digested. This causes insulin levels to rise and leads to weight gain.

Resistant starch, as its name implies, is resistant. It is not digested, which is why the calories it contains aren't absorbed. This means you can eat large amounts of resistant starch without gaining weight. At the same time, good gut bacteria are nourished—a win-win situation.

Normally, about 10 percent of the starch in potatoes, pasta, rice, and bread is resistant. The resistance can be physical; for example, kernels of coarsely crushed whole grain have higher amounts of resistant starch. The starch in raw corn and green bananas is also more resistant.

A convenient way to increase the amount of resistant starch in potatoes, pasta, and rice is to cook them and then let them cool. This brings us to pasta salads, potato salad, and sushi rice. Cold potatoes make you gain less weight than freshly cooked potatoes. In the cooling process, the starch changes form, becoming more resistant to digestion. Even if potatoes, pasta, and rice are reheated after they have cooled, the amount of resistant starch they contain barely changes. That's why it's more beneficial—at least in terms of weight loss—to reheat pasta than to eat it fresh.

Other sources of resistant starch are beans, peas, millet, oats, and green bananas. In an animal study, the consumption of resistant starch showed protection against type 1 diabetes, inflammatory bowel diseases, and other autoimmune diseases.[108] Initial studies on overweight people showed improved blood lipid levels and blood sugar levels, as well as inflammation values.[109] These positive effects are probably due to the fact that resistant starch causes gut bacteria to multiply and form short-chain fatty acids. These in turn are very beneficial for gut health.

Resistant starch and fiber are very healthy for the gut flora and protect us against a number of diseases. Fibers that are particularly beneficial for the gut bacteria are called *probiotics*. There are many foods that have a strong probiotic effect: apples, chicory, black salsify, onions, parsnips, leeks, artichokes, sunchokes.

Interestingly, there is also a probiotic-free diet, especially for people suffering from irritable bowel disease (the FODMAP diet; see page 102). The paradox lies in the dynamics of gut bacteria composition. Many people who have had a low-fiber diet for years initially experience bloating and abdominal discomfort when they start eating healthy whole-grain products. After a few weeks, however, their intestine adjusts to this new diet. We have to give our body time to adapt to new conditions and stimuli. Afterward, we're rewarded with improved health—this is one of the fundamental principles of complementary medicine.

Grain

There is evidence of grain cultivation in settlements that are older than twenty thousand years.[110] But it wasn't until twelve thousand years ago, when our ancestors first settled down, that agriculture truly took hold.[111] Grain became the basis of life. Ever since then it's been: "Give us this day our daily bread." Agriculture, grain, and bread have a fixed place within religion and mythology. Deities were devoted to agriculture—for the Greeks it was the goddess Demeter; for the Romans it was the goddess Ceres.

The types of grain available today are the result of long breeding lines ensuring bountiful and resilient crops. In recent years, ancient grains such as emmer and spelt have been celebrating a comeback. Emmer has a pleasantly nutty taste and spelt is more digestible than wheat (on the other hand, spelt dries out quicker, as you might have noticed with a spelt roll left over from the day before).

Up until the nineteenth century, practically every loaf of bread was made from whole-grain flour. In the mills, the entire kernel of grain (including the bran, endosperm, and germ) were ground into flour. The disadvantage of this way of milling was that due to the oil content in the germ, the grain couldn't be stored well. With the emergence of superfine flour, in which bran and germ are removed, the shelf life increased. Unfortunately, this process also removed the healthy parts of the grain from the flour—what remained was relatively useless (in terms of health) white flour.

Wheat

In Germany, wheat is the dominant grain, primarily because of its robust yields. However, more and more people have started experiencing discomfort after eating wheat and other types of grain that contain gluten. Intolerances to certain types of wheat, or more specifically to gluten, have massively increased in recent years. These intolerances include celiac disease, wheat allergy, and non-celiac gluten sensitivity (NCGS). The rows of gluten-free products on the supermarket shelves are becoming longer and longer. This trend is even more striking in the United States, where about 20 percent of the population has a low- or no-gluten diet.[112] How is it possible that so many people are becoming gluten intolerant?

In terms of evolutionary history, grain is a relatively new food. Our immune system and intestine were faced with the challenge of developing a tolerance for this previously unknown food. For most people now, bread, grain, and gluten are easily digestible, but infections, stress, and other disorders can easily upset this immunological tolerance and cause an intolerance.

In wheat intolerance, there can be a nocebo effect—an effect that occurs because of negative expectations. Just as a placebo, a "fake" medication, doesn't actually contain any active ingredients but can still alleviate or even heal symptoms because one expects a positive effect, a nocebo can trigger a negative effect because it is feared. The currently widespread fear of gluten seems to be such a nocebo.[113]

However, I also think many people really cannot tolerate today's wheat varieties. Certain strains of wheat have been genetically modified to increase their resistance to pests and drought as well as to improve their baking properties. A side effect of these modifications is a higher amount of amylase trypsin inhibitors (ATIs, proteins found in wheat and related types of grain) and modified proteins that are more likely to trigger NCGS. Studies have shown that these ATIs can cause mild inflammation in the small intestine and false activations of the immune system.[114]

The FODMAP Diet

To follow the FODMAP diet, you should avoid foods that contain high amounts of fructose (in fruit and vegetables), lactose (in dairy products), fructan (in wheat, onions, etc.), galactans (in beans, cabbage, etc.), and polyols (in artificial sweeteners). If you plan to follow a FODMAP diet, I recommend doing it in conjunction with nutritional counseling. Continue to try different foods that you think you might be able to tolerate. In any case, opt for organic products with fewer additives, because the body often reacts adversely to those.

In addition to gluten and ATIs, there is another group of substances suspected of triggering, or at least worsening, irritable bowel syndrome: the so-called FODMAPs (fermentable oligosaccharides, disaccharides, monosaccharides, and polyols), which cause flatulence and diarrhea. A FODMAP diet can help those with irritable bowel syndrome.

If you notice that you cannot tolerate gluten and that your symptoms are alleviated when you follow a gluten-free diet, you should seek diagnostic confirmation for celiac disease. Celiac disease is the most severe form of gluten intolerance, in which even the smallest amount (one crumb is enough) can trigger severe symptoms (flatulence, diarrhea, muscle pain, fatigue, headaches, and joint pain). This systemic disease affects only about 1 in 133 Americans, or about 1 percent of the US population. Celiac disease is diagnosed with the aid of a gastroscopy or colonoscopy and/or the identification of certain antibodies in the blood. A diagnosis can also be made by typing the genetic disposition (serotype HLA-DQ2 or HLA-DQ8). Once celiac disease is diagnosed, there are good treatment options. With a consistently gluten-free diet, most patients are free of symptoms within twelve months.

The situation is a little different with NCGS, non-celiac gluten sensitivity, which affects about 6 percent of the population in the United States.[115] In this case, unfortunately, a gluten-free diet is not enough to achieve complete, immediate alleviation. However, my patients who suffer from rheumatic diseases or irritable bowel syndrome have told me time and again that they experience less discomfort with a gluten-free diet.

A wheat allergy, also known as baker's asthma, is a defect in the immune system. Instead of fighting diseases, the immune system forms antibodies (immunoglobulin E, or IgE) to fight harmless foreign substances. In a wheat allergy, the immune system reacts with disproportionate force to protein components of the wheat that are actually harmless. This causes inflammation, which is noticeable on the skin, as well as on other organs.

> Not everyone can easily digest whole-grain bread. Therefore, you should change your diet slowly, over the course of two to three months, and make sure to chew your food well. If you can't tolerate whole-grain products at first (for example, if you experience bloating, abdominal pain, diarrhea, or fatigue), you shouldn't overwhelm your body. Allow yourself products made with white flour. Oats are a whole grain that's usually well tolerated.

Regarding wheat intolerance, the preparation and baking time of the dough are also important. Wheat is rather unique within the grain family because it has the ability to produce, through the addition of water, a dough that lends itself well to baking due to the "glue protein" gluten. All other cereal flours produce bread with smaller volume and a less elastic interior; in other words, they aren't as "fluffy" inside. Dough prepared according to traditional methods, in which it is allowed to rise for a long time, causes less discomfort. In large industrial bakeries, dough is usually taken out of the oven after an hour. Accordingly, it contains more FODMAPs than it would if it had four to five hours to rise. When dough is given time to rise, it contains only about 10 percent of the problematic types of sugar.

So, it's often not even the wheat itself that causes sensitivity, but the way it is prepared. If bread is baked traditionally, with ancient or heirloom grains, wheat sensitivity can improve all on its own. Ask your local bakery about its production method, or try baking your own bread.

> To me, sprouted bread such as Essene and Ezekiel brands is an absolute treat. This bread is made from almost 100 percent sprouted grain and has a slightly sour taste.

If you've stopped eating bread, pasta, and other wheat products because of an NCGS and miss those foods, take one step at a time toward being able to enjoy them once more. First, you should stop eating products that contain gluten for a few weeks. Then you can begin to test individual types of grain and wheat, such as wild (i.e., non-GMO) wheat, spelt, and emmer. If you are unable to tolerate those, there is some consolation: Delicious foods such as corn, rice, potatoes, buckwheat, amaranth, quinoa, and oats are all gluten free.

Low-Carb Diet

For many years, a low-carb diet has been touted as a great way to lose weight and prevent atherosclerosis. When it comes to fighting the epidemic of obesity and diabetes, many consider a low-carbohydrate diet the best method. But is low-carb really all that healthy?

A 2018 Harvard study by cardiologist and nutritionist Sara B. Seidelmann sheds some light on the matter. According to her and her team, a low-carbohydrate diet can increase mortality risk just as much as a diet that is rich in carbohydrates. To understand these results, we have to consider what the study participants ate to replace carbohydrates. Almost 6,000 deaths were examined over the course of 25 years. A 50-year-old patient who derived more than 65 percent of his daily energy from carbohydrates lived for another 32 years on average. Participants who ate significantly less sugar (50 to 55 percent) lived just one year longer. This showed that, surprisingly, a lower carbohydrate intake resulted in barely any advantage for reaching an old age. How could this be? A closer look at which foods were eaten instead of carbohydrates indicated why: A vegetarian diet lowered the mortality risk by 18 percent, whereas mortality risk increased by 18 percent if carbohydrates were replaced with meat. Therefore, only a low-carb vegetarian diet is actually truly healthy![116]

Nevertheless, I generally do not recommend a low-carb diet. A vegetarian low-carb diet makes sense only for patients with diabetes or obesity.

My Conclusion on Carbohydrates

You don't have to quit carbs! But make sure to eat whole and complex carbohydrates. Instead of readily available carbohydrates, such as those in the form of cakes or sweets, you should eat foods that are rich in fiber: raw or blanched vegetables (not overcooked), fruit in its natural form, whole-grain bread (ideally coarsely ground), and whole-grain pasta.

Chapter Four

Food as a Remedy
and My Superfoods

There are a number of plant-based foods with scientifically measurable and verifiable medical benefits. Vegetables and fruits are so healthy because they contain phytochemicals that often taste bitter and are even toxic in large quantities. In low doses, however, they have enormous health benefits for the body because they trigger cellular processes—for example, by activating a tiny stress reaction. This tiny stress reaction strengthens the cell's resilience and activates self-healing.[1] This idea that a small amount of a harmful substance can train and stimulate the body in a positive way—and that the dosage is key—is called hormesis.

The effects that the phytochemicals cause in the body are as diverse as they are remarkable: anti-inflammatory, antihypertensive, cholesterol-lowering. And they have a protective effect against cancer.[2] On average, we consume 1.5 grams of these tiny yet powerful molecules with our food.[3]

There are around a hundred thousand phytochemicals. They serve plants in a variety of ways—for example, they protect against pests; attract the natural enemies of these pests, as well as bees and other pollinating insects; help transform light energy into chlorophyll; and protect plants from too much harmful sun exposure. The largest groups of phytochemicals are polyphenols, terpenes, sulfur compounds, and saponins.

Large amounts of polyphenols are contained in colorful or spicy foods such as berries, onions, garlic, grapes, and apples (especially if eaten with the skin), as well as in herbs, spices, vegetables, and nuts. Terpenes are often characterized by a pleasant taste; they are found in citrus fruit. Sulfur compounds, some of which have an unpleasant smell, are characteristic of crushed garlic and various types of cabbage. And saponins are found in roots, leaves, and petals.

The positive effect of phytochemicals on our body is linked to the theory of oxidative stress: The oxygen we breathe in serves as fuel for our cells in the production of energy. But during the process of oxidation—when oxygen is burned to generate energy—free radicals, a reactive form of oxygen, are formed as a by-product. These free radicals can damage cells and are considered the cause of cell aging. Many phytochemicals function as "radical catchers"—they bind to free radicals and make them harmless.

Fruit, berries, and vegetables that are vibrantly colored are rich in antioxidants. Red onions are healthier than white onions, red cabbage is healthier than green cabbage, purple grapes are better than green ones, deep red apples are better than pale green apples. The effect of their phytochemicals is one reason why vegetables and fruit are so healthy for us.

In the following pages, I would like to introduce you to superfoods: a group of foods that provide valuable supplies of phytochemicals.

The word *superfood* is not defined in terms of nutritional science— it's more of a marketing tool. It is often used for exotic and overpriced foods that aren't necessary for a healthy diet. Nevertheless, I still like to use the term because it expresses the exceptionality of individual

---

Everything Organic?

The NutriNet-Santé study, the largest observational study on organic products to date, found that the consumption of organic fruits and vegetables was associated with a significantly lower risk of cancer. Organic fruits and vegetables have lower amounts of pesticide contamination, contain fewer additives, and are less processed.[4]

It is much healthier to consume less-processed foods, as shown by an observational study on heavily processed foods ("ultra-processed food") published in *The BMJ* in 2018. Frequent consumption was associated with a higher risk of cancer.[5]

This is why I recommend buying and eating organic foods if it is financially possible. The health advantage is clear, and you'll be supporting sustainable agriculture.

---

foods that is often lost in phrases like "balanced diet." Indeed, there are clear differences in food, even within one group, when it comes to their health-promoting effect. Broccoli and spinach contain more beneficial substances than cucumber, and bread made from whole grains is undoubtedly healthier than bread made from white flour.

Superfoods should be the basis of our diet, not the exception. Therefore, I encourage you to eat several of these foods every day if possible:

Whole Grain

Whole grain is deliberately at the top of my list. It contains fiber and numerous micronutrients, and it's a prebiotic. In almost all of the Blue Zones, whole grain is eaten in abundance. Only those who suffer from celiac disease or who are intolerant to wheat or gluten should avoid it. If you don't suffer from these diseases, know that it's better to have too much whole grain a day than too little. Be sure to consume good grain, organic if possible. Ancient and heirloom grains such as rye, spelt, and einkorn are good for you. Whole-grain green spelt is created through a special production method in which the spelt is harvested when it's still soft and is then toasted. Millet contains large amounts of minerals and iron and benefits your hair and skin.[6] You can eat it more often as a side dish (millet risotto) or as porridge.

These days "pseudo-grains" such as buckwheat, quinoa, and amaranth are also increasingly popular. Like millet, they are a great alternative if you can't tolerate gluten. Quinoa and amaranth in particular are valuable sources of protein and are therefore especially suitable for a vegan diet. Quinoa is a staple food in South America, especially in Peru and Bolivia. Amaranth was also originally cultivated in the Andean region; its grains are harvested from the blossoms of the amaranth family. A good argument for eating buckwheat is that it is grown more locally.

Oats

Oats contain plenty of fiber, especially soluble beta-glucans. Oats have been proven to lower cholesterol levels. Cholesterol is a component of bile acids, and beta-glucans bind bile acids in the intestine and activate the formation of new bile acids from cholesterol in the liver. This means less cholesterol remains in the blood. In addition, oats block the reuptake of cholesterol in the intestine.[7]

Studies show that, interestingly, beta-glucans are also very effective in relieving hay fever symptoms. While with conventional pharmacological drugs a balance between immunosuppression (the suppression of immunological processes) and infections needs to be considered, beta-glucans seem to achieve both: They are anti-inflammatory and allergy-inhibiting. The effect seems to work via the intestinal bacteria, because oats also have positive effects on immune diseases. This makes oats a prebiotic food.[8]

Oats also have an excellent effect on diabetes, improving insulin resistance relatively quickly and normalizing blood sugar levels.[9] Additionally, eating oatmeal reduces the weight of overweight people and regenerates the liver in fatty livers.[10] Oats even seem to prevent weight gain.[11]

So let's hear it for oatmeal! It's one of the healthiest breakfast options and is easy to make. Add blueberries, a pinch of cinnamon or cardamom, and five walnuts to your oatmeal. This combination provides your body with extremely valuable nutrients in the morning. And oat days are ideal for fasting relief days.

Flaxseed and Flaxseed Oil

Flaxseed contains large amounts of alpha-linolenic acid (the plant-based omega-3 fatty acid), lots of fiber, and an above-average amount of phytoestrogens (such as the phytochemical lignan). The effect of the lignans is probably activated via the intestinal bacteria.

Flaxseed is an effective medicine for people suffering from hypertension, high cholesterol levels, as well as diabetes and inflammatory diseases such as rheumatism. There is even promising data regarding flaxseed and cancer prevention. In a study of high-risk patients, two teaspoons of ground flaxseed a day caused a regression in the early stages of breast cancer.[12]

I recommend eating two to three tablespoons of flaxseed a day. I always have a little ground flaxseed on hand in the kitchen. It goes well with oatmeal, or with salad and potatoes because of its nutty taste. But note that flaxseed needs to be ground, because if the husk is intact our body can't utilize its valuable constituents. You can buy it already ground or grind it yourself in a blender or a coffee grinder. If stored in a cool place, it will keep for months.

Flaxseed gruel helps against heartburn and gastritis as well as constipation. Most of my patients find it quite tasty. Soak two to three tablespoons of crushed golden flaxseed in 1¼ cups of water in the evening. The next morning, bring the flaxseed mixture to a brief boil and then strain it through a cheesecloth or a very fine sieve. Pour the liquid in a thermos and drink it throughout the day. But you must remember to drink an additional six to eight cups of water as well over the course of the day; otherwise the flaxseed can cause constipation.

If you don't like flaxseed or if you can't digest it well, you can ingest omega-3 fatty acids via flaxseed oil. Of all oils, flaxseed oil possesses the highest amount of omega-3 fatty acids. However, it turns rancid quickly, so it must be stored in a cool, dark place. Moreover, you should not heat up flaxseed oil—but it's great in salad or on baked potatoes.

Olive Oil

Olive oil, the hallmark of Mediterranean cuisine, is the second oil after flaxseed that deserves to be included among the superfoods. See page 55 for its health benefits.

Garlic and Onions

The phytochemicals in garlic and onions reduce arterial stiffness, lower cholesterol levels and blood pressure, and improve blood flow and viscosity.[13, 14] Anesthesiologists frequently advise patients not to eat garlic the week before surgery to minimize the risk of bleeding.[15]

Garlic appears to reduce the risk of cancer, particularly in regard to tumors in the digestive system (esophageal, gastric, and colon cancer), as well as prostate cancer.[16] Garlic also has an antibacterial effect and protects against fungi and parasites.[17] The best way to absorb its healthy effects is to eat it raw. Garlic contains the active ingredient allicin, which is released when it's chewed or crushed. You should also enjoy raw onions more often—for example, in a Greek salad.

Turmeric

Turmeric, the vibrant yellow powder that is obtained by grinding up the turmeric plant's roots, is an absolute star among medicinally effective herbs. It is used most widely in India; Indians eat about two grams of turmeric every day.[18] Many researchers attribute the very low cancer rates in India to the generous consumption of turmeric.[19] (In addition, Indians eat little meat and animal products.)

Turmeric, also called Indian saffron, appears to have a protective effect, especially with colon and prostate cancers.[20] It even stunts the growth of polyps, the preliminary stage of cancer in the intestine. In one study, participants received turmeric as well as the phytochemical quercetin, which is found in the skin of fruit, red onion, and grapes, for six months. After six months, the number of intestinal polyps had been reduced by half.[21] Moreover, turmeric has a preventive and therapeutic effect with rheumatism, arthrosis, brain disease, lung disease, and inflammatory bowel diseases such as ulcerative colitis and Crohn's disease.[22]

The main active ingredient in turmeric is the natural pigment curcumin. These days, you can buy pills containing turmeric extract. These extracts are modified by a special chemical preparation so that higher doses of curcumin can be absorbed by the body. Only 5 percent of the curcumin from natural turmeric can enter the bloodstream; the rest is broken down in the gastrointestinal tract or excreted. But you can save yourself money—instead of buying turmeric or curcumin pills, simply buy turmeric powder and consume a teaspoon of it every day mixed with some black pepper. Black pepper significantly improves the absorption of curcumin in the gastrointestinal tract.[23] However, I wouldn't recommend more than a teaspoon of turmeric with a little black pepper once a day, because as a preventive method turmeric works just like a medication.

Curry powder, by the way, is a mixture of spices that contains about 30 percent turmeric along with cilantro, cumin, cardamom, fenugreek, and various kinds of pepper. I highly recommend using curry powder generously when cooking.

Fresh turmeric root has a strong anti-inflammatory effect. But if you grate and cook with it, be mindful of your clothes—if you aren't careful, everything from your shirt to your kitchen counter and utensils will be dyed yellow. Luckily, there is an easy solution for this problem: Place the turmeric-stained item in the sun for a couple of hours, then the stain usually disappears on its own!

Other Spices

Chili Pepper

People who consume chili peppers, the small fruits of plants from the *Capsicum* genus, have the best results when it comes to longer life and fewer illnesses.[24] This might not necessarily be a causal connection—there could be other reasons for this effect. Chili lovers generally live healthier lives. But in any case, spicy dishes do satiate better and have a beneficial effect on weight loss.[25]

Cilantro

You either like cilantro or you don't. People who enjoy the taste of this herb might describe it as fresh, lemony, or aromatic, while people who don't like it might describe the taste as soapy or moldy. The reason for this vast difference in perception is genetic, as researchers have discovered.[26] Cilantro, most famous for its role in Asian cuisine, tirelessly performs cleanup operations in the human organism with its phytochemicals. It helps with gastrointestinal complaints, infections, and chronic inflammation.[27]

Ginger

Ginger is an effective remedy for nausea from motion sickness or chemotherapy. Sailors used to chew ginger root when going through rough seas. Ginger also helps with migraines and headaches. In a comparative study, eating half a teaspoon of ginger powder was as effective as modern migraine drugs.[28] I recommend a hot ginger foot bath for headaches, an Asian home remedy. For colds, ginger tea is very pleasant due to its warming properties.

Ginger is also a delicious spice praised by many chefs. I like to use it in Asian-style stir-fries with fresh vegetables. Ginger is delicious in pumpkin soup, and pickled ginger goes well with sushi.

Amla

The Indian gooseberry, amla, has an amazing cholesterol-lowering effect due to its high vitamin C content.[29] In India, amla is considered a kind of cure-all. It is even said to prevent cancer, though that has not been proven.

Spice Mixtures

In addition to curry powder, there are other great traditional spice mixes from around the world. Garam masala is a classic in Indian cuisine and has its roots in Ayurvedic medicine. This mixture contains cardamom, cinnamon, cloves, pepper, and cumin and has a warming effect. When using garam masala, heat vegetables in the pan first and add the garam masala mixture as a final step. Ras el hanout is a spice mix that has its origins in the Maghreb, in North Africa, but is also found in other Arab countries. The name ras el hanout translates to "head of the shop." Depending on the region it comes from, the mix contains up to twenty different spices, including nutmeg, chili peppers, cardamom, galangal, cloves, cinnamon, cumin, turmeric, paprika, ginger, and anise. Just one teaspoon of ras el hanout in your food will add incredible flavor. And on top of that, it will protect you from colds.

Berries

There is no healthier fruit than berries. Bright and vibrant, they have always been easy to spot and therefore have long been easily consumed by humans. This is in the interest of the fruit, because it helps ensure that their seeds are spread. The vibrant color of most berries shows how rich they are in phytochemicals—in this case anthocyanins, highly antioxidative pigments. The antioxidative power of anthocyanins can be measured and compared. For example, a serving of apple has 60 units of anthocyanins; a serving of strawberries, about 300; raspberries, 350; and blackberries, 650.[30]

Berries that have a deep, dark color and sour taste, such as elderberries, are very healthy. Personally, I think they are too sour, though I love wild blueberries. Most blueberries in the supermarkets are cultivated berries with light-colored flesh, so their healthy effect is a little weaker.

There has been extensive research into the effect of blueberries on diseases such as cancer, inflammation, hypertension, bowel diseases, and diabetes, and the results have been consistently positive.[31] In clinical studies, a cup of blueberries improved cognitive performance in older people and children.[32, 33] And blueberries have been shown to improve mobility, balance, and walking ability in elderly people.[34, 35]

Studies that measured the concentrations of phytochemicals in the metabolism and in the blood showed an initial heavy increase of phytochemicals in the bloodstream one to two hours after consuming a serving of blueberries. There were further increases after six and after twenty-four hours. The explanation for this is that intestinal bacteria process the components of the blueberries and release them into the bloodstream bit by bit.[36] For this positive effect to occur, blueberries and other berries shouldn't be eaten with cream or milk. These dairy products inhibit the positive effects of berries, just as they do with coffee.[37] Berries also lose much of their antioxidative power when they are made into jam, as a result of the manufacturing process.[38]

Anthocyanidin (the most important component of blueberries) is also found in cranberries. Cranberries are popular in North America and were a staple for Native Americans centuries ago. They are used in medicine to prevent inflammation of the bladder and urinary tract infections. The anticarcinogenic effect of berries is probably due to one component: ellagic acid, which is mainly found in raspberries and strawberries, as well as in hazelnuts and pecans.

Berries have a long tradition in complementary medicine. Their leaves are used in teas to treat diarrheic diseases. Bowel inflammations are treated by chewing dried blueberries or drinking blueberry juice.

Berries contain less fructose than other fruit. One experiment even showed that the strong increase in insulin levels caused by the ingestion of sucrose is reduced by the consumption of berries.[39] Berries that are frozen, by the way, do not lose their beneficial effects.

One important note for those who work in front of a computer screen all day: Berries improve your eyesight. As I was writing this book, I often enjoyed a blueberry-raspberry-carrot-ginger smoothie.

> Berries are undisputedly a superfood and the best "candy" you can have.

Tomatoes

Sixty million Italians can't be wrong. And indeed, many studies point to the special health benefits of tomatoes. They contain the phytochemicals lycopene, beta-carotene, and quercetin. Lycopene is fortified by heat, which is why tomato sauces and soups are healthier than raw tomatoes. Fat also increases the availability of lycopene, so you should add plenty of olive oil to your tomato sauce.[40] Ketchup, on the other hand, should be avoided, as it does contain lycopene but also far too much sugar.

The health-promoting effects of lycopene in tomatoes have a positive impact on cardiovascular diseases and a preventive effect on prostate cancer.[41, 42] If you're drinking tomato juice on a plane, you're doing something good for your body.

Tomatoes belong to the nightshade family, whose plants are rich in natural toxins. For this reason, there are doubts about whether they're healthy. Yes, tomatoes contain toxic alkaloids, but these occur almost exclusively in the roots and leaves. The alkaloids in the tomato fruit itself are eliminated during the ripening process. Only when my patients have certain skin diseases (psoriasis, rosacea, and atopic eczema) do I advise them to stop eating fruit of the nightshade family for a trial period to see whether their symptoms improve. You should also make sure to buy organic tomatoes if possible, as they contain significantly more phytochemicals.

Chocolate

The cacao tree is native to South America. The Mayans were likely the first people to consume chocolate as a food, for both pleasure and nourishment. Originally, chocolate was combined with spices and aromatic substances, not with sugar or sweet fruit. This only happened later, when the Spanish conquistadors arrived. Dark chocolate contains a large percentage of polyphenols. Studies have shown that the high percentage of cocoa in chocolate causes blood vessels to relax. Early stages of atherosclerosis can regress, blood pressure lowers, and the heart and circulation are protected.[43] Chocolate has a healthy effect starting at a cocoa content of 55 percent.[44] Therefore, healthy dark chocolate doesn't necessarily have to be bitter.

Nuts

There is a beautiful walnut tree in my garden. Every fall, I look forward to harvesting the walnuts. Nuts are an ideal, energy-rich winter food—not just for squirrels but also for humans. For many diseases, nuts are also effective for therapy and prevention.

In the 1980s, the American Heart Association, which is dedicated to the prevention and therapy of heart diseases, warned against consuming nuts due to their high fat content.[45] Now we know that this was a total misjudgment. Nuts are among the best that nature has to offer. I have already mentioned their healthy effects; their high content of omega-3 fatty acids (walnuts) and monounsaturated fats (almonds, hazelnuts) are undoubtedly responsible for this. But we now also know about their importance to intestinal bacteria. Scientists have been able to show that the regular consumption of pistachios and almonds shifts the microbiome in favor of healthy gut bacteria.[46] Nuts are also a tasty treat to our intestinal bacteria, it seems.

Generally, nuts spoil easily due to their high fat content. When they are stored in a damp place, they may go moldy. Don't eat nuts that smell bad, have blue or black spots, or taste bitter, rancid, or rotten. If you bite into a nut that you suspect is spoiled, spit it out immediately because aflatoxins, which are toxins produced by the mold fungus aspergillus, may have formed. It's best to store nuts in sealed containers in a cool place.

Walnuts

The queen of nuts is the walnut. It has everything you would expect from a superfood: omega-3 fatty acids, fiber, and antioxidants.[47] Moreover, it's tasty. Studies have shown that walnuts have an antihypertensive effect and thus provide protection against vascular and heart diseases.[48] There's also evidence that walnuts have an anticarcinogenic effect.[49]

Pistachios

I recommend pistachios for patients with diabetes and high blood pressure. Pistachios also promote healthy gut bacteria.[50] The stool of people who regularly eat pistachios contains large amounts of the short-chain fatty acid butyrate, which is believed to have a protective effect against intestinal cancer and diabetes.[51] But make sure to eat unsalted pistachios.

Pecans

The pecan is botanically related to the walnut (and thus looks very similar). A study by Tufts University investigated the health effects of pecans in overweight people with early-stage metabolic disorders. The twenty-six participants received an identical number of calories over the course of four weeks, but one group received an additional 40 grams of pecans a day. After four weeks, the pecan eaters showed significantly better blood sugar regulation, lower insulin levels, and better cholesterol values. A handful of pecans a day could supplement the therapy for diabetes and high cholesterol.[52, 53] I like their nutty, mildly sweet taste. The only disadvantages are the high price and short shelf life.

Peanuts

Technically speaking, the peanut is not a nut but a legume. Nevertheless, like other legumes, it is very healthy. In one study, risk of heart attack in women with high cardiovascular risk was lowered by eating one tablespoon of peanut butter every day. This is why I recommend

---

How Nuts Can Help You Lose Weight

Although nuts are rich in fat and calories, they support weight loss and lower cholesterol. I often tell my overweight patients to add nuts to their diet. I know from my own experience, not just from study data, that nuts are so filling that we generally eat less afterward.

Pistachios in particular support weight loss. They need to be removed from their shells before you can eat them—this fact alone seems to give the brain enough time to send out satiety signals. In nutritional science, this psychological reaction is referred to as the "pistachio principle." The same idea also applies to hard nuts and almonds, which have to be chewed slowly and intensively. Ultimately, nuts boost the breakdown of fat; they are a true "fat burner." Because of this, I don't put any restrictions on a recommended amount.

peanut butter instead of sweetened hazelnut cocoa spread (such as
Nutella) on the breakfast table. The latter contains more sugar and also
more palm oil.

Avocados

Avocados are now finally recognized as an exceptionally healthy food.
Both avocados and olive oil demonstrate how fat can be incredibly
healthy—if it is plant based. Avocados contain monounsaturated fatty
acids, water, and fiber. The plant-based fat in this fruit is healthier than
animal fat, but also rich in calories. Therefore, at first glance, it doesn't
seem like avocado would support weight loss. But studies have shown
that people who eat them eat better overall, are less overweight, and
have lower cholesterol levels.[54]

For many years, however, this fruit was under close scrutiny. In
1975, a fungicidal toxin called persin was discovered in the leaves of
avocado trees.[55] Researchers began to examine whether this toxin could
kill cancer cells.[56] Lab studies then showed that an extract of the avocado fruit could genetically damage blood cells. However, we don't
generally have to worry about this, since most of us are not injecting
avocado extract into our veins. When we eat avocado, the harmful
substances are disarmed in the stomach by gastric acid. Lab studies
have shown that cancer cells of the esophagus, intestine, and prostate
are prevented from growing by avocado.[57] In an initial observational
study, the risk of prostate cancer dropped significantly in men who ate
at least a third of an avocado every day.[58] So, men: Let's go for some
guacamole!

From an environmental point of view, however, there is unfortunately one major flaw: Farming avocados requires a lot of water and
has already caused water shortages in a few countries. The production

of one pound of tomatoes takes about ten gallons of water; one pound of avocados, on the other hand, requires seventy-four gallons![59] So my recommendation is to eat avocados and enjoy guacamole, but not every day. And please buy certified organic avocados.

Broccoli, Cabbage, and Co.

Cabbage is the prototype of a family of vegetables known as cruciferous vegetables. The cruciform arrangement of their leaves led to this name. Members of the cabbage family have been grown for more than six thousand years; their medical effects have been described in ancient Egyptian and ancient Roman medicine.[60] The most important representatives that descended from wild cabbage are broccoli, cauliflower, brussels sprouts, and kale. Asian types of cabbage such as bok choy, as well as kohlrabi, rutabaga, radish, horseradish, arugula, rapeseed, mustard, and cress also count as cruciferous vegetables.

Broccoli

Broccoli is clearly the star among the cabbage varieties. It has a preventive effect on cancer, it is antidiabetic, inhibits inflammation, and strengthens the immune system.[61, 62] Broccoli is the most researched cruciferous plant, though that doesn't mean other crucifers aren't as healthy. Its most important components are glucosinolates. However, these take effect only when the crucifers are cut and chewed, at which point the enzyme myrosinase is released. Myrosinase breaks down glucosinolate and releases the active ingredient sulforaphane, which has an antioxidative, anti-inflammatory, and detoxifying effect. In addition to cancer prevention, sulforaphane fights the bacterium *Helicobacter pylori*, which is responsible for gastric ulcers and gastritis. That's probably why sulforaphane protects against stomach cancer.[63, 64]

When preparing broccoli, it's therefore important to make sure it isn't boiled in water for too long, because then it will lose more than half of its healthy components. In addition, the enzyme myrosinase is very sensitive—with a longer cooking time, the formation of healthy sulforaphane is prevented. Michael Greger, an American physician and nutritional scientist, has a remedy for this called "chop and wait,"[65] which means: Chop up the broccoli and let it rest on the cutting board for about fifteen minutes before you put it into the water. This ensures that myrosinase is released and sulforaphane forms. This way, you can cook broccoli for longer without depleting the healthy substances.

Another possibility is to eat broccoli raw or with horseradish, arugula, or mustard greens. All of these cruciferous vegetables contain myrosinase. Make sure to chew the vegetables well, because this makes the enzyme release better. Broccoli sprouts, which are available in organic supermarkets, are a great source of sulforaphane.

Kale

Kale can definitely go head-to-head with broccoli as one of the healthiest vegetables. It reduces cholesterol levels in the blood, among many other things.[66] While Michelle Obama was living in the White House, she planted kale in the garden and in doing so caused a kale boom in the United States.[67]

Although I don't normally recommend chips, I make an exception for kale chips—they are healthy. You can easily make them yourself: Remove the kale leaves from the stalks and put the leaves on baking paper. Toss with olive oil and then bake them in the oven for twenty minutes at 250 to 275°F. To finish, sprinkle a little salt or spice mix onto the chips—*et voilà*.

Other Cruciferous Vegetables

Brussels sprouts and horseradish are very healthy. The sharp taste of horseradish reveals the high concentration of healthy phytochemicals in it. Whether in its natural form or in the form of wasabi, horseradish is an excellent addition to meals.

By the way, frozen products are not as healthy as fresh in the case of crucifers. The process of blanching before freezing deactivates the enzymes in these types of vegetables. "Chop and wait" is no longer useful. However, the precursor of sulforaphane is still contained in frozen crucifers. So by briefly blending fresh mustard seeds, a few leaves of arugula, or a small amount of fresh broccoli and adding it to the frozen veggies, you'll activate myrosinase.

Legumes

Legumes contain the best plant-based proteins, fiber, and many micronutrients. Several studies suggest that a low rate of cardiovascular diseases can be attributed to the daily consumption of beans and other legumes.[68, 69] The American Institute for Cancer Research recommends eating whole grains or legumes with every meal.[70]

Dishes with legumes can be diverse and taste wonderful: pasta made from lentils, hummus made from chickpeas, stews made with white beans. Many people like the taste of legumes but suffer from the ensuing flatulence. But once your intestinal flora becomes used to legumes, the flatulence will decrease. Light-colored lentils and chickpeas are easier to digest than black or green. As a rule, mung beans are tolerated well. One trick to make legumes more digestible is to add spices such as curry, salt, pepper, cloves, garlic, ginger, turmeric, or bay leaves.

If you buy canned beans, which cause less flatulence than beans you cook yourself, rinse them with water to reduce their salt content. Naturally, the best option is fresh beans, which you can sometimes find in the early fall at farmers' markets.

Soy is best tolerated when it's unprocessed and fermented, like in tempeh. Tempeh is extremely delicious if you slice it and lightly fry it with soy sauce. Soy milk and tofu are already processed; about half of the good ingredients in soy are no longer contained in tofu, and even more so in soy milk. Still, both are highly recommended foods. Soy is mainly associated with a reduced risk of breast cancer.[71, 72]

Lentils are fantastic in many ways: They're powerful antioxidants, they lower blood sugar levels, contain fiber, and are a probiotic.[73, 74, 75] They cook relatively quickly, in about twenty to twenty-five minutes, and are tasty in soups and stews or added to pasta sauces. Lupines are another legume that are very rich in protein.

The positive effects of legumes, especially on insulin levels and thus on diabetes, last for a particularly long time due to the so-called second-meal effect, a kind of sustained-release meal, analogous to a sustained-release tablet that releases its active agents over the course of several hours. In a clinical study, patients were given a serving of red lentils for breakfast on the first day and a very sugary meal the next day. The following day, the insulin level was lower in the group of lentil eaters than in the comparison group. Similar to blueberries, this effect seems to be due not only to the lentils alone, but to the hard work of the intestinal bacteria. They process the lentils without haste and produce metabolites that curb the increase of blood sugar levels and thereby that of insulin levels.[76]

Beets

Beet juice is my first recommendation when patients ask for a natural supplement for treating hypertension. Data proves that consuming one cup of beet juice every day (or the equivalent amount of fresh beets) has the same effect as an antihypertensive drug.[77] Beets contain a lot of nitrate, which is absorbed into the bloodstream via the stomach. Thirty percent of the nitrate in the blood concentrates in the salivary glands. The bacteria in the mouth and tongue convert the nitrate to nitrite, and when swallowed, the nitrite is transported into the stomach, where it is then transformed by gastric acid into nitric oxide—a substance that our vessels love. Nitric oxide relaxes our vessels, thus improving circulation and reducing blood pressure. It is this process—with the aid of the mouth bacteria—that makes beets so healthy. Because of its vasodilating effect, beet juice is now recommended by cardiologists to patients suffering from heart failure.

Beet juice not only lowers blood pressure, it also acts as a natural performance enhancer: Men who drank about two cups of beet juice every day for six days showed greater endurance in subsequent fitness tests than when they drank something else.[78]

Nitrate also plays a special part in oral hygiene. Beets have a preventive effect against cavities and help locally against gingivitis and periodontitis.[79, 80]

The word *nitrate* might sound familiar. Isn't it suspected of being carcinogenic? In fact, there is always alarm when the nitrate content in groundwater increases due to the use of too much liquid manure and chemical fertilizer in fields. Smoked pork chops and other meat products are artificially "refined" with nitrites and are not considered healthy. So why are nitrate and nitrite healthy in vegetables? Nitrite itself is not carcinogenic—it only becomes so in combination with proteins such as nitrosamine. This is found in huge quantities in meat, but hardly at all in vegetables. In addition, the many phytochemicals in vegetables block the conversion of nitrite to nitrosamine. Instead, "good" nitric oxide is formed.

Leafy Greens

Leafy greens should be eaten as much as possible, daily. Be it Swiss chard, spinach, garden lettuce, endive, iceberg lettuce, or lamb's lettuce—please help yourself whenever you see green leaves. Leafy greens protect from heart disease, stroke, and periodontitis, and also increase life expectancy. They contain the magic weapon all plants have—chlorophyll—as well as other phytochemicals and omega-3 fatty acids.[81, 82] Many components are liposoluble, so you should cook spinach with olive oil or add a few walnuts or toasted sesame seeds to salad dressings. Just as with beets, leafy greens contain large amounts of nitrate.

Mushrooms

Mushrooms contain special micronutrients that specifically strengthen the immune system. There are medicinal mushrooms that are used in remedies, such as reishi, maitake, and Cordyceps. But normal edible mushrooms also support the immune system, and they have an antiallergic effect.[83] As with oats, beta-glucans are responsible for this. In lab experiments, maitake, shiitake, oyster mushrooms, and button mushrooms in particular showed an anticarcinogenic effect.[84]

Apples

I definitely want to honor the apple as a superfood; "An apple a day keeps the doctor away" still holds true. Apples are healthy because of their numerous phytochemicals. Lab experiments have shown that they have an antidiabetic and anticarcinogenic effect. Eat apples along with their peel, because beneficial quercetin is found in large quantities in apple peel.[85] In one recent study, subjects were asked to eat two apples a day during an eight-week period. At the end of the period, the researchers found beneficial effects on cholesterol, blood vessel function, and the microbiome.[86] So, while one apple a day is good, two is even better!

An apple is easy to carry around, it comes prepackaged in its own peel, you can eat it without cutlery, and on top of all this, it has a long shelf life. It's best to eat apples fresh, when they are harvested in the fall. With prolonged storage time the content of phytochemicals fades. That's when one apple a day is no longer enough to keep the doctor away.

Drinks

Water

Water is *the* superfood, or rather, *the* superdrink. Water is undoubtedly the healthiest drink and indispensable for the body. But how much is healthy?

You are probably familiar with the advice of drinking at least eight eight-ounce glasses (which equals about two liters) of water a day. It's no longer possible to determine where this idea came from. There is no scientific basis for it. Sure, after a sauna session, heavy sweating during exercise, or a loss of liquids from diarrhea, water balance needs to be restored. It has been shown that dehydration in schoolchildren leads to poor concentration and reduced performance.[87] A lack of fluids also makes you feel tired and exhausted. Patients often complain about headaches when they don't drink enough liquids.

Don't drink during meals. Ayurvedic wisdom states that one shouldn't drink during and shortly before meals so as not to weaken the digestive powers.

In people who have a healthy heart and vessels, drinking at least five glasses of water a day has a protective effect against heart diseases.[88] Being well hydrated also protects against kidney stones, chronic inflammation of the bladder, and cancer of the bladder.[89] In one study, women who suffered from cystitis at least three times a year were divided into two groups. One group was asked not to change their normal drinks for more than a year; the other group was asked to drink an additional 1.5 liters of water every day. The latter group's effort was rewarded: The number of bladder inflammations decreased by almost half in their group.[90]

It was only in 2018 that a study was conducted to determine whether drinking more fluids would relieve discomfort in people with slightly inhibited kidney function (a condition that afflicts many elderly people). Surprisingly, discomfort was not relieved. In fact, kidney function even tended to be slightly better when subjects did not drink more fluids than usual.[91]

In general, the human body seems to be prepared to use water sparingly. This makes sense given the long evolutionary history of humankind. After all, during the Stone Age, no one ran around with water bottles in their backpacks and coffee to-go cups in their hands. Constantly drinking fluids is—with the exception of the specific cases I mentioned earlier—not beneficial. Too much water can lead to a volume overload in the vessels, impair cardiovascular function, and increase blood pressure. More fluids means extra work for our kidneys, which already have a lot to do. My advice is to pay attention to the signals from your body. It is undoubtedly good to drink water when you are thirsty. But if you don't feel any desire for it, you shouldn't force yourself. (It is important to note, however, that elderly people can experience decreased thirst sensation.)

You can check your hydration levels with a simple test. Drink two glasses of water. If you then urinate roughly the same amount within an hour (and your urine is relatively light-colored), your fluid balance is fine.

WHICH TYPE OF WATER IS BEST?

Drinking water has become a rapidly growing market around the world. Major multinational corporations have long been active in the water business. For this reason alone, you should be skeptical of the health promises seen in mineral water ads.

Tap water is a good option—it is less polluted by microbes than bottled water, because our tap water is subject to stricter criteria than commercial spring and mineral water.[92] Plus, tap water is cheaper.

However, tap water in many regions has been connected to drug residue in the groundwater. These residues include hormones, benzodiazepines, antibiotics, X-ray contrast agents, and anti-inflammatory drugs such as diclofenac.[93] Despite modern wastewater treatment technology, it has not been possible so far to eliminate these residues. We can do our part to ensure the cleanliness of our groundwater by not disposing of medications in the sink or the toilet.

Many people use water filtration systems in their own homes; these are increasingly advertised, however, with exaggerated references to their health benefits. These systems, which are high quality but often expensive, effectively filter medications, heavy metals, and other undesired substances out of the water. But it's difficult to say whether this is really good for our health. Often, these filtration systems clean the water too much, removing minerals by reverse osmosis. The resulting water is low in minerals—and while this means the water has a pleasantly clean taste, those minerals are important.

I cannot recommend the more affordable systems available in drugstores. The danger of bacterial contamination is high if the filters aren't changed often enough.[94]

If you drink mineral water, buy brands packaged in glass bottles. Plastic bottles release harmful plasticizers such as BPA into the water.[95] The numerous health-damaging effects of plasticizers, particularly on the hormone system as endocrine disruptors, have been proven.[96] BPA also affects the gut bacteria. Heat in particular can cause BPA to leach out of plastic bottles and into the water. If you taste even a hint of plastic on the first sip, you should dispose of it immediately.

There's a great diversity of mineral springs around the world, so try to drink regionally sourced water if you can. And water from natural springs, where the water reaches the surface without drilling, is particularly refreshing.

> Drink enough water, but trust your sensation of thirst. Don't force yourself to drink if you are not thirsty. Choose tap water or mineral water from glass bottles; don't drink water from plastic bottles. Drink the water that you like best.

Coffee

Coffee has undergone a spectacular metamorphosis in the eyes of medicine. In the nineteenth and early twentieth centuries, it was highly valued as a "tonic" and was believed to provide strength and vitality.

This was followed by a long phase in which coffee fell out of favor because of its caffeine content. But for the past two decades it has been experiencing a grand comeback. There is even talk of coffee as a universal remedy. That is surely an exaggeration, even if, according to the current data, an impressive number of diseases can be prevented with this drink. These include Parkinson's disease, type 2 diabetes, cardiovascular diseases, kidney disease, liver disease, hepatitis, gout, gallstones, disruptions of pulmonary function, depression, colon cancer, breast and prostate cancers, and even early-stage dementia.[97] What is most impressive is that coffee may have a life-prolonging effect. In a study from 2018, even eight cups a day could still contribute to this effect. You don't have to aim for eight cups of coffee; the optimal dose is three to four cups a day.[98] Incidentally, it doesn't matter whether you drink caffeinated or decaffeinated coffee—even decaf supports health.[99]

But coffee also has undesirable side effects. This can be observed clearly in therapeutic fasting when many people (including myself) refrain from drinking coffee as they usually do and end up suffering from headaches as a result of caffeine withdrawal.

It's not advisable to drink coffee if you suffer from sleep disorders. And high coffee consumption in stressful times often has an undesired effect. The expectation that the caffeine will push you and make challenges easier to tackle masks an urgent need for rest. Excessive coffee consumption in these situations ultimately promotes exhaustion and the risk of burnout.

Consuming coffee during pregnancy increases the chance of a premature birth and is associated with lower birth weight in infants.[100] And for many people, coffee can cause an upset stomach. This irritation can often be traced to the way the coffee is roasted. Roasting coffee beans for a mere one to two minutes at very high temperatures (to speed up the roasting process) causes many bitter-tasting compounds and acids to form. A slower and gentler roasting process makes the coffee easier on the stomach and more digestible. For beans that have been roasted quickly, a dash of milk can improve tolerability, but unfortunately the beneficial effects of the coffee are inhibited by the milk. Drip coffee is often well tolerated. The oils contained in the coffee beans (cafestol and kahweol), which are responsible for a slight increase in cholesterol, get caught in the coffee filter.

Coffee has a different effect on different people. A friend of mine can't sleep if she has a cup of coffee after two o'clock in the afternoon. Personally, I sleep well even if I have an espresso at nine p.m. Indeed, there are fast and slow coffee metabolizers.[101] The way it is metabolized, however, has no influence on the positive health effects of the beans, as shown in a 2018 study that examined the genes of coffee drinkers and their metabolic activity.[102]

Proponents of an alkaline-rich diet often believe that coffee poses an acidic burden for the body. But the opposite is true—coffee itself is alkaline.[103, 104]

Italy is the El Dorado of coffee. Even at a run-down gas station you will still find a wonderful stainless steel machine from the 1970s that makes amazing espresso. Those are entirely different worlds of taste compared to the fully automatic machines in the rest of the world. If you love coffee as much as I do, you should invest in a really good machine. Classic models last twenty to thirty years if you regularly maintain and clean them. And of course, it is advisable to grind coffee beans freshly for every cup of coffee and to buy beans that haven't been roasted for too long. They are usually more agreeable to the stomach.

> Coffee supports a healthy diet. How you prepare the coffee is irrelevant to the medicinal effect. Two to four cups a day is ideal. Drink your coffee black or with almond, soy, or oat milk, and opt for medium-roast beans.

Tea

Herbs prepared as teas have been used in complementary medicine for centuries. Most of us are familiar with drinking chamomile tea or herbal teas when we are sick. But I would like to talk about *Camellia sinensis*, the tea shrub, which can grow to the size of a tree. It produces the leaves that are harvested for traditional types of tea. White, green, and black tea are all produced from this plant—it's how the leaves are processed that determines whether they become green, black, or white tea.

Both green and black tea have beneficial effects on our health. I highly recommend green tea in particular. Two to three cups a day can lower blood pressure, cholesterol levels, and blood sugar, and support weight loss.[105] Green tea is also believed to have a protective effect for autoimmune diseases such as multiple sclerosis, lupus erythematosus, and some types of cancer, including breast and prostate cancers.[106, 107] In Asian countries, where large quantities of green tea are consumed, breast cancer rates are remarkably low (although this could also be linked to soy).[108] Green tea is also linked to positive effects in regard to allergies and hay fever.[109] And it de-stresses: EEG tests show more relaxed brain wave activity mere minutes after green tea has been drunk.[110]

I think the combination of various components is what makes tea so healthy. Currently, extensive research is being conducted on the phytochemical epigallocatechin gallate (EGCG), which is believed to be the main factor responsible for the positive effects of green tea. In experiments with fruit flies, EGCG has proven itself to be life-prolonging.[111] Green teas from Japan generally contain larger quantities of phytochemicals, especially EGCG, than those from other countries. If you would like to drink green tea for medicinal benefits, you need to leave it to steep for a longer period, not just one to three minutes, as is usually recommended. The active substances develop fully only after ten minutes, even though that makes the tea taste bitter and more intense and makes it resemble actual medicine. There are one hundred times more polyphenols in a cup of Japanese green tea that has been steeped for a long time than in a cup of Chinese tea that is brewed quickly.[112, 113]

Drinking matcha, a powdered green tea, is also highly recommended. Personally, I prefer sencha, a delicate, pleasant green tea from Japan. Just a few leaves per cup are enough to create a wonderful taste adventure.

I discourage using green tea extracts, because of potential side effects on the liver. Tea in its natural form has hardly any side effects, except that, just as with coffee, the caffeine it contains can lead to insomnia if you drink it at night. And black tea can stain your teeth.

The same applies to both tea and coffee: Drink it without milk, which cancels out the health benefits.

Smoothies

If you prefer drinking fruit to chewing it, you should blend it. This way the valuable phytochemicals such as anthocyanins and polyphenols are retained. These phytochemicals are bound to fiber, dissolved by the intestinal bacteria, and released into the bloodstream. A juicer removes the best parts of the fruit. Pulp in juices or smoothies is desirable; that's why you should drink cloudy fruit juices rather than clear ones. Make sure the smoothies don't end up being too sweet. Mix sweet and sour fruit or add vegetables and spices (leafy greens, celery, ginger). Berries are preferable.

Drink smoothies in moderation (just one a day). A liter of smoothie, which is the equivalent of ten pieces of fruit, is unhealthy. That amount of fructose puts stress on the stomach and intestines and can facilitate the development of a fatty liver.

Alcohol—Just Say No

Even low alcohol consumption poses health risks. This conclusion was reached by the authors of the largest study to date on drinking behavior and alcohol-related harm, the 2018 Global Burden of Disease study. The study showed that alcohol does more harm than good from the first drop. One or two alcoholic drinks a day lowers the risk of dying from certain heart diseases. However, this seemingly positive effect pales in comparison to the number of diseases and deadly events (cancer, liver cirrhosis, hypertension, tuberculosis, car accidents) that are alcohol-related. Alcohol consumption ranks third behind smoking and hypertension in the list of the most common causes of death and health restrictions.[114]

This presents us with an enormous problem, because alcohol consumption is so deeply rooted in our everyday lives. But 10 grams of alcohol (which is roughly equivalent to a glass of wine) a day increases the risk of alcohol-related disease by 0.5 percent; two glasses of wine, by 7 percent.[115] This calculation ends at dizzying heights.

Alcohol facilitates the development of cancer. Ethanol, which is absorbed with alcohol, is converted into acetaldehyde by the biocatalyst alcohol dehydrogenase (ADH). It is assumed that this intermediate product (acetaldehyde) damages the genetic material, the DNA, when metabolized.[116] A recent British study showed that even drinking only moderate amounts of alcohol three times a week results in brain damage. A further survey study, published by The Lancet in 2018, found that alcohol shortens life expectancy. In the survey, 83 studies from 19 prosperous countries containing data on roughly 600,000 people who consumed alcohol regularly were gathered. The findings showed that starting from an amount of 100 grams of alcohol per week (about 1.5 glasses of wine a day), alcohol reduces life expectancy for both men and women. If 350 grams of alcohol is consumed per week, life expectancy is shortened by about four to five years (!).[117] The Guardian published the headline: "Extra glass of wine a day 'will shorten your life by 30 minutes.'"[118] My advice is this: Less is better, and zero alcohol is best.

The highly effective phytochemicals resveratrol and quercetin, which
are the basis for red wine's great reputation, are found in the peels of
grapes. They are indeed very healthy. These healthy substances, however, are more readily available if you don't consume them with alcohol.
Therefore, eat grapes or drink grape juice, but avoid red wine. In general,
alcohol has no health-promoting effects. Even its supposed heart-healthy
effect has come into question. According to *The Lancet*, the health effects of alcohol that had been touted for so long can probably be traced
back to statistical errors (or good marketing).[119]

Try nonalcoholic beer or wine. Remember, we are creatures of habit,
and with a little patience, any habit can be changed.

Salt

You might be surprised to find salt included in the superfoods. It's well
known that we shouldn't eat too much of it. Still, salt is a fundamental
part of our diet; it's not for nothing that wars were fought over it.

Salt is a prime example of how complex nutritional science is.
Contradictory research findings are published all the time, and most
doctors have become cautious about giving any recommendations regarding the consumption of salt. We undoubtedly eat too much of it,
but the problem is not the saltshaker on the table, but the many food
products rich in salt. At the top of the list are sausages (unfortunately,
so is organic sausage, because it is free of other preservatives), cheese,
as well as all ready-made products: Pizza, bouillon cubes, mustard, and
ketchup all contain too much salt.

The salt in miso and soy sauce can be tasted immediately, but in
these cases its unhealthy effect is balanced by the beneficial qualities
of the fermented soy. I recommend that all patients with autoimmune
diseases such as rheumatism and multiple sclerosis adopt a low-salt

diet. With hypertension, it's important to proceed on a case-by-case basis. About a third of the world's population is sensitive to salt—which means they react to it with an increase in their blood pressure. This means that for the remaining two-thirds of the population, salt has no effect on blood pressure. That's why it doesn't make sense to flat-out forbid all hypertensive patients from having salt. I recommend a four-week self-test—use hardly any salt and eat as little bread as possible, because bread is a major source of salt. Measure your blood pressure throughout these four weeks. If it becomes lower during this time, then you are likely salt sensitive and should indeed adopt a low-salt diet. But if your blood pressure doesn't drop, then salt likely has no effect on it, and you don't need to adopt a low-salt diet.

The body has evolved to retain even small amounts of salt very well in the kidneys. When people started to preserve food—for example, by pickling—our salt consumption suddenly increased and our problems with salt began.

Is All Salt the Same?

The variety of salt available these days is impressive. Chemically speaking, which salt you eat may not matter much, because ultimately it is made up of about 97 percent sodium chloride. But there are huge differences in taste. Conventional table salt often tastes dull, because anticaking agents are added to prevent it from sticking together. I prefer pure sea salt that is gathered from seawater in salt evaporation ponds. One disadvantage of sea salt is that it contains increasing amounts of microplastic—even the high-quality and expensive fleur de sel. Rock salt is gathered in underground saltworks. This salt is, technically speaking, also sea salt, which was created by dehydration processes millions of years ago. But at least the seas were clean in those days. Therefore, it's probably better to consume high-quality rock salt than sea salt.

> Use herbs instead of salt in the kitchen. If you cook without salt for a while and use a lot of tasty spices instead, you'll notice that you actually don't need much salt.

Food Supplements

An actual lack of individual vitamins and minerals is rare in the developed world, so we don't usually need to take supplements. But there are a few exceptions:

- People who follow a vegan diet should take vitamin B12 supplements (in the form of a pill, toothpaste, or an injection from the doctor).
- Women with heavy periods and a resulting iron deficiency should take iron tablets or consume whole-grain cereals and vegetables rich in iron in combination with vitamin C.
- If you are suffering from kidney insufficiency, you should take vitamin D supplements. The addition of vitamin D is not necessary for most other diseases, unless blood levels are significantly depleted.
- Pregnant women should take folic acid as a preventive measure.
- Elderly people and people with serious illnesses (such as cancer) might have increased vitamin or mineral requirements.

Apart from these exceptions, I do not recommend taking dietary supplements. Choose the natural option of fruits, vegetables, whole grains, and spices. If you would still like to take a dietary supplement, you should discuss this with your doctor.

Healthy Foods Don't Have to Be Expensive

Fast food offers calorie-packed foods for as little money as possible. But calories aren't the only thing that matter. What about nutritional value? At first glance, healthy foods seem to be more expensive than fast food. But if you realize the true value of the treasures from the produce section, you'll keep finding bargains.

For example, vegetables seem to be more expensive than ready-made meals, but they have many times the health value.

If you want to get a lot of nutrients for your money, you should buy legumes, nuts, soybeans, and whole grains, and leave meat and dairy products on the shelves. Invest your money in a healthier and longer life. The return is worth it!

Eat Better, Live Longer

WE SHOULD FOLLOW THESE FIFTEEN IMPORTANT RULES:

1) Eat a lot of (green) vegetables.
2) Eat a lot of legumes.
3) Eat healthy fats: nuts and plenty of healthy oils.
4) Eat lots of fruit, preferably in season.
5) Consume less salt and more spices, onions, garlic, and herbs.
6) Eat more whole grains and less white flour.
7) Reduce your consumption of sugar and sweets.
8) Avoid meat and eggs.
9) Avoid milk and other dairy products.
10) Eat very little or no fish.
11) Don't snack between meals.

12) Drink coffee, tea, and water; avoid alcohol, soft drinks, and sugary drinks.

13) Avoid industrially processed foods.

14) Practice good eating habits (eat slowly and mindfully, chew thoroughly).

15) Practice easy fasting (intermittent fasting on the majority of days; therapeutic fasting occasionally).

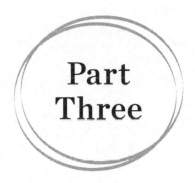

Part Three

Fast Easier, Live Longer

The Healing and Preventive
Effect of Therapeutic Fasting
and Intermittent Fasting

Chapter Five

Why Fasting Is So Important for Us

Seventy percent of all chronic diseases today are caused by a poor diet.[1] In the developed world, this has nothing to do with malnutrition, let alone undernutrition; it's an excess supply of food that is making us sick.

For millions of years, hunger was our daily companion. Our bodies were designed for long periods of not eating. But modern humans eat constantly—we consume calories up to ten times a day. Not only do we eat at mealtimes, but we also consume snacks throughout the day.

Our metabolism is overwhelmed by this constant intake of food. For decades, there have been discussions about what we should eat, yet we've failed to address the question of when and how often we should eat. The answers to these questions are of immense importance. Research from the past two decades shows that all organisms that fast regularly can prolong their life span by 20 to 30 percent.[2, 3] Even though much of what we currently know is based on animal studies, and human studies are ongoing, the fundamental research is groundbreaking: Through fasting we can improve all metabolic parameters in our organs and tissues in an impressive way.[4] No drug can achieve this life-prolonging effect!

The benefits of fasting, both therapeutic and intermittent (also known as interval fasting), are obvious: Both are easy to implement, cost little money, and are very effective in treating and preventing diseases. Fasting is very well tolerated and has an overall positive effect on health, vitality, and, in the long run, even on weight. And finally, both therapeutic fasting and intermittent fasting ultimately lead to more mindfulness and enjoyment when eating.

The Difference Between Therapeutic Fasting and Intermittent Fasting

Therapeutic fasting and intermittent fasting are two different methods. I define therapeutic fasting as a prolonged fasting period that lasts for at least five days. During that time, you consume a small number of calories every day—usually in the form of vegetable broths and juices. Intermittent fasting, on the other hand, is an eating pattern that cycles between shorter periods of fasting and eating. One of the most popular forms of intermittent fasting is the 16:8 method, in which you eat whatever you want within an eight-hour window every day and then fast for the next sixteen hours, and so on.

Fasting Does Not Mean Starving

One misconception people have about fasting is that it's antithetical to enjoying life and food, that it's akin to starvation. But fasting is by no means the enemy of the enjoyment of food. On the contrary, it can actually lead to a heightened appreciation of food. As in all parts of life, diet is about balance. Both eating *and* fasting contribute to that.

We must not confuse fasting with starving. They are somewhat re-lated but ultimately quite different. Here's an example to illustrate this: Fasting is to starving as a pleasant morning jog is to fearfully running away from a tiger. Fasting is always voluntary. Starving isn't.

Most of us have not spent a great deal of time being mindful of the different sensations of hunger. We might consume snacks or entire meals without reflecting on whether we're actually hungry. Often we eat simply because it's pleasurable. The American researcher Brian Wan-sink coined the term "mindless eating" to describe the inattentive hab-its that go into the way we eat.

When do you feel hungry? What does that hunger feel like? Try to observe your feeling of hunger from a bird's-eye perspective. When you fast, you'll learn to differentiate true hunger from appetite and other sensations.

How Fasting Activates Self-Healing

Fasting is highly effective for both therapy and prevention. In other words, it can alleviate or cure existing disease symptoms, and prevent the development of many diseases. In therapeutic fasting, this promise is contained within the term itself: Fasting can indeed be a therapy. Therapeutic fasting is the type that has been established the longest. In the past, it was sometimes derided as a luxury cure for overweight or wealthy people, but now therapeutic fasting has become one of the most important therapies in complementary medicine and innovative nutritional medicine. According to current studies, therapeutic fasting has even more health benefits than intermittent fasting.[5, 6, 7]

Many specialized clinics have been successfully using therapeutic fasting to treat rheumatism and chronic pain diseases for years. It's ef-fective in treating diabetes, hypertension, fatty liver disease, and ele-vated blood lipid levels. It can also significantly alleviate symptoms of food intolerance, irritable bowel syndrome, inflammatory bowel diseases, allergies, and even neurological diseases such as multiple sclerosis; furthermore, it can slow down the progression of these diseases. At the Immanuel Hospital Berlin, fasting is currently being researched as a complementary therapy for cancer patients undergoing chemotherapy.

I am always amazed at how easily my patients are able to adapt to fasting, considering how central food is in our daily lives. Most of us are familiar with the experience of overindulging in a heavy meal (Thanksgiving turkey comes to mind), and as a result feeling groggy and lethargic. This state is called food coma or post-meal coma for a reason. When my patients fast, they often report improved moods. Some of them even experience the so-called fasting euphoria. These positive effects lead to very good adherence; in other words, patients follow the fasting procedure as recommended.

Everyone should try fasting at least once. It can be quite powerful to discover that you are able to enjoy life even without eating regular meals for a certain period of time. After that experience, you'll approach eating with more awareness and therefore be much healthier.

How Fasting Came into My Life and My Medical Practice

In my opinion, fasting is the most effective therapeutic method in complementary medicine (I'm referring to prolonged therapeutic fasting first and foremost). I'm not alone in this opinion. Gustav Riedlin, a German doctor and a pioneer of therapeutic fasting, called it "surgery without knives."[8] Otto Buchinger, the founder of the most renowned fasting technique in Europe, called it "a royal road to healing."[9]

In my youth, I would see my father eating only wheat germ during his weekly fasting days. Fasting was an essential part of his approach to complementary medicine—which is why I was surprised to discover that during my medical training and even through the first two years of my internal medicine residency, fasting was never mentioned. This finally changed when I started a fellowship at the department of complementary medicine headed by Malte Bühring at the Free University of Berlin. On the first day of training I noticed that the majority of patients, who were suffering from various chronic diseases such as hypertension, diabetes, rheumatism, and bowel irritation, were prescribed therapeutic fasting for seven to ten days. The most astonishing thing was that the fasting period seemed incredibly easy to implement. I didn't witness a single patient asking to switch back to a regular diet, or sneaking food from the hospital cafeteria. It was more like this: After one to two days, when the (admittedly somewhat tough) initial adjustment was over, the fasting patients seemed to experience a good mood and an alleviation of symptoms.

Professor Bühring taught me to observe the effects of fasting during medical examinations. Fellows like me were asked to examine the tongues of our fasting patients every day; it didn't require much expertise to notice some impressive changes. Over a few days of fasting, a patient's tongue would start with a shockingly thick coating, which initially grew heavier, but then the tongue would change colors until it was eventually an uncoated, beautiful rosy tongue. The same thing could be observed with the skin and the connective tissue. We often saw troubled skin, which, over the course of a few days, would become clearer and more delicate. In patients with chronic pain, such as back pain, I could see the softening of the subcutaneous tissue. By observing fasting patients day after day, I could see how their connective tissue loosened up and became more elastic; many pain syndromes improved through fasting alone. But what I found most interesting was the change in people's faces. Most patients arrived at admissions with very tense faces—which, considering their severe symptoms, was understandable. Patients with hypertension or diabetes often presented with puffy faces, fluid retention, dark circles under their eyes, or severe erythema and eczema. But after only a few days of fasting, these symptoms disappeared or at least improved considerably. During our rounds, we regularly heard statements like: "My husband says my face looks youthful, relaxed, and joyful again."

Over the course of my training I came to know physicians at renowned fasting clinics and within the Medical Association for Fasting and Nutrition. I remember my first conference at the prestigious Buchinger Wilhelmi Clinic in Germany very well. Physiologists, biochemists, and doctors from many different countries—all of whom specialized in fasting—presented their case histories and findings in quick succession. I remember thinking to myself: It's shocking that so much medical experience is being ignored by conventional medicine.

Fasting Is the Supreme Therapeutic Discipline

Due to its quick and distinctly positive effect on blood pressure, blood sugar levels, inflammatory markers, and patients' subjective well-being, therapeutic fasting can be regarded as a restart or reset.

In the medical world there is a term called *self-efficacy*, which is the conviction that one can master a difficult situation on one's own. Anyone who is able to fast successfully proves to themselves that they are self-sufficient, and they can rightfully be proud of that. This self-efficacy makes it easier to then sustain long-term healthy diet and exercise changes.

In our department of internal and complementary medicine at Immanuel Hospital Berlin, about a thousand of the fifteen hundred inpatients annually fast as part of their medical therapy. In medicine, there is often the possibility of replacing certain treatment methods or medications with others that are similarly effective. As a doctor, I wouldn't want to miss fasting—it is indeed a supreme therapeutic discipline.

In one of my first studies on fasting I conducted during my time at the Essen-Mitte hospitals, I compared the dietary and lifestyle habits of roughly eighteen hundred patients. One group underwent therapeutic fasting for an average of seven days during their inpatient stay; the other received a normal-caloric diet. The results showed a clear difference between the two groups of patients after the study: Those who had fasted ate healthier and exercised more, even six months later.[10]

A patient described this effect very succinctly in a letter I received a few weeks after he was discharged: "In May, I spent some time at the department for complementary medicine at Immanuel Hospital for pain treatment and therapeutic fasting. I consider this experience of therapeutic fasting as a momentous, positive event in my life. In addition to weight loss, an improvement of my blood values, and pain relief, all my senses became *heightened* and I now perceive the taste of many dishes, the smell and sound of nature as a completely different, positive experience."

As recently as the 1970s, the typical American would eat three meals a day without consuming anything in between. I remember growing up and hearing my grandparents say things like: "Meals are eaten at the table" or "Don't spoil your appetite for dinner." It was completely normal not to eat anything for hours during the day.

This has changed. Today, the typical daily food intake for many people looks something like this: We eat breakfast, perhaps toast with jam or honey, or croissants, and drink sweetened coffee. At ten or eleven we might have a prelunch snack. A little later we'll have lunch, which isn't necessarily healthy, especially when it's eaten at a cafeteria. Around three in the afternoon we feel a little peckish and we might quench that feeling by eating something sweet. Then we have dinner. Later in the evening, in front of the TV, we might nibble on chips or chocolate. All in all, we end up consuming about six to seven meals a day—plus drinks such as coffee, alcohol, and other sweet beverages.

A study conducted by Satchidananda Panda, the renowned researcher of intermittent fasting at the Salk Institute for Biological Studies, has shown that Americans currently consume an average of seven
to nine meals a day.[11] Constant eating is a symptom of our modern
times, and so it's not at all surprising that obesity, diabetes, hypertension, and bowel diseases have become such an enormous problem
around the world.

Seven Misconceptions About Fasting

1. Fasting means hunger.

When people prepare properly and follow an established fasting technique such as the Buchinger method (see page 159), most feel little to
no hunger after the first or second day of fasting. If hunger occurs at
all, it is usually felt more in the evening. That's why if you're not fasting
in a clinic, it might be a good idea to plan something to distract you
in the evening (such as watching a movie) or go to bed early.

That said, people react in different ways, and some do indeed feel a
strong and frequent sensation of hunger during fasting. What I can say
for comfort here is: The longer and more often you practice therapeutic
fasting, the more your body gets used to it. After the third or fourth day
the hunger disappears. And if you try fasting for a second or third time,
you'll be able to overcome the sensation of hunger much more easily.

2. Fasting leads to vitamin deficiency.

This is simply not true. The body can fast effortlessly for one to four
weeks without developing any vitamin deficiency. The fasting technique I recommend, the Buchinger method, also involves consuming
a certain amount of vitamins and minerals via juices and broths.

3. Fasting is a starvation diet.

There are types of fasting, especially in the United States, in which nothing but water and unsweetened tea are allowed. However, with the European fasting techniques that I prescribe to my patients, we avoid solid food but purposefully allow small amounts of calories to be ingested in the form of juice or vegetable broth. This helps calm the stomach, and the consumption of this small number of calories prevents muscle loss.

4. When fasting, you can drink as much juice as you want.

You can, in fact, drink as much water and unsweetened tea as you want during fasting, according to your thirst. But you must limit the amount of vegetable or fruit juice you drink to 100 to 150 milliliters (about half a cup) a day. I remember two patients who complained about how they did not lose any weight even after a couple of days of fasting. When asked, one patient told me that she drank four to five large smoothies throughout the day. Hearing that, I was no longer surprised that she wasn't shedding any pounds. Fruit contains fructose, and a smoothie often contains many pieces of fruit—especially high-calorie fruit such as bananas. Four to five smoothies amounts to about 1,500 to 2,000 kcal! The other patient explained that she liked to sweeten her fasting tea with honey. When I asked her how much honey she used she said that one jar of honey lasted her roughly two days. Now, a little honey is allowed during fasting, but by "a little" I mean about two tablespoons a day—not half a jar of honey a day. One hundred grams of honey has about 300 kcal, and with 500 grams to a jar, my patient had been ingesting about 750 kcal a day in honey. When you add those calories to the calories ingested through broth and juices, this amounts to 1,110 kcal a day. You could call this a reduction diet, but it no longer counts as fasting.

5. Fasting is dangerous because it causes loss of heart muscle.

This misconception is based on studies conducted in the 1970s, in which severely obese patients were put on starvation diets for months to cure their obesity. There were indeed isolated cases of death due to cardiac arrhythmia. But this kind of prolonged crash diet is to therapeutic fasting what a leisurely stroll is to a triathlon. I do not recommend months-long starvation diets. Tens of thousands of patients fast in clinics every year, and they're no more likely to experience cardiac side effects than non-fasting guests staying at hotels or resorts.

6. Fasting purges and detoxes the body.

Detox (detoxing and purging) is frequently used as a buzzword to advertise fasting methods. And indeed, many blood values, including blood sugar and cholesterol levels, are improved by fasting. This result can be viewed as a kind of detoxification. But there is no proof that heavy metals such as lead and mercury, which can form deposits in the fat tissue, are removed from the body through fasting. Nevertheless, we can be grateful for the fact that autophagy, the cell's repair and self-cleaning processes, is boosted during fasting. These processes are much more relevant from a medical standpoint than the idea of purging or the nebulous "detox."

7. Fasting can lead to a yo-yo effect.

Our body is constantly burning energy, since all the organs and somatic cells do their work around the clock. The energy needed to maintain these normal processes even when we are sleeping or hanging out on the couch is called the basal metabolic rate. Early studies attest to the fact that bodily functions are reduced to these basic energy requirements during phases of prolonged therapeutic fasting or hunger.[12, 13] That's when the metabolism enters starvation mode. We can observe this in ourselves during fasting—you might notice a slower heartbeat and a tendency to be cold. The body temperature is lowered in order to save energy.

When we start to eat again after prolonged fasting or a longer period of hunger, the metabolism remains in the reduced basal metabolic rate for a while. If we were to resume eating the same amount of food we were eating before fasting, this would undoubtedly result in a yo-yo effect. In practice, however, this effect is extremely rare. From my experience I can say that almost all people who fast for a prolonged time change their dietary habits. Hot dogs and french fries are no longer as appealing, or at least not as often. That's why the large fasting clinics, especially the Buchinger Wilhelmi Clinic, did not see any yo-yo effect in their long-term data. This effect is a myth and by no means fact.

In terms of intermittent fasting, the yo-yo effect can be ruled out completely. Recent data even shows the opposite—during intermittent fasting the basal metabolic rate *increases*. An early study on intermittent fasting showed that this type of fasting increases fat burning significantly. This means the body cranks up the burning of fat permanently when intermittently fasting![14]

Fasting and Autophagy

In 2016, the Japanese scientist Yoshinori Ohsumi was awarded the Nobel Prize in Physiology or Medicine for his research on autophagy (from Greek, meaning "self-devouring"). Ohsumi discovered that somatic cells possess a kind of recycling program that enables them to deconstruct old, damaged cell components and then rebuild them into new complexes.

When we fast, we trigger autophagy. The molecular scientist Frank Madeo, one of the world's leading researchers on fasting and autophagy, has closely examined the cellular processes that change during fasting and found that fasting boosts the incredible process of self-healing through autophagy. He says, "No event changes the microstructure of the metabolism as extraordinarily as fasting, not even pregnancy or the most difficult heart surgery."

The Body's Reactions to Eating and Fasting

When we eat, we take in more energy than we need right at that moment. But the body manages its resources very wisely by storing excess energy. This makes sense, because for millions of years our ancestors didn't know when their next meal would be. We're able to store excess calories through glycogen, the storage form of sugar in the liver. The amount of glycogen that can be stored, however, is limited. As soon as the storage capacity is exhausted (i.e., when the reserve is full), the body begins to build fat reserves in other places. These reserves are the notorious "love handles" and "beer belly." In other words, surplus carbohydrates are stored in the form of body fat.

This process is controlled by the hormone insulin, the levels of which increase during meals. Insulin has two functions: One, it enables the sugar created through digestion and the breakdown of carbohydrates to enter the somatic cells directly. These cells draw their energy from the sugar. Two, insulin ensures that excess energy is stored as body fat, as described. The extent to which insulin levels rise depends on the food we eat. Carbohydrates, especially pure sugar, make insulin rise the fastest. By now we know that proteins make it rise as well, albeit more slowly. Fats, on the other hand, are absorbed directly and have little effect on insulin level.

Basically, the body knows only two states of being: the satiated state (high insulin levels) and the fasting state (low insulin levels). We either store the energy derived from food or we burn it. It's important that both states occur in a balanced manner; otherwise we inevitably gain weight (at least, that is the case with most people).

If we don't eat but are in need of energy, the glycogen reserves in the liver are the first to be used up. According to current research and estimates, this takes about 16 to 24 hours for men, and probably a little less for women (14 to 20 hours).[15] As soon as the glycogen reserves are emptied and the body needs more energy, it will start to break down amino acids, or proteins, to create sugar in a complicated process. At the same time, the body begins to boost lipolysis, or fat breakdown, in which the fat reserves are broken down in order to extract energy. These reserves are commonly found as so-called visceral fat, which surrounds the organs in the abdomen and is also on our hips. The fatty acids gained from this process provide energy that can be used by most body tissues directly.

The only exception to this is the brain, because fatty acids can't pass through the blood-brain barrier. This barrier is a kind of protective filter for the brain and wards off dangers (pathogens, toxic metabolites, drugs). That's why the brain needs sugar in order to function. If no sugar is available, other brain energy providers need to be found. These include the so-called ketones, which start to build up rather quickly during fasting. The advantage: They can reach the brain and be metabolized there. Today we know that ketones are beneficial to the brain and to health. There are growing indications that they are linked to improvements for certain neurological diseases such as multiple sclerosis, Parkinson's disease, and even dementia.[16]

How Long Can You Fast?

First and foremost, fasting simply means not eating. The body only has two programs—fasting and eating—at its disposal. The logical consequence is that we fast every time we don't eat. The English word *breakfast* means the breaking of a fast. Without realizing it, we fast every day in some form or another, particularly during the night—usually from after dinner until breakfast. This shows us that fasting isn't unusual or bad, but that it is already a positive part of our everyday life or that it can become one if we decide to do intermittent fasting.

Fasting therefore doesn't lead to a detrimental lack of energy, because the body is well prepared and can, if the reserves are right, fast for many weeks at a time. The fasting period, however, depends on the fat reserves that are available. Very thin people are going to have a hard time fasting for more than ten days, because that's when the reserves start to run low, which means putting stress on the body. An overweight person, on the other hand, can fast for two, three, or even six weeks with the appropriate medical supervision. They are even going to feel better and better with every passing day. But their reserves will eventually run low too. When this happens, the fasting person will start to feel that they aren't doing well physically or mentally. Fatigue and performance loss are further symptoms. That's the body giving the signal: Enough, now—time to break the fast!

Neither therapeutic fasting nor intermittent fasting has a clearly or scientifically defined standard duration. My recommendation is that therapeutic fasting should be done for at least five and a maximum of twenty-eight days at a time, and, depending on the conditions, not more than two to four times a year.

Therapeutic Fasting—the Main Methods

Fasting nearly faded into obscurity in the world of Western medicine, but two physicians—a German and an Austrian—played important roles in reestablishing it as a therapeutic method.

The Otto Buchinger Method

Picture this: Germany, 1920. World War I ended just two years ago. War, bad harvests, and hunger are plaguing the country. Meat, bread, and flour are coveted. People eat anything they can get their hands on. But in the small town of Witzenhausen, a physician named Otto Buchinger is using fasting cures to treat patients. Though he's mocked and criticized, Buchinger's fasting method is successful, and word gets around. More and more people flock to him, wanting to experience the astounding fasting cure firsthand. Within a few years, Buchinger's fasting clinic becomes one of the most important places in the life reform movement, a social movement that emphasized a return-to-nature lifestyle (and that later influenced the hippie movement in the United States).

Otto Buchinger was born in 1878. As a child and teenager, he suffered from poor health with chronic colds, tonsillitis, and flu. He studied medicine and became a doctor in the navy. There, confronted with the sailors' unhealthy diets and the widespread consumption of alcohol, Buchinger began to explore nutritional therapy and the possibilities of lifestyle medicine. After sixteen years of serving in the navy, he was forced to retire in 1917. He fell ill with severe arthritis and kidney disease. Soon, he could walk only with the aid of a stick. He was advised to go see the fasting physician Gustav Riedlin, who had been influenced by American fasting physicians and who considered fasting the most powerful therapy in complementary medicine. Riedlin believed that "hunger is the best chef, fasting the best doctor." After fasting for nineteen days under Riedlin's supervision, Buchinger experienced a healing and an awakening: "After fasting for nineteen days, I was thin, but I was able to move all my joints like a young man again."[17]

From that time onward, Buchinger continued to fast regularly until the end of his life. He also adopted a healthy diet. Buchinger, who had been a sickly child and was forced to end his military service due to illness, was healthy right up until old age. He died at eighty-eight. He dedicated his medical practice to therapeutic fasting and, together with the Austrian Franz Xaver Mayr, became one of the defining figures of German fasting medicine. Today, his clinics—the Buchinger Wilhelmi in Germany and Spain—remain beacons of clinical fasting.[18]

In the fasting method that Buchinger developed, a certain number of calories are consumed daily in the form of liquid food. This number amounts to 200 to 300 kcal and, with possible supplements, a maximum of 500 kcal, so as not to slow down the breakdown of fat in the liver. Solid food is strictly forbidden to avoid encouraging a sensation of hunger caused by chewing. This modified version of fasting developed by Buchinger is currently the most commonly employed method in Europe; it is sometimes also called juice fasting.

This therapeutic fasting method is designed as part of a diverse therapeutic program. Therefore, the method doesn't only consist of a limited intake of calories, but is embedded in a holistic treatment that includes various forms of therapeutic exercise and learning relaxation techniques.

Fasting is most effective when it's accompanied by both exercise and relaxation. It's not absolutely necessary, and many people continue to go to work while fasting. However, I recommend an extensive relaxation and exercise program while fasting, for more intense health benefits.

The Buchinger method of therapeutic fasting also focuses on concepts such as cleansing, purification, and drainage, which is sometimes referred to rather exaggeratedly as detoxification. Fasting is complemented by treatments such as sweating at low temperatures in the sauna, receiving liver packs, and drinking large quantities of water and tea—this supports regenerative processes and helps drain harmful substances from the somatic cells. In our clinic, fasting patients receive one liver pack a day (we place a warm, damp cloth on the skin over where the liver sits, and on top of the cloth we place a hot-water bottle for half an hour), because it is believed that the liver is forced to work harder during fasting, and its blood flow is stimulated by warmth. A study conducted in Freiburg, Germany, recently proved this effect.[19]

The F. X. Mayr Method

Franz Xaver Mayr was born in 1875 in Gröbming, an Austrian mountain village. As a teenager, Mayr observed animals and concluded that diet and digestion have a significant effect on health. At the time, he was focused on a topic that is trending today: the intestine. During his medical training and while practicing medicine, he noticed how terrible people felt when something was wrong with their digestion. So he developed a therapy that focused on calming the intestine with easily digestible food and fasting. Since he recognized that hastily eaten and badly chewed food are possible causes of digestive problems, he developed a fasting technique that is accompanied by "chewing training."[20] He was influenced by the American "chewing guru" Horace Fletcher, a businessman born in 1849, who had become rich in the cheese trade. Fletcher was severely obese and suffered increasingly from health problems. Advised by an acquaintance, he began to chew all food until it was almost completely dissolved in his mouth. This technique, combined with intermittent fasting—Fletcher took to eating only once a day—led to him losing fifty-five pounds within a short period of time. In addition, he started to exercise. Some days, he cycled for more than sixty miles, increasingly without experiencing joint pain and building up stamina. His own positive health success story made Fletcher famous, and he became a proponent of thorough chewing. Through other contemporaries of Fletcher, such as Will Keith Kellogg, the inventor of cornflakes, the practice of "Fletcherism"—that is, chewing thoroughly—spread.[21, 22]

Mayr incorporated chewing as a central element of his fasting therapy. With the Mayr method, fasting patients should chew and insalivate a bite of bread (ideally day-old bread) thirty to forty times in the mouth before swallowing the masticated food with a small sip of a drink (Mayr recommended milk). This process lightens the intestine's workload and supports digestion as the food is predigested by the enzymes in the saliva. Moreover, the deliberate and slow chewing teaches patients to eat mindfully and consciously, and to experience the feeling of being full. That's at the heart of Mayr's fasting method: to stop eating as soon as you feel full. This feeling of satiation happens sooner when food is chewed slowly, which helps us eat less.

The Mayr method includes ingesting grain and tea as well as easily digestible foods (such as white rice, white bread, and cooked vegetables like carrots, zucchini, and potatoes). Mayr recommended milk as the drink to wash down the soft-chewed bread, but I do not recommend it because animal proteins cancel out many of the beneficial effects of fasting, as shown by recent scientific data. Instead, I recommend a modern alternative: soy, almond, or oat milk.

The Healing and Preventive Effect
of Therapeutic Fasting

Fasting shows us how much can be achieved with diet and lifestyle changes when it comes to disease. Of course, not all diseases can be treated or prevented with nutritional therapy, exercise, and stress reduction. The effect on many noteworthy diseases, however, is astonishing.

In chronic diseases such as hypertension and type 2 diabetes, the combination of therapeutic fasting and subsequent intermittent fasting is powerful. Moreover, fasting leads to healthy and reliable weight loss.

The current state of research on fasting, especially data from laboratory studies, is impressive. Though many questions remain unanswered (for example, beneficial effects seen in animal experiments cannot be assumed to be true for humans without further study), the wide spectrum of beneficial results is valuable data for us doctors to consider. Caution is advisable when it comes to fasting and cancer. But the unambiguously positive effects of fasting have been proven for the following diseases in particular:

Hypertension

For most people, blood pressure falls by about 25 to 30 mmHg during fasting, which is far more than can be achieved with antihypertensive medications. On the topic of the antihypertensive effect of fasting, I would like to mention a study conducted by Alan Goldhamer, who has been running a fasting clinic in California for many years and has treated tens of thousands of patients. His fasting is pure water fasting—that is, a starvation diet—which we don't recommend in quite the same form at our clinic. Still, Goldhamer's results regarding the improvement of blood pressure through fasting are remarkable. Blood pressure levels of 174 patients were compared before and after fasting. The participants fasted for eleven days, followed by a six-day nutritional buildup period. The systolic pressure value decreased on average by 37 mmHg; in severely hypertensive patients (stage 3), by as much as 60 mmHg (from 190 mmHg to 130 mmHg).[23] These results are very difficult to achieve with medication—and with medication comes side effects. In addition, these positive effects on blood pressure and metabolism reduce the risk of future vascular diseases such as heart attack or stroke.

If I see comparable results with one of my fasting patients as their supervising physician, then I know that a lot can be achieved later on, after fasting, with a vegetarian, whole-food diet in combination with exercise. It's very likely that the patient will be able to stop taking certain medications in the future. On the other hand, if fasting shows little or no effect on the patient's blood pressure, then medication remains indispensable.

Rheumatism

The effect of fasting on rheumatism was proven as early as 1991 by a group of Scandinavian researchers led by Jens Kjeldsen-Kragh. Their research showed that almost all symptoms of rheumatism improved significantly during the ten-day fasting period. Symptoms documented before the fasting started—such as swollen hands, signs of inflammation in the blood, and pain—were registered in graphs and showed a steep downward trajectory.[24] This corresponds with Otto Buchinger's firsthand experience, and I too regularly observe these results in my patients. The effectiveness of therapeutic fasting on rheumatism has even been proven in a meta-analysis, which is a study that compares the results of various studies.[25]

Osteoarthritis of the joints is currently a widespread disease. It's generally caused by lifelong overexertion and distress; in other words, it's the result of wear and tear (unlike rheumatoid arthritis, which is an autoimmune disease). Nevertheless, osteoarthritis also has an inflammatory component. Accordingly, many patients suffer from swelling and sometimes redness of the joints. Therapeutic fasting has a good effect here; the inflammatory component in particular improves. In addition, fasting makes a subsequent change in diet easier, which is associated with weight loss, which in turn relieves the joints even further. Therefore, fasting should be part of a multifaceted therapy for osteoarthritis. If joint and muscle pain are alleviated during fasting, chances are very high that medication for this disease can also be reduced (for example, the dosage of pain medication).

Diabetes

Fasting has a very valuable medical effect on people suffering from type 2 diabetes. For patients who normally need insulin injections, the insulin requirement is almost always reduced during fasting. And a healing effect persists long after the fasting period has ended. This is beneficial because even though insulin lowers sugar levels, it exaggerates the weight gain caused by the diabetes. Insulin is essentially fattening. One of its main tasks is to transport glucose from the blood to the cells so that the cells can derive energy from the glucose (sugar). In type 2 diabetes with insulin resistance, the cells no longer respond to the insulin, which is why the sugar can no longer be channeled into the cells and therefore remains in the blood. As a reaction to this, the body produces even more insulin, because high blood sugar levels are the trigger for insulin release. This leads to constantly increasing insulin levels in order to be able to clear away the sugar. The increased insulin levels prevent the breakdown of fat in the body and also promote inflammation and cell aging.

This sets the vicious cycle of diabetes in motion: Since the cells have become resistant to insulin, the body releases increased amounts of the hormone, which is then even less effective. Increasing the dosage of insulin in the syringe is barely sufficient then, because we know it makes no sense to increase the dosage when resistance has developed. This is similar to a resistance to antibiotics. Initially, it can be broken with a larger dosage of the antibiotic drugs. But this doesn't work for long and only amplifies the vicious cycle of antibiotic administration and the development of resistance. The solution can only be found in the opposite action: The use of antibiotics must be drastically restricted so that resistant bacteria can no longer multiply.

Similarly, fasting breaks the vicious cycle of diabetes: The cells recover, and insulin is suddenly more effective again. We can observe this phenomenon in the fasting patients in our clinic by looking at the necessary doses of insulin before and after one week of fasting. Before fasting, diabetic patients often need to inject 80 or 100 units of insulin every day. After the fasting period, this number drops to 20 or 30 units. Some patients are even able to omit the insulin altogether. No drug-based therapy can achieve anything like this!

For many years, we have been observing the fantastic effects of fasting on type 2 diabetes in our clinic. We were able to show in an initial small study that blood pressure, the important hemoglobin A1c value (which indicates the average blood sugar level of the past three months), and other risk factors are lowered quickly and effectively through fasting.[26] In two further studies with overweight patients with type 2 diabetes, we were able to show that after just one week of outpatient therapeutic fasting, blood sugar regulation improved significantly and the effect persisted for several months.[27, 28] The famous gerontologist and fasting researcher Valter Longo, director of the Longevity Institute at the USC Leonard Davis School of Gerontology in California, has presented even more astounding results in mice. In a spectacular paper, he showed how repeated fasting in some animals even *cured* type 1 diabetes by regenerating the insulin-producing cells in the pancreas that had been destroyed by the disease.[29] I'm not sure that this miracle could be reproduced in humans, but it's possible the insulin dose for patients with type 1 diabetes can be largely reduced through fasting. We are currently exploring this question in an ongoing study conducted in cooperation with Witten/Herdecke University.

Fasting can be helpful for many diabetics. Unfortunately, diabetes and insulin resistance have become very common, and the numbers of these diseases are ever increasing. There were hardly any diabetics in Europe after World War II, but now there are about 8 million people who suffer from type 2 diabetes.[30, 31]

An Important Note for Patients with Type 2 Diabetes

During fasting, the insulin intake must either be paused or the dosage reduced. This should always be done under medical supervision. A very commonly prescribed diabetes drug, metformin, must not be taken during fasting.

Patient History: Type 2 Diabetes

Christina F. (57), a nurse in early retirement from Munich, suffers from type 2 diabetes, rheumatism, and polyneuropathy (PN), a disease that damages the nerve fibers and manifests itself in severe, recurring pain in the limbs. She combats her symptoms with therapeutic fasting and a change in diet.

"For me, fasting has broken the vicious cycle of symptoms."

That our diet can influence our entire body is something I have experienced firsthand. I have had type 2 diabetes, rheumatism, and neuropathic pains in my arms and legs, called polyneuropathy, for thirty years. Over the years, my insulin units had to be increased to such an extent that I kept putting on weight—because the additional hormones not only regulate blood sugar levels, they also increase one's appetite. At some point, I weighed 185 pounds at my height of 5'1". Naturally, the weight made the joint pain even worse.

That was when I started reading a lot about nutrition—and dropped carbohydrates such as pasta, rice, and potatoes from my meals. This was surprisingly easy for me and I lost almost eleven pounds within a few weeks. But something else disappeared as well: my neuropathic pains! Until then, they could not be tamed by any drugs and had always flared up again and again. But all of a sudden, they were simply gone! Unfortunately, in the midst of this success a great mental strain arrived, because my mother became care-dependent. She first lost her hearing in one ear, then became blind in one eye. My joints were in great pain; I could barely get out of bed in the mornings. My rheumatologist, whom I had told about the successful change in my diet, asked me whether I wanted professional help at the Immanuel Hospital Berlin.

I said yes—and became an inpatient at the clinic for two weeks. On day one of the therapeutic fasting treatment, I ate only rice and vegetables. On day two I received 150 milliliters of vegetable juice three times a day, and for lunch and dinner, a thin fasting broth with the occasional piece of carrot or potato. This was accompanied by water and thin tea. My insulin medication was initially reduced, then omitted wholly. Fasting was surprisingly easy for me. I was never really hungry, though I did worry about my blood sugar. It did indeed react; during nights I tended to become hypoglycemic. To be on the safe side, a nurse came to measure my blood values every night at two a.m., and sometimes I was given a little dextrose. Fasting worked wonderfully for seven days, after which I was asked to stop, because a little fluid was being retained in my legs.

Still, the success I achieved through fasting was enormous! I had arrived at the clinic at 163 pounds and left at 152 pounds. I only needed a quarter of my former insulin dosage, was pain-free, and didn't need to take any antirheumatic medication. Some of the symptoms returned when I was back home, but they were less intense—and you can't expect miracles, after all! But for me, fasting has broken the vicious cycle of symptoms. I have maintained my no-carbohydrate diet and am currently trying to switch to a vegetarian diet. So far I have often eaten sausage and meat, but I have learned that they fuel the inflammatory nature of my rheumatism. I haven't succeeded in dropping meat completely, but I experiment with tofu, flaxseed patties, and vegetarian spreads from the health food store. My goal is to limit how much meat I eat and to lose two to four pounds every three months. It's going really well so far!

When the neuropathic or joint pains come back, I counter them with other things I learned at the clinic: cold Scotch hose treatments and dry brushing. To be honest, I wouldn't have time to do anything else if I "checked off" all the valuable advice and implemented everything I learned; that's just impossible. . . . You want to live, after all, and not just fulfill a checklist. But I have noticed my body reacting very positively to certain treatments—and those I do regularly. Warm liver packs, for example, help me calm down at lunchtime and get some rest. And it seems to help my liver, which is now able to regulate my metabolism better due to the things I have improved in my diet. The liver filters out toxins—and I really feel cleaner and healthier now.

Allergies

Several scientific studies on the connection between fasting and allergies are currently being conducted. Through my clinical experience, I've witnessed many patients who were suffering from an allergy show significant improvement in their symptoms after fasting. This applies to hay fever as well as allergic asthma. I remember a fruit farmer who came to our clinic while he was suffering from a very severe allergic episode with asthmatic symptoms. To his surprise, he was completely symptom-free by the third day of fasting. The trick, of course, is to find a form of nutrition that can be used in the everyday lives of patients and that can stabilize this effect.

Skin Diseases

Just as patients with rheumatic diseases show great results when fasting, so do patients with psoriasis. The positive effects of fasting apply to both the symptoms of psoriasis, which affect the skin itself, as well as inflammatory diseases of the joints, such as psoriatic arthritis. I advise every patient with psoriasis to try fasting and a wholesome vegetarian diet as a complementary therapeutic measure.

With neurodermatitis, rosacea, and other skin diseases, the effectiveness of fasting is not so clear. We very often see good improvements in rosacea, which causes redness and visible blood vessels in the face, but in cases of neurodermatitis the progress is erratic. Nevertheless, in these cases it can be worth testing whether regular fasting can alleviate the symptoms on an individual basis.

Bowel Diseases

Some bowel diseases can be improved through therapeutic fasting. These include chronic inflammatory bowel disease (IBD), Crohn's disease, and ulcerative colitis, as well as irritable bowel syndrome. We now know that an unbalanced microbiome (intestinal flora) can be the cause of at least one of these bowel diseases. The diversity of the microbiome— that is, the types of bacteria in the intestine—increases after fasting and can therefore have a long-term positive effect on IBD. But another reason why fasting might be so effective for bowel diseases could have to do with the intestinal mucosa, which regenerates during fasting. This mechanism was discovered by the famous French penguin researcher Yvon Le Maho. Penguins share parental care, so one parent looks after the chick while the other searches for food. The latter fasts for weeks as it hunts for food for the partner who remains behind. Maho discovered that the penguins who fasted experienced major changes, particularly in the intestinal mucosa.[32, 33, 34] To some extent, we could call this a self-cleaning mechanism.

Neurological Diseases

Mark Mattson, one of the world's leading neuroscientists at Johns Hopkins University, has demonstrated the positive effects of fasting on the brain and nerve cells. When Mattson fed mice a diet rich in fats and fructose, they not only became excessively overweight, they also became less intelligent. Learning difficulties and memory problems appeared even in young animals. But the animals were able to recover (losing weight and regaining intelligence) through fasting.[35, 36]

The preventive effect that regular fasting and intermittent fasting

have on chronic neurological diseases such as dementia, multiple sclerosis, Parkinson's disease, stroke, and epilepsy has been documented in
countless laboratory experiments.[37] This effect is due to the fact that
fasting leads to an increased release of the growth factor BDNF (brain-
derived neurotrophic factor), which has neuroprotective qualities. This
factor not only prevents brain cells from dying, it also stimulates the
formation of new nerve cells, particularly in the hippocampus, the area
of the brain that is responsible for memory and spatial memory.[38]

Why does the hippocampus react to fasting by growing? It might
seem counterintuitive, but from an evolutionary biology standpoint, it
makes sense. When you live in an area where there is little food and
you're constantly suffering from hunger, being able to remember where
there might be food and how you avoided danger the last time is an
advantage. There are numerous changes on the metabolic level during
fasting, in addition to the increased release of BDNF, that are advantageous for the brain. I would like to mention ketones in particular
here, metabolic products that are produced from fatty acids during
fasting. For diseased brain cells that have trouble processing sugar,
ketones form a kind of "therapeutic food."[39] That's why the ketogenic
diet is used specifically for patients with epilepsy, for example. Through
both therapeutic fasting as well as intermittent fasting, you can provide
your brain with more ketones.

Due to his remarkable lab results on intermittent fasting, Mark
Mattson is fairly certain that we can prevent the brain diseases I mentioned before with regular fasting—even if there is a genetic disposition. However, only studies on humans will bring definitive results.

In the world's first-ever clinical study of this kind, conducted by my
research team together with the department of neurology at the Charité,
headed by Paul Friedemann and Valter Longo's team, we were able to
show that therapeutic fasting (and a ketogenic diet) has a positive effect

The Ketogenic Diet

The ketogenic diet (also known as the keto diet) forbids carbohydrates almost completely, so in that sense it is a kind of "sugar fasting." Just as with fasting, the ketogenic diet boosts autophagy and the regeneration of mitochondria.

There is increasing evidence that the ketogenic diet has a therapeutic effect on neurological diseases. It is used in the treatment of epilepsy, especially in children.[40] There, it is undoubtedly effective and can help bridge difficult treatment situations. For other neurological diseases, the effect of this diet has not yet been sufficiently documented in studies.

But the ketogenic diet also has glaring disadvantages: The near-total omission of carbohydrates also means omitting healthy carbohydrates from whole grains—and with them, healthy fiber. This not only increases the risk of vascular diseases in the future, it's also bad for the intestinal bacteria. Problems for the vessels and the heart are aggravated if a lot of meat and dairy products are consumed, because this means the direct ingestion of large quantities of unhealthy saturated fats and pro-inflammatory animal proteins. For this reason, we have tried in our own studies on the ketogenic diet to develop a version that supplements plant-based foods rich in fat to as great an extent as possible. But every ketogenic diet, even one that is predominantly plant based, is ultimately an unbalanced diet.

In some online forums, the ketogenic diet is hailed as a "cure-all," even though there is insufficient knowledge about what actually happens in the body with permanent ketosis. Could there be disadvantages for the cells and the metabolism? Without a doubt, the ketogenic diet is useful for the specific situation of therapy-resistant epilepsy. And a slight regular increase in ketones, which happens during therapeutic fasting and intermittent fasting, seems to benefit the cells. But more studies need to be done in order for us to know whether omitting carbohydrates to such a great extent is generally health-promoting.

on the quality of life of patients with multiple sclerosis.[41] We hope to confirm these effects in a currently ongoing large-scale study.

Unfortunately, one very serious neurological disease can't be influenced by fasting. On the contrary, it tends to get worse. It's amyotrophic lateral sclerosis (ALS), which was brought to global awareness by the "ice bucket challenge," a fundraising campaign to support the fight against this disease, in 2014.

Neurological pain syndromes such as fibromyalgia, on the other hand, improve during fasting. In one study, we were able to document that a fasting treatment achieves better results for patients with fibromyalgia than the standard treatment with cortisone and other pain medications.[42]

Migraines and Headaches

Migraines and chronic headaches are common and debilitating illnesses. They're often treated with medications that ensure that large amounts of serotonin are made available in the brain. The painkillers aspirin and ibuprofen are widely prescribed. The problem with these drugs is that above a certain threshold, they themselves can cause or amplify headaches.

To alleviate headaches or migraines, to heal them in the long run, or to decrease the frequency with which they occur, fasting has been recommended by many doctors, to great success. Two things happen in the brain during fasting: One, more serotonin is made available to the brain; this effect lasts long after fasting has ended and is also the reason for its mood-enhancing effect. Two, fasting is also a kind of withdrawal, a "detox" from addictive pain medications. For this reason, headaches or migraines caused by pain medication withdrawal can occur at the beginning of the fasting period. When this happens, we support our patients intensively with naturopathic remedies. It's important that this pain is overcome in order to break the pattern. Because if patients are able to get through the first few days and finish their fast, their migraines and headaches usually occur much less frequently than before fasting—and often for a long time.

Mental Illness

The mood-enhancing effect of fasting, which can even lead to fasting euphoria, is a well-known phenomenon. It is probably caused by serotonin, which I already mentioned, but also by the increased release of other mood enhancers produced naturally in the body, such as endorphins. In our own studies, I was able to observe this mood-enhancing and antidepressant effect again and again.

> **Important:** Fasting should only be tried by patients suffering from mild or moderate depression, never by those with severe depression.

Fasting and Cancer

Fasting has a rather unique role in the context of cancer treatment. Current data from animal experiments indicates that short-term fasting has a preventive and therapeutic effect in cases of cancer. This effect can be explained by the complex differences in the ways a healthy somatic cell and a cancer cell respond to fasting. The ketones produced during fasting can be processed well by healthy somatic cells, but only to a limited extent by cancer cells. As a result of this and because of the loss of growth signals from insulin, mTOR, and IGF-1, the degenerated cancer cells find themselves in a disadvantageous metabolic situation, whereas the healthy somatic cells transition to a fasting metabolism that has existed for centuries.

There's been ongoing research on the effects of fasting for sixty to eighty-four hours while undergoing chemotherapy. In an initial pilot study, we were able to determine significant effects on fatigue and quality of life in cancer patients who fasted while undergoing chemotherapy, in comparison to cancer patients who were on a normal diet during chemotherapy. The effectiveness of seventy-two-hour fasting as a supplement to chemotherapy is currently being examined by our research team in two larger clinical studies.

One of the greatest challenges with chemotherapy and the reason it has such severe side effects is that it attacks not only the cancer cells but also healthy somatic cells. But Valter Longo discovered something incredible. After conducting research on yeast cells and bacteria for years, he made a pioneering achievement: He found that healthy cells and cancer cells have very different reactions to fasting.

We have known for a long time that healthy somatic cells are genetically programmed to switch to a kind of hibernation mode when energy derived from food is no longer available. Essentially, when no food is available, healthy cells go into a protective mode in which all cell functions are stifled and protein synthesis is curbed. As a result, nothing much happens in the cell anymore, but due to this mechanism, it is protected from adverse external factors and toxins.

On the other hand, the cancer cell possesses mutated genes, so-called oncogenes. They ensure that the cancer cell can grow even without external stimulating signals. Oncogenes make the cancer cell more prone to damage by toxins because all its gates are open in this state. In other words, when starved, cancer cells don't go into a protective mode. Instead, they remain hungry and consume any type of food without inhibition, including the harmful cytotoxin administered during chemotherapy.

Longo described the situation for the body as a "differential stress resistance." Food deprivation causes stress—which makes the cancer cell vulnerable—but the healthy cell is able to manage this stress beautifully. The healthy cells enter a protective mode—they take cover and concentrate on life-sustaining measures such as self-cleansing and thus become more resistant to toxins such as those administered during chemotherapy. Cancer cells, on the other hand, stay active and keep dividing, as is characteristic for them—and this is what makes them vulnerable to the toxins administered with the chemotherapy. Cancer cells are thus severely decimated by chemotherapy.

In his decades of experimental laboratory tests, Longo was able to substantiate the differential stress resistance time and again. But of course, lab and animal experiments aren't enough; the human organism is much, much more complicated.[43]

ON THE CURRENT STATE OF CANCER RESEARCH

In 2014, my team and I started our own study on fasting and chemotherapy. Fifty patients with breast or ovarian cancer who were planning to undergo chemotherapy were included in the study. While the patients were undergoing chemotherapy, we recorded their quality of life, mood, overall well-being, and side effects of the treatment. Since some women discontinued the therapy, received other treatments, or no longer had time for the extensive questionnaires, we received data from thirty-four patients all together. All of them fasted in half of their four to six chemotherapy cycles. Fasting started thirty-six hours before chemotherapy was administered and was continued for twenty-four hours afterward, which adds up to more than sixty hours overall. And indeed, our results confirmed Longo's hypothesis: When patients fasted, they tolerated chemotherapy much better, with fewer adverse effects on their quality of life.[44]

Still, I advise caution on fasting during chemotherapy. Oncologists are indeed right when they argue that it's too early to recommend it.

It's very important to check all the prerequisites, to control the patients' weight continually, and to monitor the fasting very closely. At the moment, we are taking these requirements into consideration in a larger study. Our colleagues in Los Angeles are also continuing their studies in this field. We hope that in two to three years we can tell more accurately whom fasting could help during chemotherapy.

Whether fasting has additional benefits in fighting cancer can, for now, be tested only in animal experiments. To be able to starve cancer cells into oblivion would be a dream, but unfortunately it's not that simple. Nevertheless, a combination of a healthy diet and periodic fasting could be a good method to support cancer therapy. By now it has been proven that breast and colon cancer, for example, occur less often if the overall diet is healthy.[45]

> **Important:** If you are suffering from cancer, fast only under medical supervision and, ideally, within the framework of a study. Make sure you don't lose too much weight; being underweight has to be avoided at all costs.

We recommend that cancer patients as well as patients with chronic diseases switch to a mostly plant-based, low-sugar diet after fasting. This strengthens their immune system in the fight against the disease. Recent scientific data suggests that fasting foods such as broth and gruel should be kept free of animal protein and refined sugar as much as possible.[46, 47] This is why vegan fasting methods such as the Buchinger fast are advantageous. When choosing the juices to drink while you fast, you should make sure to drink vegetable rather than sweet fruit juices to avoid a high fructose content.

THE FASTING MIMICKING DIET

After researching fasting for many years, Valter Longo discovered that there is a way to mimic the effects of fasting without actually fasting. He noticed in experiments that part of the effect of fasting can be traced back to omitting animal products as well as sugar. If both animal products and sugar are left out of a diet, there is a significant decrease in the concentration of insulin, IGF-1 (a marker for future cancer risk), and mTOR (an enzyme that promotes inflammatory growth in the cells)—just as occurs in "proper" fasting.[48]

This observation motivated Longo to develop the fasting mimicking diet. Traditional fasting can be difficult for many people, and the fasting mimicking diet allows people to eat while also enjoying the benefits of fasting. In order to make this diet available to people, Longo created a fasting mimicking food product line, in which proceeds from product sales go toward a foundation dedicated to fasting research.[49]

Two of the products available are Chemolieve and ProLon. Chemolieve is a four-day meal program designed to support patients undergoing chemotherapy treatment. ProLon is designed for anyone who wants to achieve the beneficial effects of fasting. It consists of a five-day, ready-made meal program based on the fasting mimicking diet. The drawback to ProLon, of course, is that it's expensive. The advantage is that you don't have to worry about shopping, caloric content, and meal preparation. Everything you'll eat for five days is prepared. Soups, bars, snacks, drinks, vitamins, and supplements make up the daily rations—and they're all vegan and low in sugar.

I participated in what is, to date, the largest clinical study on humans that was designed to review this fasting program. We examined one hundred volunteers from California. Half of the test subjects received ProLon for five days at a time over the course of three months;

the other group was asked to eat normally. After three fasting cycles (one five-day fasting cycle per month), the fasting mimicking diet showed good results. The participants lost weight, their blood pressure dropped, their blood lipid values improved, and their levels of the growth factor IGF-1 were reduced.[50]

Is the fasting mimicking diet the future? Even though I don't care for the amount of packaging and the lack of freshness, I think it may be exactly the right thing for certain therapeutic situations. This includes fasting during chemotherapy. During this time, it's easy and convenient for patients and oncologists to receive all the ingredients for fasting in one single package. The ingredients are precisely defined— patients no longer need to worry about getting fasting advice and time-consuming shopping. But for healthy people or those with only mild illnesses, who would like to use fasting as a preventive method or who would simply like to try it for themselves, traditional fasting with self-prepared juices and broths may be a more cost-effective approach.

Additional Effects of Fasting

Strengthening the Immune System

Valter Longo and other researchers have repeatedly observed the beneficial effects of fasting on the immune system, inflammation, and stem cell production in the body.[51] Moreover, in recent years scientists from all disciplines have discovered that the immune system is essentially controlled and influenced by the type and composition of the intestinal bacteria, the microbiome.[52] In 2016, an Austrian study researched whether any changes in the microbiome could be detected after one week of fasting according to the Buchinger method. And indeed there was an increase in diversity, or the variety of bacteria strains.[53] This is essential for a healthy immune system.

There are also increasing indications that fasting can be a good supplementary treatment for other diseases of the immune system, such as collagenosis, allergies, and chronic neurological diseases such as multiple sclerosis.[54, 55]

The Effect on Colds and Chronic Infections

Fasting often helps against recurrent common colds. A cold can even be a good entry point into fasting. Many of us are familiar with this: When we're plagued by a cold, we naturally tend to not have as much of an appetite. In this situation, I highly recommend following your instincts. Follow up the cold with a short-term fast of three to five days, which strengthens your immune system in the long run. Fever is also a good entry point into fasting. And remember that fasting in general curbs inflammatory processes.

Fasting and Weight Loss

Naturally, many people are deeply interested in what happens to their weight when they fast. There's a big misconception that the main benefit of fasting is weight loss. I wouldn't recommend fasting to anyone who is exclusively interested in losing weight and doesn't intend to change any of their dietary or lifestyle habits. That said, people often commit to fasting throughout their lives after giving it a try, so it can be a great way to begin adopting a healthy lifestyle.

The causes of obesity are complex. Yet it is generally true that in most cases the main causes for obesity are excess caloric intake and/or insufficient calories burned (meaning inadequate exercise). There are exceptions, of course, such as hormonal causes like pregnancy, thyroid disease, or the use of certain medications.

From a physiological standpoint, the amount of weight we can lose during fasting is predetermined: The body breaks down fat to make energy available. One gram of body fat provides roughly 9 kcal of energy. We normally burn 2,000 to 3,000 kcal a day, depending on our activity; women generally burn about 400 kcal less than men. This means that on average we burn 300 to 400 grams of fat per day of fasting. More is not possible.

Still, most people who fast lose a much greater amount of weight. The explanation: The omission of salt, the increase of dehydrating hormones, and the low insulin levels cause most fasting patients to lose a lot of fluids—since normally insulin causes the retention of salt and water in the kidneys. Incidentally, this is one of the reasons why low-carb diets often make us lose increased amounts of fluids initially; the weight loss, therefore, is a loss of fluids at first. But don't be disappointed by that, because this drainage is definitely a good thing.

Some protein is broken down in the first few days of fasting. It's unclear whether this is protein that is already damaged or if it is useful protein. In any case, protein provides less energy, only 4.1 kcal per gram. At 30 grams of protein breakdown per day of fasting, there is initially an additional slight weight loss.

As a result of the hormonal change, a lot of sodium is exuded from the first day of fasting onward, which takes with it fluid retained in the body. Fluid retention in the legs, swelling in the hands, and even a "puffy" face recede. In patients for whom fluid retention is a medical problem, the weight loss can reach up to twenty-two pounds in one week. Most people who fast are impressed when they are told that the pounds they shed come from excess fluid in the body. It's important to know this in order to prevent disappointment. At least some of the fluid lost is retained again when we return to eating normally, especially if we continue to eat food rich in salt. But often, fasting changes our sense of taste, and many people use less salt following their week of fasting. As a result, some fluid retention will permanently disappear. Nevertheless, weight loss shouldn't be the focus of fasting. To me, fasting is primarily about other health benefits; weight loss is merely a pleasant side effect.

From time to time, I hear complaints from my patients like, "I only lost five pounds after fasting for a week while my roommate lost ten." I comfort them by explaining that when it comes to shedding pounds—that is, the reduction of fat during fasting—everybody is dealing with the same issue. Depending on their basal metabolic rate and physical activity, everybody loses between four and seven pounds of fat per week. No more. Any other weight loss comes from body fluids. Still, therapeutic fasting is key for weight loss. I like to call it the "kickoff" for people suffering from obesity and the consequent problems that are often already present. Fasting offers us a new beginning.

The Effect on Sleep

During fasting, sleep patterns also change. But the way sleep patterns change is very different from person to person. Many fasting patients feel like they need less sleep, or they wake up more often during the night without finding it unpleasant. But there is sometimes also the reverse effect: Some fasting patients need more sleep, and their sleep isn't as restful. In my experience, this tends to apply to people who suffer from severe exhaustion at the beginning of the fasting period.

Fasting Has a Mood-Enhancing Effect

People often describe feeling in a good mood during prolonged fasting. I wanted to find out if this was really true, so I conducted some research among my patients with prepared mood scales and questionnaires. With great curiosity, we asked the patients who were fasting to evaluate their mood every day. And indeed, their mood improved, on average, by the fourth day of fasting at the latest. The good mood didn't turn into euphoria for all of them, though this phenomenon exists (and is actually not rare). It has been scientifically proven that when a person is fasting, large amounts of the "happiness hormone" serotonin are available in the brain, and other mood enhancers (endorphins) are increasingly produced.[56] There is an evolutionary explanation for this. If our ancestors had stayed holed up in their caves and been depressed because they had run out of food, they would likely not have survived—and all of us probably wouldn't exist now.

As a doctor, I have learned from years of experience with fasting that on average, overweight people tend to experience better moods than thin people during fasting. This is probably due to the greater change in hormones. In overweight people, the change in metabolic hormones is usually more pronounced during fasting.[57] Ketones, which are produced when fat is broken down, are also thought to be responsible for improving mood. And finally, it's a wonderful experience for our bodies and souls to experience how well we can cope without food; we lose weight and become healthier. This effect of fasting should not be underestimated, and it lifts the spirits profoundly.

The Effect on Sexuality and Fertility

There are many myths and legends surrounding the effect of fasting on sexuality. There is unambiguous proof that there is a decrease of the sex hormones testosterone and estrogen during fasting. We also know that a prolonged state of malnutrition is more likely to cause infertility.[58] This is all understandable: If the body is busy maintaining its basal metabolic rate, it doesn't focus on procreating. But when the fasting period ends, the situation completely changes. Many patients report having a lively libido after the fasting period.

Fasting Protects Our Health

Fasting is not just an effective way to treat existing health problems; it's also a wonderful method of prevention.

Thousands of healthy people fast every year in groups under the guidance of instructors or doctors. Together with my team, I examined the results of this type of outpatient fasting in healthy people and published our findings in the journal *Research in Complementary Medicine* in 2013. Thirty women participated in this study after their fasting instructor told them about it. Of course, men would have also been welcome, but women are often much more motivated and committed when it comes to their health (if you are a man reading these lines, please excuse my criticism of our gender). About our study: All thirty women—who were on average forty-nine years old—underwent extensive medical exams before and after fasting. We measured blood lipid levels, blood pressure, and hormones as well as blood sugar metabolism. After the week of fasting, we saw strong effects: On average, the women who were overweight lost roughly 13 pounds, systolic blood pressure was lowered by 16 mmHg, LDL cholesterol levels dropped by 30 units, and insulin levels dropped from 14 to 3 mg/dl. In addition, mood, mental health (depression and anxiety), fatigue, and quality of sleep all improved dramatically.[59]

Another benefit of fasting is the regeneration of fatty liver.[60] Research from recent years has shown that fatty liver disease plays an adverse role in the conservation of too much weight and the negative consequences associated with that.[61] When I first conducted ultrasound examinations of livers twenty-five years ago, I used to say to my patients: "You have a fatty liver, but that's not dangerous." I would not say that now. On the contrary: We now know that fatty liver contributes to the development of diabetes and hypertension.[62]

All three of these—insulin, salt-hormone metabolism, and fatty liver—can radically recover within a few days of fasting. In several studies I carried out with my team, I was able to show that after seven days of therapeutic fasting, the cells become sensitive to insulin once again, and that blood pressure drops quickly.[63, 64] In another study, conducted with the physician and fasting expert Françoise Wilhelmi de Toledo and Stefan Drinda, both from the Buchinger Wilhelmi Clinic, we found that patients with a fatty liver showed significant improvements after fasting. Fasting didn't just affect weight loss but also led to a "leaner" liver.[65]

Who Should *Not* Try Therapeutic Fasting

Children, Adolescents, Pregnant Women, and Breastfeeding Mothers

Life phases during which a lot of energy is required for growth are not suitable for fasting. That's why children and adolescents shouldn't fast. Pregnant women and breastfeeding mothers also should not participate in therapeutic fasting. Pregnant women, breastfeeding mothers, and teenagers over the age of seventeen can try moderate intermittent fasting, but only if they don't lose any weight doing so.

People Who Are Underweight or Have a History of Eating Disorders

People who have suffered from eating disorders such as anorexia or bulimia should not fast for several days at a time; it might cause their eating disorder to flare up again. So I strongly advise that people with this background do not fast.

Therapeutic fasting is also not advisable for people who are underweight or who have recently lost a lot of weight due to other causes. Most fasting doctors consider the lower limit for fasting to be a body mass index (BMI) of 19. When in doubt, you should always have a discussion with your GP.

If fasting is recommended as a supplementary therapy for a medical disease despite the patient being underweight, it is absolutely mandatory to fast under supervision in a clinic.

People Who Are Morbidly Obese

People who are moderately overweight have a particularly easy time with fasting. Since they often lose weight while fasting, typically these patients are then motivated to change their diet afterward, which leads to additional weight loss. All data that has been collected from clinics on slightly overweight patients who practice fasting shows that there is generally no yo-yo effect.[66] However, when patients are morbidly obese (with a BMI above 45), therapeutic fasting should be considered carefully. Severe obesity is often the result of complex causes, and in these cases it may make more sense to focus on healthy, regular eating habits or intermittent fasting, or to think about other medical treatments such as surgery (bariatric surgery or gastric banding). I recommend talking to your GP or a specialist.

You Shouldn't Fast When Suffering from These Diseases!

There are diseases for which I do not recommend prolonged therapeutic fasting, since side effects are more likely to occur. These include:

- **Gout:** If you've experienced attacks of gout in the past, fasting can cause a renewed attack. Refraining from eating and initiating the fasting metabolism causes uric acid levels in the blood to increase and can induce another attack of gout. If you have elevated uric acid levels but have never experienced an attack, you can attempt fasting—but only in a clinic where uric acid levels can be monitored.

- **Biliary colic and gallstones:** If you suffer from biliary colic and gallstones, you should be careful with fasting. If colic has occurred recently or in the past few months, I advise against fasting. Colic may occur during fasting or right afterward. If gallstones are visible on an ultrasound but they don't cause any discomfort, fasting can be carried out as an inpatient treatment and under supervision.

- **Heart disease and severely impaired liver or kidney function:** People with severe heart, liver, or kidney impairments should not fast, or should do so only in specialized clinics that can provide monitoring. For some liver diseases (such as severe fatty liver disease), fasting is a good therapeutic treatment, but medical supervision is necessary.

- **Retinal detachment:** In cases of retinal detachment, acute thyroid disease, and rare genetic metabolic disorders, fasting should never be performed. During fasting, water content in the retina is reduced and thus may deteriorate the situation.

- **Type 1 diabetes:** While fasting is a very good therapy for type 2 as well as type 3 diabetes, patients with type 1 diabetes should fast only in exceptional cases. Even though there are individual patients with type 1 diabetes who have had positive experiences with fasting, this only occurred with the approval of a specialist and as part of an inpatient program.

- **Depression:** Fasting helps with mild forms of depression, but those with severe depression shouldn't fast because it means a change of body and mind and, particularly during the first days, sensitizes the system—that is, it makes it more susceptible. Severe depression could worsen with fasting.

Can You Fast While on Medications?

If you have to take medications regularly, you should fast only under medical supervision, and ideally your first time should be in a clinic. This is because some medications need to be stopped or reduced significantly during therapeutic fasting. These include antidiabetic drugs such as metformin, diuretic antihypertensive drugs, and anticoagulants such as Marcumar. The effect of the birth control pill can also be weakened. Pain medications could irritate the stomach more than usual. All vitamins and permanently taken thyroid medications, other antihypertensive drugs, and antidepressants can be continued.

If you're practicing intermittent as opposed to therapeutic fasting, you don't have to worry about adjusting medication, except when diabetes is treated with insulin. In that case, the insulin dosage needs to be adjusted accordingly.

> **Important:** Taking or discontinuing medications during both therapeutic and intermittent fasting should always be discussed with your doctor.

Chapter Six

Therapeutic Fasting—
The Practical Program

Before fasting for the first time, you'll likely have a lot of questions: What can I expect? How will it feel to eat nothing? Will I be okay? Am I going to be very hungry? Will I lack strength? Does fasting have side effects?

After supporting patients through tens of thousands of rounds of fasting, my team and I know the answers to all these questions. Of course, there is always the individual experience, which can vary from one end of the spectrum to the other, but for most people we can predict what fasting is going to feel like.

Therapeutic fasting is the most thorough reprogramming of the body we can achieve naturally. Since even minor stimuli and challenges, such as a visit to the sauna, a bike ride, or a cold, can have a significant impact on our general well-being, it's clear that therapeutic fasting can effect great change. In order to make it easier to switch from eating to not eating, one or two relief days should be carried out before fasting. These relief days are followed by the fasting days, fast breaking, and finally, three buildup days.

Enemas—Are They Necessary?

People who suffer from constipation or irritable bowel syndrome know that we usually feel better when our bowels are emptied. Fasting creates a rather unique situation for this digestive organ. Usually, evacuation of the bowels, the bowel movement, is stimulated mainly by eating. Everybody has experienced this. A few minutes after eating breakfast or lunch something starts to move and we visit the bathroom. Doctors call this the gastrocolic reflex: A stomach that is full passes this information to the intestine via the nerves in the abdominal cavity in order to make room for new food, so to say, in the lower part of the digestive system. This reflex is no longer activated during fasting, since there is no food coming in. That's why some of the intestinal contents from the days before you started fasting may remain in the bowels for longer. This feeling is not very pleasant, and so it makes sense to help the bowel movements along a little during fasting.

Accordingly, most fasting techniques begin with a bowel cleanse— an evacuation of the bowels—with the aid of a laxative salt such as Glauber's salt or Epsom salts. In addition, regular enemas are recommended during fasting. The Buchinger method, for example, recommends an enema every two days during fasting. In the United States, where the topic of bowels, defecation, and enemas is still rather shameful, an evacuation of the bowels is usually not part of the fasting program. US fasting experts often consider it unthinkable to recommend enemas for their patients.

However, many patients in our clinic who have tried fasting both with and without an initial bowel cleanse plus subsequent enemas report that they feel less hungry when they fast with a bowel cleanse and enemas. This makes fasting more pleasant and easier to manage. Headaches, fatigue, and discomfort, which are quite common in the first two days, are also relieved by enemas. In our clinic, we therefore recommend traditional fasting methods with laxatives and enemas, but only if the patient is willing to do them. By no means is fasting unsuccessful if you decide to forgo these practices.

Intermittent fasting does not require any accompanying laxatives or enemas. And during therapeutic fasting over the course of several days, no further enemas are necessary if you continue to have spontaneous bowel movements. It may sound surprising that you'd have to go to the toilet even if you haven't eaten anything. But the intestine continues its work in many people even when they haven't eaten for days. After all, the intestine is not just a passive tube through which food simply slides down and is digested. Instead, fluids inside the body are still actively secreted into the intestine. The intestinal mucosa cells are regenerated. In addition, the intestinal flora also changes after a few days.

Fasting with laxatives and enemas is traditionally established in Europe, but depending on individual preference and digestion, you can fast with or without these methods.

Enemas

An enema cleanses the rectum and part of the large intestine. It is mostly administered on the third and fifth fasting days, and can help alleviate hunger and headaches during fasting. To administer an enema, you will need an irrigator (a plastic enema bag attached to a tube). Fill the bag with one liter of lukewarm water and hang it on a towel rack or something that is the height of a doorknob. Kneel on the floor and insert the lubricated tube about eight inches into your anus. The tube should contain only water and no air so that the latter can't get into the intestine. Then, open the tube and let the water run into your intestine. Try to keep the water in your intestine for a few minutes before using the toilet. Enemas can also be carried out with the aid of an enema bulb.

How Is a Fasting Treatment Structured?

Relief Days

It's important to ease slowly into the fasting program. So I recommend beginning with one or two relief days. For these days, you should consciously eat less than usual and stop drinking coffee. You can have rice, vegetables, and plenty of fruit, such as apples, pears, or oranges. Chew your food slowly and mindfully. The function of relief days is to only leave food remains in the intestine that can be digested easily during the subsequent fasting phase. Fruit, vegetables, and rice can all be easily digested during the fasting phase, which is why I recommend these foods for relief days. Meat, sugary foods, and bread (especially made from white flour) start to decompose and fester when their passage through the intestine is slowed down, as is the case during fasting. This can cause flatulence and stomach pain and significantly affect your well-being.

Nothing much else happens on the relief days. You will feel a slight sensation of hunger, especially in the evenings. If you drink coffee regularly, you'll most likely experience a headache due to the caffeine withdrawal. But this pain will stop. You can use naturopathic remedies such as rubbing peppermint oil on your temples and your forehead to alleviate the pain. Many people who fast report that their headaches improve after enemas.

Even though coffee is now considered healthy and is recommended as a preventive measure against diabetes, liver disease, and Parkinson's disease, the withdrawal headache shows that excessive coffee consumption can also be a type of addiction. So in my opinion it's good to disrupt this habit once in a while. The good news for all lovers of coffee is that after fasting, your espresso is going to taste even better.

First Day of Fasting

The first day of fasting should start with a bowel cleanse, because an empty intestine dulls the sensation of hunger. Of course, you can skip the bowel cleanse if you're not comfortable with it, but it does make the fasting process much easier. Multiple bowel movements can cause minor circulatory problems, so be careful and take it easy. Rest and relax as much as you can.

> For the bowel cleanse, dissolve 20 grams (for people who are of average or below-average weight) or 30 grams (for people who are of above-average weight) of Glauber's salt in half a liter of water. It's best to drink the Glauber's salt solution quickly in one go; you can drink a little lemon water afterward to cleanse the palate. If you have a sensitive intestine or otherwise quite frequent bowel movements, 30 grams of Epsom salts is preferable to Glauber's salt. Alternatively, instead of Glauber's salt or Epsom salts, you can also try over-the-counter bowel-cleansing products that are designed to be used before a colonoscopy.

Without food intake, the body begins to adjust. Over the next twelve to twenty-four hours, the sugar reserves in the liver are used up, and the body switches to using fat as a replacement fuel via an orchestra of hormones and control signals. This means the fat reserves, mainly from visceral fat (which surrounds the inner organs), are broken down.

Some people who fast—including myself—experience strong, temporary back pain during this time. One theory for the cause of this pain has to do with the loss of fluids, which affects the intervertebral discs. This explanation, however, has not been scientifically proven. So basically, there is no explanation for the back pain. It's important to know that it will pass. Many people who suffer from chronic or frequent back pain experience slightly more intense pain during fasting. However, they are often pain free for a long time following the fasting period. This reaction has also been documented in patients who suffer from migraines: While fasting, an uncomfortable migraine attack may occur initially, but after fasting a long-term protective effect sets in.

Second or Third Day of Fasting

The second or third day of fasting is usually the "day of crisis." It's the period when a massive change in metabolic processes takes place within the body. You will feel tired, listless, and hungry, and your mood probably won't be the best. But stay strong! This day will pass, and from then on it will be easier. And it's worth it!

Third or Fourth Day of Fasting

Usually, the third or fourth day of fasting ushers in the stable phase. Now the pleasant and positive medical effects appear. The joints hurt less, water retention and feelings of tension decrease, elevated blood pressure is normalized, and mood improves. A slightly sour breath may occur, but that can be mitigated by drinking tea or sucking on lemon wedges. Sometimes the skin becomes dry.

A few people who fast experience visual disturbances, the most common being muscae volitantes, blurring in the vitreous humor of the eye, which is perceived as threads or shadows. It is harmless and only occurs temporarily. From the fourth day of fasting onward, most people feel quite well; many even notice a fasting high (fasting euphoria).

I generally recommend that people fast for longer whenever they can. Because once you've worked your way through the difficult first few days, the rest is easier. If you fast for five days at a time, you have to get through the first one to three tougher days again and again. So overall, you gain more if you fast for ten days at a time and not just for five.

Fast Breaking and Buildup Days

Fast breaking (ending the fast) is an elementary and essential part of good and correctly done fasting. If it's done sensibly, your relationship to food will be transformed, and you will not experience a yo-yo effect. After my first fast, I wasn't necessarily a role model—I overindulged in sweet, salty, and greasy foods immediately after my fast, and felt terrible. Therefore, I strongly caution patients against breaking their fast with unhealthy foods such as pizza or chocolate cake. During the buildup days, start with a single apple in the morning, which you should chew slowly and with relish. After the apple in the morning, you should have simple soups for lunch and dinner (detailed meal suggestions are outlined on pages 199–223).

Should I Fast Alone or in a Group? How Long Should I Fast?

Therapeutic fasting can be done at home or in a clinic. As a rule of thumb, healthy people can fast alone or in a group, at home or as outpatients. People with an illness should, at least for their first time, fast in a clinic that has experience with the process. The duration of the fast can vary. For healthy people, I recommend fasting for at least five days and up to seven or even ten days. For people who are seeking to treat an illness, longer fasting periods are necessary, up to fourteen, twenty-one, or even twenty-eight days. However, these longer fasting periods (anything over ten days) should be done in cooperation with a physician or fasting instructor, or at a fasting clinic. The duration of the fast often depends on individual fat reserves—this applies to both healthy as well as sick people.

Therapeutic fasting isn't hard. Still, jokes about expensive fasting clinics ("where they make a lot of money with water and tea") aren't really fair. Fasting is like a highly effective medication, or rather, it's more effective than medication. Fasting as a therapy requires a certain amount of medical know-how. If it could be turned into a pill, it would be *the* bestseller; billions in profit would be guaranteed.

It's Surprisingly Easy to Stick with the Treatment

Therapeutic fasting is surprisingly easy to stick with once you get past the first or second day. Not eating anything is, in many ways, easier than eating a little because our bodies have evolved to go for long periods without eating. Forgoing food is part of our primeval behavior.

Of course, when fasting, a certain degree of self-discipline is necessary. You need to fight your weaker self—especially during the first two days. Over the course of many centuries, cultures across the world have developed different rituals around the conscious renunciation of food. These rituals are part of almost all the world religions and spiritual ways of life.

My Tips for Perseverance

Distract yourself with activities you enjoy (except for eating and drinking). Exercise. Try to fast in a group, so you have other people to help hold you accountable. If you feel hungry, drink a cup of herbal tea. Think about all the health benefits you'll gain and how proud you will be of yourself if you persevere.

My Recommended Fasting Schedule

A 10-DAY PROGRAM

Two Relief Days, Five Fasting Days,
and Three Buildup Days

Day One and Day Two

FIRST AND SECOND RELIEF DAYS

Meal Plan

Throughout the day: Drink plenty of fluids—at least 2.5 liters of non-carbonated water or unsweetened herbal tea.

> Drink a variety of herbal teas; choose whichever ones you prefer. I recommend rosemary tea for low blood pressure, lavender tea for anxiety and restlessness, chamomile tea for indigestion, and sage tea if you have an unpleasant taste in your mouth.

Breakfast: Oatmeal

> Measure out ½ cup of dry oats. Cook with water. Add cinnamon and grated apple.

Lunch: Vegetables with rice or millet

Steam or gently sauté 1 cup of vegetables and herbs (such as broccoli, tomatoes, carrots, zucchini) with not too much salt and some olive oil.

Measure out ¼ cup of raw brown rice or millet and then cook.

Dinner: Pumpkin soup or vegetable soup

Pumpkin Soup

1 liter water

1 Hokkaido pumpkin, chopped

1 leek, sliced

1 potato, chopped

1 tablespoon olive oil

½ teaspoon sea salt

Pour the water into a pot. Add the pumpkin, leek, and potato to the water and bring to a boil. Let simmer uncovered for about an hour. Add the olive oil and salt, then puree the soup—make sure the soup is no longer boiling. This will make two to three servings.

Vegetable Soup

1 liter water

2 to 3 carrots, chopped

1 celery root, chopped

1 potato, chopped

1 leek, sliced

6 tablespoons herbs (e.g., parsley, chives), chopped

4 bay leaves

½ teaspoon sea salt

Pour the water into a pot. Add the carrots, celery root, potato, leek, herbs, and bay leaves to the water and bring to a boil. Let simmer uncovered for about an hour. Then remove the bay leaves, add the salt, and puree the soup—make sure the soup is no longer boiling. This will make two to three servings.

Supportive Measures

- Mentally prepare yourself for fasting with relaxing activities such as meditation.
- Move or exercise in the fresh air.

What's Happening to My Body?

By eating these low-salt, light meals, you're:

- Draining the body
- Preparing the body for fasting
- Relieving the digestive organs

Day Three

FIRST DAY OF FASTING

Meal Plan

Throughout the day: Drink plenty of fluids—at least 2.5 liters of non-carbonated water or unsweetened herbal tea.

Breakfast: Purge using laxative salts such as Glauber's salt or Epsom salts (dissolve the salt in 500 ml of warm water and drink quickly) and drink one liter of peppermint tea.

Lunch: 250 ml vegetable juice

You should opt for tart vegetable juices, such as tomato, beet, carrot, kale, spinach, celery, fennel, etc. You can either buy or make the vegetable juices yourself. If you're buying, make sure to buy organic, not-from-concentrate juice.

Drink the juices and broths slowly. Take about the same amount of time that you would take if you were eating a normal lunch or dinner. Drink everything sip by sip, using a spoon.

Dinner: 250 ml vegetable broth

Vegetable Broths

Pumpkin broth

5 cups Hokkaido pumpkin	6 bay leaves
1½ cups potatoes	6 juniper berries
1 leek	½ teaspoon sea salt
6 cups carrots	

Wash the vegetables thoroughly, chop them, and bring to a boil in 1.5 liters of water. Leave to simmer uncovered on low heat for at least 60 minutes. Strain out anything solid and serve with a garnish of very finely chopped parsley, basil, or chives to taste. This will make approximately 2 to 3 servings.

Beet broth

3½ cups beets	1 cup tomatoes
1½ cups potatoes	6 bay leaves
1 leek	4 cloves
1½ cups celery root	½ teaspoon sea salt

Wash the vegetables thoroughly, chop them, and bring to a boil in 1.5 liters of water. Leave to simmer uncovered on low heat for at least 60 minutes. Strain out anything solid and serve with a garnish of very finely chopped parsley, basil, or chives to taste. This will make approximately 2 to 3 servings.

If you are pressed for time, instead of making broth you can briefly heat up a vegetable juice. Another alternative to homemade broth is to mix 150 ml of tomato juice with 150 ml of warm water.

Supportive Measures

- Start the fast with a bowel cleanse (using laxative salts).
- Light gymnastic exercises at home will promote bowel movements.
- Incorporate periods of rest into your day.
- Ideally around noon, stimulate liver activity with one liver pack for thirty minutes.
- If there has been no bowel movement at all today, use an enema in the evening.

Liver Packs

Fill a hot-water bottle with hot water. Then, take a linen cloth or towel and fold it so it's about eight by twelve inches. Soak it in hot water. Let it cool slightly and wring it out. When the cloth is still hot but tolerable enough to place directly on your skin, lay it over your liver (right upper abdomen). Immediately after, place a dry cotton sheet (about sixteen by twenty inches) on top of the moist cloth. Then, lay the hot-water bottle over the dry cloth. Finally, wrap yourself in a large cotton or wool blanket. Rest for about thirty minutes. It's important that the moist compress directly on your skin does not become cool—if it does, remove it.

What's Happening to My Body?

- Bowel evacuations help the body adapt to nourishment from within.
- The body breaks down glycogen reserves (glucose) in the liver.
- The continual draining of fluids lowers blood pressure.

Day Four

SECOND DAY OF FASTING

Meal Plan

Throughout the day: Drink plenty of fluids—at least 2.5 liters of non-carbonated water or unsweetened herbal tea.

Breakfast: 150 ml vegetable juice

> If you can, try to vary the juices you drink over the course of your fast. For example, you might have carrot juice for breakfast and beet juice for lunch.

Lunch: 150 ml vegetable juice

Dinner: 250 ml vegetable broth (see page 206)

Supportive Measures

- In the morning, try a dry brush massage to stimulate blood circulation.
- Do some light exercise.
- Incorporate plenty of time to rest throughout the day.
- Ideally around noon, stimulate liver activity with one liver pack for thirty minutes.

What's Happening to My Body?

- The glycogen reserves are now quite empty; your body is switching to a fasting metabolism.
- Ketone bodies are being created from body fat—it's possible that this change causes mild weakness.

GRUEL FASTING

If you discover that you're experiencing stomachaches during fasting, you can try having gruel instead of broth and liquids exclusively. You can have oat or flaxseed gruel two to three times a day, instead of broth and juices. It might not be to everyone's taste, but the gruel protects the stomach mucosa very effectively.

If you're still experiencing hunger or stomachaches with gruel, try a flaxseed soup instead.

Flaxseed Gruel

1 serving

Boil 2 tablespoons of golden flaxseed (ground is ideal) in 250 ml of water for 5 minutes. Strain the mixture and drink only the liquid.

Oat Gruel

1 serving

Boil 2 tablespoons of oats in 250 ml of water for 5 minutes, strain out the oats and drink the liquid.

Flaxseed Soup

1 serving

Boil 2 tablespoons of golden flaxseed (ground flaxseed is ideal) in 250 ml of water for 5 minutes. Consume the flaxseed soup with the ground flaxseed.

Day Five

THIRD DAY OF FASTING

Meal Plan

Throughout the day: Drink plenty of fluids—at least 2.5 liters of non-carbonated water or unsweetened herbal tea.

Breakfast: 150 ml vegetable juice

Lunch: 150 ml vegetable juice

Dinner: 250 ml vegetable broth (see page 206)

Supportive Measures

- Ideally around noon, stimulate liver activity with one liver pack for thirty minutes.

- Do a bowel cleanse with an enema.
- Increase your tongue and mouth hygiene.
- Incorporate exercise into your day, such as a brisk walk for at least thirty minutes.

What's Happening to My Body?

The body is now operating in fasting metabolism:

- Repair processes are ongoing.
- Metabolic products are increasingly exuded, such as acetone via the lungs, which may cause an unpleasant sensation in the mouth or a discolored tongue.
- Bowel cleanse supports regeneration of the intestine.

Day Six

FOURTH DAY OF FASTING

Meal Plan

Throughout the day: Drink plenty of fluids—at least 2.5 liters of non-carbonated water or unsweetened herbal tea.

Breakfast: 150 ml vegetable juice

Lunch: 150 ml vegetable juice

Dinner: 250 ml vegetable broth (see page 206)

Supportive Measures

- Ideally around noon, stimulate liver activity with one liver pack for thirty minutes.

- Increase your tongue and mouth hygiene.
- Incorporate exercise into your day, such as a brisk walk for at least thirty minutes.
- Incorporate relaxing exercises, such as yoga or qigong.
- Try sauna sessions to stimulate blood circulation.

What's Happening to My Body?

Your body will feel lighter and your mind will feel more relaxed.

- The parasympathetic nervous system is now active (creating a sense of relaxation), and serotonin (a.k.a. the happiness hormone) has an increased effect.
- The cellular cleansing process (autophagy) is taking place—your cells are recycling damaged components, deriving energy from that, and becoming stronger.

Day Seven

FIFTH DAY OF FASTING

Meal Plan

Throughout the day: Drink plenty of fluids—at least 2.5 liters of non-carbonated water and/or unsweetened herbal tea.

Breakfast: 150 ml vegetable juice

Lunch: 150 ml vegetable juice

Dinner: 250 ml vegetable broth (see page 206)

Supportive Measures

- Ideally around noon, stimulate liver activity with one liver pack for thirty minutes.

- Do a bowel cleanse with an enema.
- Increase your tongue and mouth hygiene.
- Incorporate exercise into your day, such as a brisk walk for at least thirty minutes.
- Incorporate relaxing exercises, such as yoga or qigong.

What's Happening to My Body?

Five days of fasting has, among many others, the following beneficial effects:

- Lower blood sugar levels
- Lower hormone levels (insulin, IGF-1)
- Better blood lipid values
- Reduction of inflammation parameters
- Breakdown of glycated proteins (AGEs)
- Reduced blood pressure

Day Eight

FIRST BUILDUP DAY

Meal Plan

Throughout the day: Continue drinking plenty of fluids.

Breakfast: Raw or steamed apple. If you're feeling particularly hungry, you can also have flaxseed soup (see page 211).

Steamed Apple

Peel and cut one apple into thick slices. Then stew or steam it in a little water for four minutes. Eat with some cinnamon and/or cardamom.

Lunch: Vegetable soup (see page 202)

Dinner: Vegetables with rice or millet (see page 202)

Supportive Measures

- Eat foods that are high in fiber and low in salt.
- When you eat, eat slowly, chew your food thoroughly, and be mindful of feeling full.
- If necessary, drink lactic-acid-fermented sauerkraut juice (250 ml).
- Apply a liver pack.
- Do only mild exercise and incorporate periods of rest throughout the day.

Sauerkraut Juice

Sauerkraut juice is a mild laxative, thus supporting bowel cleansing. It is also a probiotic with beneficial bacteria that improve the microbiome. Finally, it is rich in vitamin C. You can buy bottled sauerkraut juice at the grocery store. You can also get sauerkraut juice by buying or making sauerkraut and then straining the liquid out. Another option is to put sauerkraut in a blender or processor.

What's Happening to My Body?

- A diet that is sugar free, high in fiber, and low in salt is good for the regeneration of the intestinal flora, or the microbiome.
- The metabolism adjusts again. Ketone production is reduced.
- Your sense of taste will be heightened.

Day Nine and Day Ten

SECOND AND THIRD BUILDUP DAYS

Meal Plan

Throughout the day: Continue drinking plenty of fluids.

Breakfast: Oatmeal

> Measure out ½ cup of dry oats. Cook with water. Add 1 apple or ½ cup of berries with cinnamon.

Lunch: Salad, or potatoes with vegetables

Dinner: Vegetable soup (see page 202)

Salad

¼ cup lamb's lettuce, arugula, or spinach

2–3 tomatoes, chopped

½ bell pepper, chopped

½ bunch cress

4 walnuts, chopped

1 tablespoon flaxseed oil or olive oil

black pepper to taste

herbs, chopped

Toss everything together and serve.

Potatoes with Vegetables

1 cup potatoes, chopped

1½ cup vegetables (e.g., broccoli, tomatoes, carrots, zucchini), chopped

1 teaspoon curry powder

1 tablespoon flaxseed oil or olive oil

black pepper to taste

herbs

Steam or gently sauté all the ingredients together. During relief days, the meals should be simple and light, not too complex or flavorful.

Supportive Measures

- Eat foods that are high in fiber and low in salt.
- When you eat, eat slowly, chew your food thoroughly, and be mindful of feeling full.
- If necessary (for example, if you're experiencing constipation, or have not had a bowel movement in three days), drink lactic-acid-fermented sauerkraut juice (250 ml).
- Apply a liver pack.
- Incorporate exercise.

What's Happening to My Body?

- The body starts to retain fluid once more and weight increases.
- The sensitization of the taste buds through fasting makes previous habits easy to change.
- The new experience strengthens self-confidence. Fasting brings inner mental strength and a more mindful attitude.

How Often Can You Do Therapeutic Fasting?

Traditionally, fasting was often based on religious rules. In Islamic tradition, it takes place during Ramadan, the ninth month of the Islamic lunar year. In Buddhist tradition, some monks and nuns stop eating after twelve p.m. In Jewish tradition, Yom Kippur is the major day of fasting. And in the Christian tradition, fasting happens in spring, during Lent—from Ash Wednesday to Easter Sunday (forty days all together). Since fasting is related to new beginnings and new resolutions, and since sensitivity to cold also increases during fasting, late spring is a good time for it due to the warmer weather and longer days. But other times are also possible. In the Christian tradition, a fasting period before Christmas is common as preparation for the holiday.

Nowadays, scientists consider fasting more than once a year to be a positive thing. I recommend therapeutic fasting once or twice a year for five to ten fasting days at a time. People who can and want to fast for a longer period should do so once a year (instead of two shorter fasts).

However, your initial weight is ultimately a decisive factor. People who are overweight and want to continue to normalize their weight after fasting can fast more often. There is no reason not to have four to six fasting periods a year (consisting of five fasting days each time). People who tend to be underweight should be more cautious—fasting more often could result in physical weakness and an increased susceptibility to infection.

Feeling Cold During Fasting—Should I Be Concerned?

Constantly feeling cold during fasting is an indication that the body is lowering its temperature in order to save energy. This is nothing to worry about; the body is just cooling off a little.

However, if you feel very cold, I don't recommend a prolonged phase of therapeutic fasting, because this could permanently lower the basal metabolic rate. When the basal metabolic rate is permanently lowered, the body uses less energy, fat reserves are depleted further, and losing weight after fasting has ended could be difficult. If you are overweight, it would be better for you to incorporate intermittent fasting into your daily routine. It doesn't lower the basal metabolic rate—in fact, according to some preliminary findings, it may have the opposite effect.[1,2]

> If you feel very cold during fasting, you should ask your GP to check your thyroid function.

Rare Complications After a Prolonged Period of Fasting

Refeeding syndrome is a rare medical complication that can occur after a prolonged fasting period, at the moment when you start eating again. This syndrome is also a problem for patients who have been in the intensive care unit for a long time, as well as those with anorexia nervosa who start to eat normally again; it is due to malnutrition, often over the course of many years. The cause of refeeding syndrome is the empty electrolyte reserves, which are lacking phosphorus, but magnesium deficiency can also be a critical factor. If you eat too much after fasting, your insulin levels will suddenly elevate, which causes the kidneys to retain salt and water. Not only does this put a strain on the heart, it also causes water retention in the tissues (including swollen ankles). This is also called refeeding edema. Refeeding syndrome became widely known through the performance artist David Blaine, who locked himself in a Plexiglas box above the Thames in London in 2003 and didn't eat solid food for forty-four days. Not only did he lose fifty-five pounds during this time, but he also lost a lot of muscle and bone mass and damaged his health. It goes without saying that one shouldn't undergo fasting while locked in a plexiglass box.

Refeeding syndrome is very rare, and we have never seen it in any of our thousands of patients who fast. If this is something you're concerned about, we recommend taking vital minerals during fasting, for example in the form of alkaline powders, and to rely on a diet that is rich in bases and minerals during the buildup days.

Be Well-Prepared for Your Fast—Practical Tips

For healthy people who can practice fasting outside of a clinic, five fasting days are ideal to start with. Longer fasting periods are necessary to treat a disease. They should always be carried out in close consultation with a physician and/or a fasting instructor. For fasting periods of two or three weeks, supervision in a fasting clinic is necessary.

It makes sense to think about the start date and length of the fast beforehand, and it helps to coordinate this period with your work schedule as well as your family's or partner's schedule. Most people like to start their fast on a Friday or Saturday so that they can adapt to the first, more challenging days without stress. This, of course, only applies to those who don't have to work on weekends. You should also prepare yourself mentally. Don't make too many appointments for the first week of fasting, at least nothing stressful or strenuous. You might respond well to the fast and feel vibrant and full of energy, but it's also possible that the opposite will be the case, and you'll want time to rest and recover.

Before fasting begins, it's best to be done with all the shopping (including the ingredients for the relief and fasting days). Take your time in choosing your food and pay attention to quality. Since you won't be ingesting large quantities of juices, soups, or oatmeal, try to buy high-quality, organic products. Since you're buying a smaller quantity of food than usual, you won't have to spend too much more money on groceries than you normally would. Try to give up coffee during the fasting period. Thanks to its tannins and bitter compounds, coffee has a stimulating effect and can cause appetite to increase and irritate the stomach lining. Teas, on the other hand, are great. Due to their wide range you can have great variety without any calories. On cooler days I appreciate ginger or fennel tea, which will warm your body. In the summer I prefer mint tea and lemon verbena tea. But you don't have to force yourself to drink liquids. Just trust your thirst.

You should also say good-bye to sweets and alcohol. Give away the cookies in your pantry and empty your fridge as much as possible. Removing these temptations can make it easier to stick to your fast. This is not necessary to guarantee a successful fast—I know many mothers and fathers who cook for their families while fasting and sit at the dinner table without being tempted. But this requires a lot of inner strength.

Finally, you also need laxative salts, a hot-water bottle for the liver pack, and an enema kit if you wish to use it. You can make the juices yourself or buy them freshly squeezed. However, homemade juices have a significantly more intense taste because they haven't been heated up. You should opt for tart vegetable juices (such as spinach, celery, beet, fennel) instead of sweet varieties (such as grape, carrot, apple, prune, peach, apricot). Studies in our clinic have shown that the insulin-like growth factor IGF-1 decreases to a significantly lesser extent when sweet juices are consumed. As a result, the overall desired fasting effect is weakened.

Fasting Helpers

- Hot-water bottle for the daily liver pack
- Dry brush with natural bristles for better circulation

- Tongue scraper to thoroughly clean the tongue
- For the initial bowel cleanse at the start of the fasting period, 30 grams of Glauber's salt or 30 grams of Epsom salts mixed with a half liter of water (this helps with gastrointestinal sensitivity and those who tend to suffer from headaches or migraines)
- Enema kit with a flexible tube for bowel cleansing during fasting
- Lemon water to gargle with and maybe oil pulling for oral hygiene

Exercise and Wellness Program

To increase your well-being during the fasting period, treat yourself to sunlight and walks in nature. Long showers and baths (I like to recommend a lavender bath in particular) are also wonderful. Make

---

Kneipp Scotch Hose Therapy

Kneipp Scotch hose treatment is a water therapy I highly recommend for many people. After taking a normal shower, you can try a Scotch hose treatment on yourself. First, you want to make sure that you have a showerhead attachment that can send out a targeted jet of water. Adjust the water temperature so that it is cold. Start by applying the jet of cold water to the outer side of your right foot. Then move the water up along the outer side of your right leg to the groin, and back down on the inside of the right leg. Repeat the same procedure on the left foot and left leg (moving from the outer side of your left foot and up along the outer side of your left leg to the groin, etc.). Following that same principle (outer and up, then inner and down), guide the water along your arms, followed by circular motions across the chest and face. Finish off by dousing your back. If you feel tired or exhausted, a short version of the Kneipp treatment will suffice—you can just apply the jet of cold water from your feet only up to your knees. Not only does this help stimulate blood flow, it also often helps against headaches.

sure your bath isn't too hot. Afterward, get out of the bathtub carefully, since circulatory problems can occur due to lower blood pressure during fasting. If you get out of the tub too quickly, you might
get dizzy or faint.

Using a dry brush on your skin—you can do this in the bathtub,
before you shower or bathe—will stimulate your circulation. Scotch
hose treatments (see page 228) with cold water are also a good way
to stimulate blood flow and relax leg muscles.

Last but not least, fasting and meditation go very well together, as
each reinforces the other's beneficial effects. You must try it.

Weighing

You can certainly weigh yourself every day and keep a weight log while
fasting, but don't be disappointed. Weight loss during fasting is also
caused by water leaving the body. If you would like to weigh yourself,
it's best to do so in the morning without wearing many clothes or even
naked, and after a bowel movement (if you're still having those) or
after urinating.

Side Effects of Fasting

The typical side effects of therapeutic fasting are common but usually
mild and, most important, temporary. During the first days, you might
suffer from headaches, minor circulatory problems, nausea, tiredness,
restless sleep, a grumbling stomach, or back pain.

Potential stomachaches during fasting can be avoided by having
gruel instead of broth and juice exclusively. You'll then fast with the
same reduced number of calories in the form of rice, oatmeal, or a different cereal gruel. It might not be to everyone's taste, but the gruel protects the stomach lining very effectively.

These Methods Help With Side Effects

- Headache: Apply some peppermint oil externally (temples, forehead); an enema or a hot foot bath can also help.
- Back pain: Place warm pads or a hot-water bottle on the aching muscles; take a hot bath; do yoga.
- Acid reflux: Eat a teaspoon of medicinal clay, flaxseed gruel, or oat gruel.
- Unsettled stomach: Drink potato juice or chamomile tea.
- Feeling chilly or cold: Drink ginger tea or fennel tea; take a hot bath; do Kneipp Scotch hose treatments, alternating between warm and cold water.
- Circulatory problems: Do Kneipp Scotch hose treatments using cold water; brush your skin with a dry brush; move around; do an ear massage; drink rosemary tea.
- Bad breath, bad taste in your mouth: Suck on a mint leaf or a slice of lemon; make sure your oral hygiene is thorough; clean the coat on your tongue with a tongue scraper in the mornings; do oil pulling.
- Nausea: Drink ginger tea.

Chapter Seven

Intermittent Fasting—
The Brilliant New Discovery
Suitable for Everyday Life

Intermittent fasting has come into fashion surprisingly late, compared with the hundreds of dietary trends that have emerged over the past few decades. This is astonishing, since intermittent fasting is, in many ways, quite obvious. Ultimately, it simply means not eating all the time. And this should be made clear: Intermittent fasting is *not* a diet, because the aim is neither to eat less (even though this is often a side effect) nor alter what you eat. You can, of course, alter your diet while practicing intermittent fasting, but it's not a must.

Just as with therapeutic fasting, there are numerous ways to practice intermittent fasting. You can adhere to an intermittent fasting period of twelve, fourteen, or sixteen hours. You could even choose to fast for two days a week. Furthermore, you could try only ingesting 500 to 600 kcal a day. Intermittent fasting is very easy for the body to adjust to; it is the most natural form of nutrition. A return to our prehistoric heritage, so to speak: Once upon a time, our ancestors ate only when food was available. When there was no food available, the body simply had to cope with hunger. That's why intermittent fasting or periodic fasting doesn't just seem natural, it's also easy—and very healthy!

Almost all diets fail because it goes against our nature to eat very little over the course of many weeks. It's no surprise, then, that when we eventually stop dieting or take a break from it, we end up gorging ourselves, leading to the fat reserves filling up again faster than we want. But not eating anything every now and again—that's easily managed.

We don't know exactly when humans began adhering to regular times for breakfast, lunch, and dinner. We know that in Germany it slowly became a habit to have not just two but three meals a day in the Middle Ages. This depended on the social class one belonged to—nobility, for example, thought it courtly to be served only two meals a day for a long time. The timing of meals, therefore, was connected to common customs and not to a certain necessity.[1] One of the pioneers in the field of chronobiology, Satchidananda Panda, has found that twelve hundred genes are activated only in the state of fasting. And these are predominantly genes responsible for metabolic activity, as well as those that control the immune system—clear proof of our ancient biological program.[2]

In 2018, I gave a lecture on fasting in Berlin. The speaker just before me was the director of Zoo Berlin, Andreas Knieriem. In the discussion that followed he expressed how persuasive he found the concept of fasting in medicine. He mentioned the lions in his zoo, who ate sixty-six to eighty-eight pounds of meat at a time and subsequently managed without any food for days. Living beings in the wild are all slender. In other words, there are no overweight wild animals. Domestic cats and many dogs, however, now have similar weight problems to us humans.

Many years ago, when I began my research on intermittent fasting, I often had to put up with criticism from nutritionists who said that this was just another diet, and diets have been proven to be useless.

There is a major misconception with this opinion, because intermittent fasting is *not* a diet at all—all it means is turning back the clock and changing the way we think. We've been taught to feel guilty when we skip a meal—we're meant to have regular meals! Societal norms are deeply anchored within our minds.

Intermittent fasting is not a new invention but rather the norm in the history of humankind. That's why it is codified in our genes. Some people worry that they won't be able to concentrate and stay active after several hours of fasting—but the opposite is the case. Generally, intermittent fasting is much easier than most people think it will be. The feeling of hunger does not increase. Instead, it fades. We also learn to recognize and evaluate the stomach rumble, often misinterpreted as hunger, as a temporary phenomenon.

The Origins of Intermittent Fasting

Many religious texts mention intermittent fasting. For example, Luke 18:12 in the Bible reads: "I fast twice a week." Originally, fasting or partial fasting in Christian culture was done twice a week, in addition to Lent. Wednesday commemorated the betrayal of Jesus, and Friday the crucifixion. But this kind of remembrance and rite of humility disappeared almost completely over the course of the centuries.[3] At my house, however, it was at least partly preserved—on Fridays our family did not eat meat. Instead, we ate only vegetarian dishes or fish (and nothing sweet).

Intermittent fasting is practiced during Ramadan, the fasting month of Islam. Followers of Islam will fast from sunrise to sunset, and can eat and drink only before sunrise and after sundown. But people sometimes overindulge when they're not fasting. This seems to be a contributing factor to why Ramadan fasting, for example, isn't as medically successful as other forms of intermittent fasting in many studies.[4]

But overall, fasting during Ramadan does show health benefits. On average, body weight drops slightly, and blood lipid values and cholesterol levels improve.[5] Nevertheless, it's difficult to examine Ramadan fasting scientifically because depending on the geographical location and the time of year, the daily fasting period can vary between nine and twenty hours. In our facility we conducted research into a religious type of fast quite similar to Ramadan fasting, the fasting of the Baha'i religion, which has its origins in Iran. Under the direction of my colleague Daniela Liebscher, we made some interesting discoveries: There was a significant improvement in mood as well as a shift of the circadian rhythm of almost an hour and a half. In other words, fasting can help readjust disrupted circadian rhythms.

Seventh-day Adventists in Loma Linda, California, form one of the Blue Zones. On average, they live seven to ten years longer than other Americans who don't belong to this church.[6] The excellent health of the Adventists is mainly due to their vegetarian diet and their healthy lifestyle, but interestingly most of them have their last meal for the day in the afternoon. This essentially means that they practice TRE (time-restricted eating) with a prolonged night fast. Within the scope of the Adventist Health Study, data on this factor was unfortunately not gathered, but it's possible that it contributes to the significantly longer life span.[7]

Intermittent fasting has been known in the world of medicine for some time. Edward Dewey, born in 1839, was a pioneer of fasting as a cure in the nineteenth century. He himself didn't have breakfast and described his improved mood and more energetic condition in his book *The No-Breakfast Plan and the Fasting-Cure*. In the mornings, he only drank a cup of coffee, because he was convinced that breakfast was just a habit that weakened the nerves. He believed that having just one or two meals a day, eaten slowly, was a cure for chronic diseases. By fasting in the mornings, one would both lose weight and gain muscle strength. These early observations are impressive, because they were confirmed by scientific research 150 years later. Dewey formulated another intelligent dietary principle: You shouldn't eat when you are tired—instead, you should rest. You've probably experienced this before. You arrive home exhausted, from a long day of work or some sort of strenuous activity. That's when you might feel a sensation of hunger, so you eat voraciously and end up eating way too much. I second Dewey's advice. Rest for twenty minutes after you get home. Eat afterward, and make sure to eat slowly. Once you've tried this, you'll notice that you'll eat in a more relaxed manner and therefore eat less.

Intermittent Fasting in Complementary Medicine

Intermittent fasting has long had a place in complementary medicine. Intermittent or partial fasting is used as a way to prepare for therapeutic fasting, after fast breaking, or for patients for whom therapeutic fasting would be too strenuous. It allows eight hundred to twelve hundred kcal a day. The fasting effect is predominantly achieved by the reduced intake of salt, fat, and protein.

The concept of eating only when you are hungry (or eating less) can be found in many cultures; for example, in Japan (where people practice hara hachi bun me, eating only until you are 80 percent full) or in traditional Chinese medicine (TCM). There are also religious traditions that occasionally practice a day of fasting, such as in the Mormon religion. The Intermountain Heart Collaborative Study was an interesting cardiological study conducted at Brigham Young University in Utah many years ago. The study was able to show that among forty-five hundred participants, Mormons have a significantly lower rate of cardiovascular diseases compared with other demographic groups.[8, 9]

A follow-up study of 448 participants examined the monthly fast, which is practiced by this religious community, more closely. Researchers inquired about and documented the practice of the monthly fasting days of all patients who had undergone a cardiac catheterization. Roughly 30 percent of the heart patients practiced intermittent fasting. The results showed a lower frequency of coronary heart disease and diabetes mellitus in the participants who fasted, regardless of all other risk factors.[10]

My team and I have been advising patients on the topic of intermittent fasting for two years now. Almost all the feedback we get has the same positive message: Patients who fast intermittently lose a significant amount of weight, especially if they are very overweight. Blood sugar and blood fat levels drop, and sleep also improves significantly. During the day, the patients who fast intermittently feel less tired. Some patients may initially experience mild headaches. From a general health standpoint, I would absolutely recommend incorporating intermittent fasting into your daily life.

Intermittent Fasting—A Pleasant Way to Reduce Calories

The foremost question that doctors and researchers have long been preoccupied with is one that is as old as humanity itself: How can we live longer, healthier lives? This question is becoming increasingly important in medicine, since we're now living longer than ever before, but a major share of the chronic conditions we suffer from—such as arthrosis, dementia, hypertension, diabetes, Parkinson's disease, heart attacks, strokes, and cancer—occur more frequently with age. Researchers in the field of biogerontology, a specialty that deals with aging and human longevity, have made one of the biggest discoveries on caloric restriction.

In the 1930s and 1940s, animal researchers made a spectacular observation: All living beings they examined—whether it was round-worms, mice, rats, or dogs—lived significantly healthier and longer if they did *not* receive food regularly and if they did *not* receive a lot of food (their feed quantity was reduced by 20 to 30 percent). Even in old age, there were no noteworthy diseases. Since then, this observation has been studied again and again in different organisms and animal species. The result has been the same every time: Less food every day prolongs life.[11, 12, 13]

But figuring out how to apply this research to humans is tricky. Daily caloric restriction as a method of prevention and therapy? Most people would probably decide against such a recommendation despite the possibility of a prolonged, healthy life, because a permanent restriction of calories sounds like a tedious and unpleasant way to live.

Even so, there are people who practice this kind of permanent caloric restriction. The American gerontologist and pathologist Roy Walford developed a concept of strict caloric restriction for humans called CRON (Calorie Restriction with Optimum Nutrition)—and found followers.[14, 15] But the so-called CRONies are not only very thin, they don't appear to have an abundance of joie de vivre. They are very sensitive to cold, often wearing multiple layers of sweaters even in moderate temperatures. CRONies suffer from infections more often and most of them have a very low sex drive.[16] The limited zest for life alone can have a negative impact on the immune system and thus increase susceptibility to infections. Despite excellent cholesterol, blood pressure, and blood sugar levels, pneumonia could end one's life early. Such a radical restriction of calories produces mixed results.

Intermittent fasting is a much more pleasant form of caloric restriction. Valter Longo, Mark Mattson, Luigi Fontana, and other scientists have been pursuing this approach in their work for a long time. In their studies, they did not reduce the number of calories consumed, but only started feeding the animals at intervals. Astonishingly, the results were the same as with CRON: improved cholesterol, blood pressure, and blood sugar levels. In the natural world, there are hardly any animals who divide a limited food supply into three meals voluntarily. Normally, everything is eaten immediately. Then, there is nothing left to eat, which results in a long fasting interval. The highlight of intermittent fasting, therefore, is that you don't have to reduce the number of calories you consume—you just have to take breaks from eating to achieve identical health effects.

One of the key experiments on intermittent fasting was conducted by Satchidananda Panda. He fed two groups of mice the same amount of food and calories. Half the mice had 24-7 access to their feeding bowls. The other half was forced to take a sixteen-hour break from feeding. Up until now, one incontrovertible rule of research on nutrition and weight research had been: Whether someone is thin or large depends solely on the number of calories they consume. In Panda's experiments, however, something entirely different began to take place: The mice in the first group became overweight, developed fatty livers, inflammation, and diabetes, and became exceedingly lethargic. The mice in the second group (who fasted for sixteen hours) maintained a normal weight and stayed healthy and energetic despite the identical type of food and number of calories consumed. Their livers were healthy, there was less inflammation in the body, the amount of bile ensured perfect digestion, and their cholesterol levels sank. The mice who fasted also appeared to be livelier and more dynamic—in other words, younger.[17] It's clear that what is important is not the overall number of calories consumed, but the fasting period!

Panda and other researchers made another big step beyond this groundbreaking discovery. They found out that all the metabolic, digestive, and energy processes in the body are controlled by so-called clock genes. These genes switch on and off, depending on daylight. This made the scientists realize that there is another important factor to consider in addition to the number of calories and the energy content of the food, which is timing. The question of what time and how often we eat our meals is also crucial. For this reason, Panda called this type of intermittent fasting "time-restricted feeding."[18, 19] Since we humans feed ourselves and aren't being fed, at least for most of our lives, the phrase "time-restricted eating" is more suitable in my opinion.

But more research needs to be done to clarify whether all these findings can be fully applied to us humans. "Mice tell lies" is one opinion among critical scientists. The final results on intermittent fasting in humans are therefore eagerly awaited.

What Are the Methods for Intermittent Fasting?

In therapeutic fasting, the main variant is the number of days you choose to fast. But for intermittent fasting, there exist many different approaches. You can choose different ways to space out the intervals during which no food is consumed. In the following sections, I'll introduce you to several different approaches to intermittent fasting.

At the moment, it's not possible to say whether one method is superior to the others. My recommendation is to try to see what suits you, what you can easily incorporate into your everyday life, and what feels good to you. Keep an open mind and try out different approaches. I meet many patients who initially reject intermittent and therapeutic fasting. They argue that skipping even a single meal makes them feel weak. They don't think they'll be able to withstand the feeling of an empty stomach. These same people are completely stunned when they discover that after overcoming their initial discomfort, they can handle fasting surprisingly well.

Alternate-Day Fasting

One method of intermittent fasting is called alternate-day fasting (ADF). It is also called the eat-stop-eat diet (ESE) or up-day, down-day. With the ADF method, you consume only 25 percent of the normal amount of food (a "normal" amount is about 2,200 kcal per day for men and 1,900 to 2,000 kcal per day for women) on fasting days, and on non-fasting days you eat as much as you want. You alternate between days: one day of fasting, one day of eating, one day of fasting, and so on. Krista Varady, a nutritional scientist at the University of Illinois at Chicago, was the first to conduct research into ADF in humans and wrote a book about it: *The Every Other Day Diet*.

A couple of small clinical studies on the ADF method showed weight loss similar to that of daily caloric restriction (CRON), even with slight advantages in terms of insulin levels and a reduction in fat mass.[20, 21] The explanation is obvious: If you're following the ADF method, even on non-fasting days, when you're free to eat as much as you want, it's difficult to eat enough food to make up for all the calories omitted the day before. It's not easy to eat two days' worth of food in one day. In intermittent fasting, the overall caloric intake is lowered and as a result, weight is lost in the long term.

There hasn't yet been enough research on whether ADF carries additional health benefits. I do want to say that it's not easy for most people to fast and eat in a two-day cycle. In addition, it's difficult to practice in everyday life because of our family life, social life, weekends, holidays, and so on. In the largest study on the topic, roughly 40 percent of subjects in the group that fasted this way terminated their participation.[22] However, in a recently published research project at the

University of Graz (InterFAST study), led by Frank Madeo, the ADF method was successfully introduced to one hundred volunteers. The participants remained highly motivated.[23]

The 2-Day Diet

After ADF came the 2-Day Diet. It was developed in 2011 by the British nutritional scientist Michelle Harvie, who works at the University Hospital of South Manchester, together with the oncologist Tony Howell at the University of Manchester, with the aim of facilitating weight loss. This diet was originally designed for women with breast cancer: A maximum of 600 kcal is consumed per day on two consecutive days each week. For those days, the focus is on a low-carb diet with dairy products, tofu, vegetables, fish, fruit, and eggs. For the other days, a Mediterranean diet is recommended.[24]

The 5:2 Diet

This fasting method, created by British doctor and science journalist Michael Mosley, is based on Michelle Harvie's concept and fueled by his bestseller *The Fast Diet*. With 5:2, on two non-consecutive days only 600 kcal are eaten per day, ideally divided into two meals of 300 kcal each. Most people have an easier time with this kind of food restriction. Mosley recommends eating mainly vegetables and whole grains on the fasting days as well as drinking plenty of fluids. In addition to her research on the 2-Day Diet, Harvie has conducted the most clinical studies on the 5:2 version. She was able to prove that this form of intermittent fasting is equal to continuous caloric restriction regarding weight loss, but that it shows better compliance: People participate better.[25]

Time-Restricted Eating

Another method of intermittent fasting is known as time-restricted eating (TRE) or time-restricted feeding (TRF). Shifting the daily rhythm of eating is a very attractive method for many people. But so far it is unclear which interval of regular fasting periods brings the maximum therapeutic benefit. The TRE method assumes that a daily fasting period of fourteen to sixteen hours is ideal (some people extend it as far as twenty hours). The liver's glycogen reserves are the key factor that determines when our metabolism switches to the fasting state. When this switch happens, the body shifts from relying on glucose as its primary energy source and instead begins to break down body fat and start the production of the substitute fuel, ketones. It's important to note that the point when this metabolic switch happens varies from person to person, depending on gender and individual differences. In women, glycogen reserves appear to take about 12 to 14 hours to be depleted, whereas in men glycogen reserves generally take a bit longer, around 14 to 18 hours, to be depleted. So for women an initial spike of ketone levels in the body could begin after only 12 to 14 hours of fasting, whereas for men that initial spike would likely begin after 14 to 18 hours of fasting.[26]

In practice, TRE means taking advantage of our natural night fast (when we sleep we're fasting, since we're not eating). You can either skip breakfast altogether or eat later in the morning. Or you could skip dinner. For example, if you plan to have breakfast at eight a.m., you would eat at six the night before in order to get a fourteen-hour break from eating. This form of intermittent fasting is generally very practical, since you don't need to drastically change the overall number of calories you're consuming. Clinical studies are showing that simply having two meals a day instead of three usually results in a reduction in energy intake for most people, and that pounds are shed as a result.[27]

You should decide on the rhythm you adopt—early dinner and breakfast or late dinner and no breakfast—based on your individual habits, your circadian rhythm, and your social life. If dinner is the most important shared meal for you and your family, it doesn't make much sense to leave it out. It is crucial to eat your last meal of the day three hours before going to bed, to coincide with the release of the sleep hormone melatonin, which sets in with nightfall.

Personally, I usually skip breakfast or have it later, when I'm already at work. Many people aren't hungry in the mornings, which naturally facilitates this form of intermittent fasting. And luckily, even if you skip breakfast, coffee and tea (as long as you leave out milk and sugar) are allowed.

> One popular form of time-restricted eating is 16:8 intermittent fasting, which involves fasting for a sixteen-hour period and then eating whatever you want for the other eight hours.

Relief Days (Rice, Fruit, and Oat Days)

One other way of practicing intermittent fasting is through relief days once or twice a week, which alleviate health issues such as diabetes and hypertension.[28] On relief days, you should eat nothing but rice, oatmeal, or fruit.

Rice has great health benefits. A 2009 study examined 113 patients with high blood pressure. They were asked to follow either the usual antihypertensive diet (DASH diet) or the CALM-BP program. The CALM-BP program includes, in addition to healthy lifestyle recommendations, a special vegetarian diet with brown rice. After four months, both groups showed a significant decrease in blood pressure, but patients who had been eating brown rice could discontinue their antihypertensive medications more often.[29] Other, smaller studies showed beneficial effects from eating rice, particularly an improvement in sugar metabolism and increasing suppleness of the vessels in patients with diabetes. The vessels became biologically younger again.[30, 31]

RICE DAYS

When talking about rice, we must tell the story of the German physician Walter Kempner, who immigrated to the United States during the Nazi era. To this day, almost every US hypertension specialist knows the Kempner diet. Kempner specialized in nephrology—kidney care and treating diseases of the kidneys—which is closely connected to hypertension therapy. He was frustrated by the modest treatment options in his specialty, because at the time there were few antihypertensive drugs. Then he had an idea for an extremely simple therapy, based on the following physiological fundamentals: If the kidneys no longer work correctly, salt, water, and acids are insufficiently discharged with the urine. The amounts remaining in the body cause blood pressure to rise, and a high blood pressure in turn prevents the kidneys from working properly. The blood pressure continues to rise, the heart is forced to pump harder, and heart disease is the consequence. Kempner thought, why not break this cycle with a radical diet that reduces salt and protein, thus relieving the kidneys?

Based on this idea, Kempner prescribed an extremely low-salt rice diet, along with a little fruit juice, to his seriously ill patients. Although his diet could not be considered fasting because it added up to about 2,000 kcal, it had a fasting-like effect due to the low content of salt, protein, and fat. The success was spectacular. In a large number of patients, blood pressure, blood lipid, and blood sugar levels normalized after several weeks, and heart function also improved.

Nevertheless, Kempner suffered the fate of many pioneers who venture on new paths off the beaten track. He was treated with hostility for his method. Critics claimed it was impracticable, that patients had neither the interest nor the discipline to cure their disease by changing their diets.[32] This turned out to be a misjudgment. I find rice days to be an excellent supplement after therapeutic fasting, and so rice diets are still used whenever required in our clinic.

Around 2010, it became known that rice contains arsenic and therefore has the potential to increase the risk of cancer. Indeed, the arsenic content in rice is ten times higher than in other grains. It is especially high in processed products such as rice crackers, rice cakes, and rice milk.[33, 34] However, the arsenic content in rice can be reduced in a simple way: Wash the rice thoroughly before you boil it. Rinse the rice with fresh water at least twice (wash once, drain out the water, wash again with fresh water). Opt for brown rice rather than white rice. Even though brown rice contains even more arsenic, it also has a larger amount of fiber. If this fiber is metabolized in the large intestine, less arsenic enters the body via the bloodstream. One type of rice with a low arsenic content is basmati rice.

I recommend occasional rice days, but I do not recommend a weeklong rice diet. In any case, such a diet tastes so bland that it's out of the question for most people anyway.

OAT DAYS

As a supplement after therapeutic fasting, oat days are another great option instead of rice. Oats were used to treat diabetes decades ago, but this method has faded into obscurity. Oat has a vitalizing effect and contains large quantities of fiber such as beta-glucans, along with polyunsaturated fatty acids, B vitamins, iron, and calcium. Particularly due to its high content of beta-glucans, oats lower cholesterol and blood pressure and improve sugar metabolism. It's a valuable source of food for the microbiome in the intestine. Oats are, in other words, an all-arounder.

In fact, oat days reduce blood sugar so drastically that you should consult your doctor if you are taking diabetes medication and you plan on trying oat days. On the other hand, oat days are great for improving blood sugar regulation during a hospital stay. In the departments for internal medicine in large hospitals of anthroposophical medicine, oats have been successfully used for many years.

This Is What Your Rice or Oat Day Could Look Like

Rice Day

Have a rice day before fasting or as a weekly relief day after fasting: Boil three servings of rice (¼ cup of dry rice per serving) without salt; a little unsweetened stewed fruit or applesauce is also allowed (but no more than 1 cup a day).

Oat Days

Two consecutive oat days is ideal. Boil ¾ cup of whole grain oats per serving for breakfast, lunch, and dinner in water or unsalted vegetable broth. Suitable spices are pepper, curry, turmeric, cinnamon, and fresh herbs. One teaspoon of shaved almonds is allowed. In addition, you can eat raw vegetables (such as cucumber or kohlrabi).

Which Method of Intermittent Fasting— Alternate-Day, 2-Day, 5:2, or Time-Restricted Eating—Should You Choose?

Even though the study results on alternate-day fasting and the 5:2 diet aren't bad, I believe that both of these forms of intermittent fasting would be challenging to incorporate into a daily routine in the long run. This belief is based on the relatively high rate of dropouts from the studies on these methods.[35] Based on everything I've seen, I recommend time-restricted eating in combination with one relief day every week or two. The relief day can be incorporated as a weekly ritual or as a follow-up to more opulent, calorie-rich days.

But how long should your fasting period be for TRE? And should you skip breakfast or dinner? Or should you have not just two but two and a half meals, as Valter Longo suggests? There are currently no limits to the speculation. Indeed, it's difficult to give clear and precise answers. While at a conference with fasting experts in 2018, I had a discussion about this with Satchidananda Panda. I asked him why he had decided on sixteen hours of fasting and eight hours of feeding in his animal studies. He grinned and looked at me cheerfully before replying, "This was due to the family situation of my PhD student." This PhD student was the one responsible for moving the test animals from the cages with unlimited access to food to the cages without access to food every day. Since he had just become a father and wanted regular working hours, it was decided that the feeding time of the animals would be limited to eight hours a day according to an eight-hour workday. It's important to remember that science is sometimes influenced by very human factors.

In any case, according to the latest findings, you should wait for an hour after getting up before having breakfast. This is when melatonin levels drop properly. Since insulin and melatonin influence each other, you should definitely wait that one hour.[36, 37] Measurements also show that carbohydrates or carbohydrates in combination with protein are best metabolized between ten a.m. and twelve p.m.[38] That's why for the 16:8 intermittent fasting method, I recommend eating between ten a.m. and six p.m. You should have lunch no later than twelve thirty p.m., and make sure this is the highest-calorie meal of the day.

The neurologist Mark Mattson has pointed out that the fasting-induced formation of ketones is particularly important for achieving a good effect on neurological diseases. These ketones are created only when glycogen, the reserve sugar in the liver, is used up. Now, nobody can say precisely how many hours it takes for glycogen to be depleted. Mattson believes it takes fourteen to sixteen hours, and I agree.[39]

Based on my experience with intermittent fasting, I advise against painstakingly counting the hours. For success to be achieved, it seems more important to me that the intermittent fasting fits well into your daily routine and rhythm of life. Twelve hours of fasting is a good start; fourteen hours is even better. But if more time without food is causing you stress, you should not torture yourself. The same thing holds true for the question of whether it's better to skip breakfast or dinner.

When Satchidananda Panda planned his pioneering study, the first thing he noticed was how dramatically few people in California even had an eating rhythm to begin with. He later used this observation as an opportunity to prescribe a short period of intermittent fasting of fourteen hours to the most chaotic eaters. He let the participants of this small follow-up study decide for themselves when they wanted to take their daily fasting break. After sixteen weeks, the test subjects had on average lost eight pounds, they felt more energetic, and they enjoyed more restful sleep. Panda's method of leaving the rhythm to the individual fasting person is a better solution than a generic schedule predetermined for everyone.

From a physiological standpoint, however, there is unambiguous proof of the benefit of eating at certain times. Numerous studies show that the metabolic response to food in the morning hours as well as around noon achieves the greatest benefit. This metabolic response results in less fat buildup and lower blood sugar levels.[40] In her lectures, the Czech diabetologist and intermittent fasting researcher Hana Kahleová urges people to eat a substantial breakfast and practice intermittent fasting by having an early dinner or skipping dinner altogether.[41,42] But as I said, I don't want to recommend rigid solutions. If dinner is the highlight of your social life, as it is in some Mediterranean countries, it doesn't make sense to omit this meal.

Almost all the traditional healing methods, such as Ayurveda, recommend eating a rich lunch. Ayurveda uses the image of the digestive fire (Agni) to explain this. The Agni is strongest at noon, so the meal will be digested in the most effective manner at that time.

A 2013 study proved this by looking into how much participants ate, when they ate, and their risk of obesity. In fact, the risk of obesity was the lowest in people who ate more than a third of their entire daily caloric intake around noon. The risk for people who tended to overindulge in the evenings, on the other hand, was twice as high.[43, 44]

Don't be fooled by press reports claiming that skipping breakfast is harmful to your health. In one study that was widely reported on in the media, participants who skipped breakfast were observed over the course of several years. In some of them, a heightened risk of cardiovascular diseases was noticed.[45] Many newspapers presented the result with headlines like: "Omitting Breakfast—Dangerous for the Heart." Upon examining the study more closely, however, my colleagues and I found that the parameters that could be responsible for a heightened risk of cardiovascular diseases to a much larger degree than skipping breakfast weren't sufficiently adjusted. The participants— employees at a major Spanish bank—had a lot of other risk factors, such as stress, smoking, and an unhealthy diet. A quick cigarette often replaced breakfast.

Intermittent fasting made easy—all you need is a watch!

THE METHODS OF INTERMITTENT FASTING

Alternate-Day Fasting (ADF)

Fast for a day, eat the next day, then fast the following day, and so on.

- On fasting days eat only 25 percent of the recommended daily calorie intake, which means limiting yourself to roughly 500 kcal on fasting days.
- On non-fasting days eat a "normal" amount of food, about 2,200 kcal per day for men and 1,900 to 2,000 kcal per day for women.
- Alternate between fasting and non-fasting days.

2-Day Diet

Every week, on two consecutive days, eat only 600 kcal per day of low-carb foods.

During the remaining days of the week, follow a Mediterranean diet.

5:2 Diet

Every week, choose two nonconsecutive days to fast. On those fasting days eat only 600 kcal each day. For one day of fasting you might have two meals that are each 300 kcal. For example:

- Monday: A 300 kcal lunch that includes vegetables and whole grains. A 300 kcal dinner that includes vegetables and whole grains. Plenty of fluids throughout the day.
- Tuesday and Wednesday: A "normal" diet each day (approximately 2,000 kcal)
- Thursday: A 300 kcal lunch that includes vegetables and whole grains. A 300 kcal dinner that includes vegetables and whole grains. Plenty of fluids throughout the day.
- Friday, Saturday, and Sunday: A "normal" diet each day (approximately 2,000 kcal)

Time-Restricted Eating (TRE)

Take breaks from eating that last 14 to 16 hours. Take advantage of the time you're sleeping:

- If you are a morning person: Eat between 7 a.m. and 3 or 4 p.m., or between 8 a.m. and 4 or 5 p.m.
- If you are an evening person: Eat between 10 or 11 a.m. and 7 p.m., or between 11 a.m. or 12 p.m. and 8 p.m. It's easiest for most people who practice TRE to skip breakfast and have an early lunch as their first meal of the day.
- Another option: Eat between 10 a.m. and 6 p.m.

The Healing and Preventive Effect of Intermittent Fasting

The Effect on Weight

Intermittent fasting almost always leads to good and sustainable weight loss. This is important because conventional diets and weight loss programs don't work in the long run. An impressive example of this was the Women's Health Initiative. This study observed fifty thousand women over the course of seven years. One group of women received a low-fat, low-calorie diet with a lot of grains, fruit, and vegetables, in which the women reduced their overall caloric intake by more than 350 kcal a day. At the same time, they were asked to exercise more; 14 percent of the women in this group complied with these requests. The other group was asked to continue their lifestyle and dietary habits as before. The scientists were hoping that the group who exercised and followed a low-fat diet would lose thirty-five pounds a year. The result surprised everyone and, frankly, was shocking: The actual difference between the two groups was less than three pounds of weight lost. In fact, waist circumference increased among the women in the diet-and-exercise group.[46]

Diets are challenging because that slight feeling of hunger is constantly present, and the body possesses defense mechanisms that fight back against the small amount of food being consumed. But these challenges aren't present when patients practice intermittent fasting; the body is basically tricked. And intermittent fasting doesn't result in people becoming underweight, which is a disadvantage we see in the permanent caloric restriction of the CRONies. With intermittent fasting, there is only weight loss or weight normalization. Furthermore, intermittent fasting is easy to practice, since during the periods when you're not fasting, there are no restrictions on what you can eat and how much you can eat, allowing you to enjoy food with total pleasure. Since you're not starving but rather are adapting the mealtimes to a new rhythm, this means intermittent fasting doesn't lead to a lowering of the basal metabolic rate, making it optimally suitable for weight loss.

I deliberately did not emphasize weight loss when discussing therapeutic fasting earlier, since weight loss is less of an aim there but is instead a pleasant side effect. Sustainable weight loss as part of therapeutic fasting always depends on subsequent dietary habits too.

It's different with intermittent fasting. Here, there is almost always a noticeable weight loss after several weeks and months. First, less food is eaten overall. Second, the mechanism of fat reduction through the depletion of the sugar reserves takes effect. The same calorie, therefore, creates less fat. Basically, intermittent fasting is equivalent to permanent caloric restriction when it comes to weight loss. But it has additional advantages: Muscle mass, for example, is not reduced, and muscle function even improves. For all these reasons, I think intermittent fasting is generally the best medical method for weight loss.

Does TRE lead to weight loss because most people who eat during an eight-hour window every day simply ingest fewer calories—or does this mode of eating itself lead to weight loss? The answer: both. People who follow intermittent fasting do indeed ingest fewer calories overall. But this rhythm of eating also has an effect on insulin as well as on ketone body metabolism.

So the best thing to do, of course, is to follow a healthy diet and to fast intermittently. An unbeatable combination!

Patient History: Obesity and Arthrosis

Sixty-five-year-old Dieter P., a small business owner, has lost almost thirty-seven pounds, lowered his blood pressure, and alleviated his arthrosis of the knees through intermittent fasting in the form of a daily sixteen-hour fast.

"I've experienced fasting as an asset and a good strategy for me and my health, without having to give anything up."

I have a long history of diets behind me. There is virtually nothing I haven't tried, but my weight always came back. Ever since I got married in my early twenties, I have been putting on weight. At my heaviest, I weighed 260 pounds at 5'8".

To me, the worst thing about diets was always the fact that you manage to persevere for some time, but if you make just the tiniest exception, that's it. You postpone eating better again till tomorrow, the day after tomorrow, next week . . . In the summer of 2017, I saw Dr. Michalsen on television. He was talking about intermittent fasting and said that you would lose weight doing it, no matter what you eat—the main thing is to leave a sixteen-hour break from eating within a twenty-four-hour period. I thought he was crazy and wanted to prove to him and to myself that this was nonsense.

The very next day I started what I have stuck with through today: I have breakfast at 9 a.m., lunch at 12 p.m., and dinner at 5 p.m. After that I'm strict and eat nothing at all! At lunch, I make sure that I don't eat more than 50 grams of rice or pasta, plus meat, fish, and lots of vegetables, but other than that I have always eaten whatever I felt like and until I was full. I also mostly avoided alcohol. Of course, I slipped up sometimes, had two sausages with rolls at five p.m., for example—but still, I kept losing weight. My lowest weight: 223 pounds! The best thing about fasting (which I think of as a nutritional strategy and not a diet) is that if you ever stop—on holiday, for example, or at Christmas, birthdays, or other occasions—it's easy to pick it back up again. As soon as I return to intermittently fasting, it all goes downhill again—my weight, that is!

My health has also benefited: My blood pressure is no longer at 140 over 100 but levels off at 125 over 80. My son and my daughter-in-law, both internists, are impressed. I was able to discontinue one of my antihypertensive drugs completely and reduce the dosage of the second one. And my knees are doing better too. I have arthrosis in both legs, a condition that runs in the family. During long car rides, my legs used to start hurting quite quickly. In the evenings they were often very swollen, and when I slept I couldn't cross my legs without pain and slept poorly. Since I started intermittent fasting, the swelling has just disappeared, as has the pain at night and when driving. My arthrosis is certainly not completely gone, but I'm managing much better.

I've told many people about this method, but not everyone responds to it the same way. Some people have told me that they lose only a little weight doing it. But that probably also has to do with how consistent they are. To me, this break from eating was truly a surprise, and I've experienced fasting as an asset and a good strategy for me and my health, without having to give anything up.

The Effect on Diabetes

One of the most important experiments on intermittent fasting was conducted by the diabetologist Hana Kahleová, with fifty-four type 2 diabetes patients. One group of participants was asked to split a pre-determined amount of food and number of calories into six small meals a day. The other group of participants was asked to eat the same pre-determined number of calories a day, but they were asked to have their breakfast between 6 and 10 a.m. and lunch between 12 and 4 p.m.; they were asked to skip dinner. For the second group, this amounted to a roughly sixteen-hour break from eating. After several weeks, all the participants were examined and the results were impressive: The subjects who fasted intermittently not only had improved blood sugar levels, reduction of fatty livers, and lower blood lipid levels, but they also had lost significantly more weight than the participants in the control group.[47] The idea that patients with diabetes should never skip meals and should eat many small meals, which had been recommended for years, was debunked once and for all.

Fasting researcher Mark Mattson was once asked in an interview why he believed that diabetologists came up with the idea of recommending snacks to their patients. He replied succinctly that it probably had to do with a certain convenience for doctors, because the medication was much easier to adjust with snacks.[48] To be fair to diabetologists, it should be said that patients who are being treated with medication understandably want to avoid hypoglycemia. Snacks plus insulin seem to enable a consistent, safe, and suitable setting. Today, however, we know that constant eating fuels disease. The argument that it's better to eat more often so that you don't get hungry and resort to junk food seems plausible at first. But the reality is different: Regular, frequent eating doesn't lead to people consuming less junk food. On the contrary, more junk food is consumed![49]

For the regulation of blood sugar levels through insulin, it is actually better to eat more food in the morning. The same amount of carbohydrates consumed in the evening often leads to adverse insulin levels. But keep in mind that this only applies to diabetes.[50, 51] For example, we don't know whether intermittent fasting in patients with hypertension might be better on a different time schedule.

The Effect on Hypertension and Heart Health

Intermittent fasting leads to a drop in blood pressure for most people. Data from lab experiments also shows that the heart is better protected against circulatory disorders. So there could be a certain protective effect against heart attacks. This assumption, however, has not yet been adequately confirmed by human studies.

Patient History: Hypertension and High Cholesterol

Ingrid B., age sixty-eight, a retiree, suffers from hereditary hypertension and high cholesterol. After years of treatment with medication, she has been successfully fighting both with therapeutic and intermittent fasting.

"It's never too late to take charge of your health and do something good for yourself!"

I'm quick to get fired up—and by that, I mean that when I get stressed my blood pressure spikes. This, along with my elevated cholesterol levels, is inherited from my family. My mother died at seventy-two; my sister, at sixty-eight, after several strokes and being dependent on care for a long time—when she died, she was as old as I am now! For a long time, I believed that I was at the mercy of these diseases—a slave to my genes, so to say. But that's not true. You can fight your genetic family history. It's never too late to take charge of your health and do something good for yourself!

Over the years, I have taken various beta-blockers for my hypertension. The beta-blockers triggered asthma for me; I was constantly listless and tired. At some point, I found a drug that was kind of okay. But when I was prescribed a cholesterol-lowering medication on top of that, I went on strike, so to say, and started to look for alternatives. I'm not against conventional medicine, but I believe it's good to incorporate the knowledge of complementary medicine.

In Dr. Michalsen's clinic I underwent therapeutic fasting—and from the very first day I started feeling noticeably better. On the third day, I got hungry, so I drank a lot of water and the hunger went away. When the therapy ended after five days, I was sitting in front of an apple and thought: Actually, you don't need that yet. I felt light and free, not dependent on anything. In the past, I used to often say, "I need coffee first, before I can do anything!" But actually, no, I don't need it!

I took advantage of my rejuvenated and fresh taste buds after fasting to change my diet. Though I haven't become fully vegan, as they recommended (I don't want to be that person at every party who has "special requirements"), I try my best to maintain a diet without meat and dairy products. This wasn't easy for me at the beginning, especially since I cook not just for myself but also for my husband, who likes to eat meat. Now I usually cook up a healthy vegetable dish; sometimes my husband just has that with me, and sometimes he gets a steak with it. I haven't drunk alcohol in years, because I noticed how badly it affects me.

I also fast intermittently. I take a break from eating for sixteen hours within the span of twenty-four hours. Because dinner is sacred to my husband and me—it's time that we spend sitting together cozily and chatting—I skip breakfast instead. In the mornings I only drink some tea and then I set out on my "morning rounds": three miles of brisk walking across the fields and through the small forest that surrounds our house. In the past, I used to walk this distance every day with my dog, who died, sadly—but I still stuck with the route. The walk wouldn't be as enjoyable on a full stomach. When I get home, I look forward to cooking something nice and enjoyable for lunch. Vegetable casseroles, soups—there are some wonderful dishes.

Intermittent fasting has a euphoric effect on me, similar to the feeling I get from therapeutic fasting. I'm usually in a good mood, and if I happen to deviate from my routine of skipping breakfast, drinking tea, and going on my walk—on holiday, for example—I really miss it. These days, my blood pressure is no longer at 180 over 100—it has dropped to 130. I take a smaller dose of the antihypertensive drug, and I was able to discontinue a second drug altogether. And to lower my cholesterol levels I didn't need any medication at all—my LDL levels dropped from 230 to 144.

I never imagined I'd be able to make all these health changes. "You'll never be able to do that; it's too much," I thought—but to be honest, those were just excuses. I'm responsible for myself. And now I don't consider these changes a burden but a gain.

The Effect on Autoimmune Diseases

Cases of autoimmune diseases such as multiple sclerosis, rheumatism, Crohn's disease, polymyalgia rheumatica, and type 1 diabetes have been increasing for many years.[52] The causes for this haven't been conclusively identified, but there are many indications that diet, the makeup of the microbiome, and stress play a role.[53, 54] Fat cells also produce pro-inflammatory messenger substances such as interleukin-6 and TNF-alpha.[55] Thanks to new medications that block exactly those substances (TNF-alpha blockers and IL-6 blockers), these diseases can be treated better now than they could only a few years ago. The medications, however, only control the symptoms and don't cure the underlying disease. If the medication is discontinued due to side effects, the symptoms come back, sometimes even stronger than before.[56]

In addition to fat, salt determines the autoimmune inflammatory processes in the body.[57] When we promote fat loss and salt reduction through therapeutic fasting and intermittent fasting and follow a healthy diet, it's a good therapeutic combination to curb the inflammatory processes in the body.

The Effect on Bowel Diseases

During intermittent fasting, we can observe the "housekeeper reflex," a habit of the small intestine of cleaning itself when no food has arrived for several hours. This is very useful for keeping bowel function healthy. Intermittent fasting could therefore also have a positive effect on intestinal diseases.

The Life-Prolonging Effect of Fasting

We've gained many valuable insights into intermittent fasting from research on mice. However, we need to keep in mind that the life span of mice is much shorter than that of humans. Twenty-four hours of fasting is much longer, relatively speaking, for a mouse than for a human. Accordingly, the mouse loses more weight during that time than a human, specifically 25 to 30 percent of its body mass.[58] Mice are also quicker in their reactions—for example, they switch to a fasting metabolism more rapidly. That's why we need to bear this factor in mind if we want to transfer these research findings from mice to humans. I believe we don't need any further animal tests on the subject of fasting. Now it's time to conduct more research on humans, to confirm and ideally optimize earlier findings.

Chapter Eight

Intermittent Fasting— The Practical Program

However you decide to carry out intermittent fasting, lunch should *always* be your highest-calorie meal. That's why you should ensure that you are eating a healthy lunch. It would be ideal if you ate not just bread but vegetables as well; warm food is generally good. From the very start of intermittent fasting you should get used to a rhythm that you can sustain. That way, the body and the mitochondria in the cells are "trained."

Rhythm is the crucial point here. We know from chronobiology that the suprachiasmatic nucleus, which is part of an area of the brain called the hypothalamus, determines our circadian rhythm (in other words, our body clock—when we sleep and when we wake). The suprachiasmatic nucleus is mainly controlled by light—through the recognition of light and dark, that is. All our organs and body structures, down to blood cells, are based on our circadian rhythm. In addition, our biorhythm is heavily influenced by the timing of our meals.[1, 2, 3] You should build up a very firm rhythm at least for the first few weeks before you start intermittent fasting, so that your cells won't get confused and suffer from jet lag.

Once your new eating rhythm is introduced and you are managing

it well, you can disrupt it at a later stage. In other words, if you stick
to an eating rhythm for five days a week, you can enjoy an opulent
brunch on the weekend and forget about the rhythm. But you shouldn't
make exceptions too often. Instead, handle it like travelers who have
to be in another time zone for one or two days. They usually stay in
their normal rhythm in order to avoid jet lag. In that sense, changing
mealtimes too often means eating "against" the light for the body and
therefore is a kind of metabolic jet lag.

Of course, it's ideal if you know your biorhythm. This is the field
of research of my colleague Achim Kramer at Charité. Kramer and his
colleagues determined the activity of twenty thousand genes over the
course of the day and identified twelve that reliably indicate the individual's circadian rhythm.[4, 5]

In the future it will likely become possible to "personalize" intermittent fasting by determining your chronotype beforehand. We will
soon be conducting a study designed to find out if this knowledge will
make intermittent fasting even more effective. Until then, it's helpful
to ask yourself whether you're more of a morning person or an evening
person. As an evening person, it doesn't make sense for you to force
yourself to eat a rich breakfast. For the morning person, however, a rich
breakfast would be suitable.

I'm often asked, "Is intermittent fasting disrupted if I skip breakfast but still add milk and sugar to my coffee?" Here's my answer: It
depends on the amount. Adding a small shot of frothed milk to your
unsweetened coffee doesn't interfere with fasting; drinking a cappuc-
cino with two spoonfuls of sugar, on the other hand, does.

In the evening, you should avoid drinks that contain calories.
Many people forget about alcohol here. It's not for nothing that beer
is sometimes called "liquid bread." If you are fasting in the evenings
or follow the rule of not eating anything three hours before going to
bed, you should make sure to leave out alcohol.

Who Should *Not* Try Intermittent Fasting

I would not recommend intermittent fasting for children and adolescents, especially not the form of intermittent fasting in which breakfast is skipped. A good and substantial breakfast is important for children and adolescents, not least for their ability to concentrate and their academic performance.

Finding Your Intermittent Fasting Rhythm

It's important to try to figure out what intermittent fasting rhythm works best for you and your lifestyle. There are no known risks of any of the methods presented here, but you should still inform your GP if you are under any kind of medical treatment. This is especially important if you are suffering from diabetes.

You can find out which form of intermittent fasting suits you best by answering the following questions:

How alert do you feel in the mornings in the first half hour after waking up?

    A) Not alert at all (1 point)
    B) Slightly alert (2 points)
    C) Quite alert (3 points)
    D) Very alert (4 points)

How dependent are you on your alarm clock if you need to get up at a certain time in the morning?

    A) Very dependent (1 point)
    B) Quite dependent (2 points)

C) Slightly dependent (3 points)

D) Not dependent at all; I wake up on my own (4 points)

How hungry are you in the first half hour after waking up?

A) Hardly (1 point)

B) A little (2 points)

C) Quite hungry (3 points)

D) Very hungry (4 points)

How easy is it for you to get up in the mornings?

A) Not easy at all (1 point)

B) Not very easy (2 points)

C) Quite easy (3 points)

D) Very easy (4 points)

If you had to stay up until 11 p.m., how tired would you be then?

A) Not tired at all (1 point)

B) A little tired (2 points)

C) Quite tired (3 points)

D) Very tired (4 points)

- If you scored more than 14 points, you are more of a morning person, in which case you should follow a time-restricted eating rhythm that allows you to have breakfast, lunch, and either an early dinner or no dinner. For example, an eating window from 7 a.m. to 3 p.m. or 4 p.m. could work for you.

- If you scored 8 points or less, you are an evening person. You should follow a time-restricted eating rhythm in which you skip breakfast and have a substantial lunch. You'd also be able to enjoy dinner at a "normal" time. For example, an eating window from 11 a.m. to 7 p.m. could work for you.

• If your score is somewhere in between or you don't feel like either a morning or an evening person, eating between 10 a.m. and 6 p.m. could be a good compromise for you.

All of these are estimates. The NIH (National Institutes of Health) is currently conducting a large study designed to examine whether and for whom early or late restricted eating is better. Once the results are in, we will know more clearly which brings us more health benefits.

Be Well-Prepared for Intermittent Fasting— Practical Tips

Start your intermittent fast with two preliminary stages:

Stage 1: Don't eat any snacks in between meals. After your last meal of the day, you should not have any drinks that contain calories (for example, unsweetened herbal tea would be fine; juice would not). If you drink alcohol, you should do so only during meals. No snacking after your last meal of the day! If you feel that you must snack on something late at night, have radishes or cucumber slices.

Stage 2: Start with a prolonged night fast (twelve hours) for about four weeks. After that, you can start with the intermittent fasting method you have chosen for yourself. It is imperative that you stick with this method consistently for the first two to three weeks. After that point, one or two days in which you change the rhythm will be fine.

How Long Should I Fast This Way?

You should stick with intermittent fasting for at least six weeks. Give it this chance. The first three to four weeks are the most difficult; after that the body starts to get used to this eating rhythm. Mark Mattson compares fasting to exercise and reminds us that we need a certain training period when we start to exercise as well.[6, 7] For example, when we first start running, we might be out of breath after one lap, and the next day we'll experience muscle soreness. After a week, we can run two laps without difficulty. Through regular training, the body becomes fitter and fitter; running becomes easier and easier. It's the same way with fasting.

After six weeks you can ask yourself: Is fasting still difficult? How do I feel? How is my sleep? Has my weight changed? If the intermittent fasting method you have chosen isn't for you, try another one. Again, choose a time frame of six weeks. After that, you can decide whether you would like to stick with intermittent fasting.

> **For athletes:** Since your glycogen reserves are already almost depleted after an intermittent fast of eight to ten hours overnight, you can expedite the switch to the fasting metabolism by doing an endurance exercise of medium athletic difficulty for thirty minutes in the morning. That way, your body moves more quickly into the fasting metabolism and ketone production. Since, in my experience, intermittent fasting carries a number of performance benefits for athletes in particular (including improved sleep), I recommend a training session before eating in the morning. Exercise also has an anorexiant effect (meaning it helps suppress appetite) so that the fast can then easily be extended by an hour or two.

Patient History: Athlete

Frederic K., age twenty-seven, an athletic trainer for the German professional basketball team Rasta Vechta, uses intermittent fasting to improve his sleep and to boost his performance.

"I finally found a form of fasting that really agrees with me!"

I'll admit it: In the past, I used to think fasting was for elderly people who are sick or overweight—or both. I had heard that conscious fasting can help with illness and obesity—but it took a long time until I made the connection that what could help sick people could also benefit healthy people. But that's the way it is!

When I first worked as a trainer, my boss at the time was a yoga instructor and had a holistic view of health. That's how I initially came into contact with fasting and the Ayurvedic diet. At first, I was skeptical. Then I tried therapeutic fasting with my girlfriend as a New Year's resolution—and gave up after three days, grumpy and hungry. If you exercise every day, eating nothing is really hard. But what I did notice after that short amount of time was that two chronically inflamed areas in my body, at the Achilles tendon and at the elbow, became noticeably better. So there had to be something to fasting after all!

Next, I tried 6:1 fasting, which means not eating for one day of the week. But since I train for several hours every day, just that one day of fasting was hard for me. I could only exercise in the mornings, so by the evenings my reserves were empty; I got headaches and was in a bad mood. But I noticed that the training session in the morning was easier than on the days when I didn't fast.

In the meantime, I moved to a new city and tried intermittent fasting there. I finally found a form of fasting that really agrees with

me! I eat within an eight-hour window during the day, usually between around one p.m. and nine p.m., then I take a sixteen-hour
break. So I skip breakfast, take the dog for a walk in the morning
to get some fresh air, then I train, go to the training session with the
basketball team I work with, and eat only after that. I always eat
whatever I feel like: sometimes lunch, sometimes oatmeal with a lot
of fruit and nuts—whatever my energy levels need in the moment.
In the beginning, I often overate because I was so hungry, but after
a while, this normalized, and I found a good balance. In the evenings
I eat a lot of vegetables and legumes.

It happened almost automatically that I started to adopt a vegetarian, partially vegan diet along with intermittent fasting. I reduced
my consumption of meat by about 80 percent. Animal products inhibit the regeneration of the muscles after exercise. Now I hardly ever
have sore muscles. When it comes to dairy products, I noticed that
my sleep is not as good if I drink a protein shake with milk in the
evenings, for example. Now I just use water. Sleep is one of the big
pluses of intermittent fasting! My sleep is deeper, and I'm much more
recharged when I wake up. Also, due to the break from digesting
food, my stomach seems to be calmer. In the mornings, I drink a
mixture of one tablespoon of apple cider vinegar, two tablespoons of
water, a freshly squeezed lemon, and a dash of Himalayan salt—this
stimulates the digestion and gives me a kick of freshness.

I have been living like this for four months now and I'm realizing that my performance is improving. I'm lifting seventy-five
pounds instead of sixty pounds per side on the bench press, for example. I usually feel a little hungry during training, but that doesn't
bother me. On the contrary, it motivates me. One of my players says
that's not surprising—lions hunt better when they're starving too.

I'm constantly trying to find things that help me get better and
feel better. After all, I'm looking after the fitness of a whole team and

have to lead by example. I just recommended intermittent fasting to an injured player so that he will recover faster. There are currently numerous studies being conducted on fasting and training—and I believe this could be beneficial for many athletes.

Could There Be a Fasting Pill Soon?

Researchers are currently exploring the question of whether the strong effects of fasting could be imitated by individual molecular substances. Frank Madeo has identified one of the most promising substances: spermidine.[8] The somewhat striking name stems from the fact that spermidine was first identified in sperm cells, but it can be found in almost all somatic cells. The concentration of spermidine in somatic cells decreases with age,[9] yet healthy centenarians have remarkably high concentrations in their blood.[10, 11] In lab experiments, spermidine regenerates the genetic material, mitochondria, and various tissues. It has an anti-inflammatory and cancer-inhibiting effect, and it promotes autophagy.[12]

Interestingly, many foods such as nuts, apples, garlic, citrus, wheat germ, mushrooms, the Japanese soy dish natto, and the durian fruit also contain spermidine.[13, 14] It could be possible to achieve longevity by stimulating autophagy with the consumption of these foods. However, this is just a theory so far.

Therapeutic and Intermittent Fasting for a Longer Life

In his book *The Longevity Diet*, Valter Longo describes the enthusiasm with which he visited pathologist Roy Walford to work in his laboratory for two years. Walford was one of the researchers involved in Biosphere 2, a scientific project that explored the idea of a self-sufficient biosphere. From 1991 to 1993, Walford and a small number of other crew members lived in a building complex built in the Sonoran Desert in Arizona. For those two years, the crew had to live under difficult circumstances—including being unable to grow as much food as anticipated and thus having to survive on a calorie-restricted diet. By the end of Biosphere 2, Longo writes, the team had become frighteningly thin and irritable. Yet even though Walford and his colleagues looked emaciated, medical examinations showed that they were not malnourished. Almost all risk parameters—from blood pressure to cholesterol levels—had reached incredibly low and healthy levels.[15]

Inspired by the results of Biosphere 2, Longo decided to examine the link between fasting and aging, starting with less complex organisms: yeasts. This enabled him to better understand the mystery of aging. Longo made two simple but impressive discoveries. First, if you left the yeasts to starve by administering only very small amounts of a nutrient solution, they remained alive for twice as long. Second, if you gave them a lot of sugar, the aging and dying processes were accelerated. The reason for this was, among others, that two messenger substances—PKA and RAS—were activated.[16, 17, 18]

With that, the door to fasting research was pushed wide open and more and more scientific laboratories in the United States started to work on this topic. In addition to PKA and RAS, it was discovered that growth hormones play an adverse role in the human aging process. These growth hormones include insulin and the insulin growth factor IGF-1. When we lower insulin levels, we help facilitate the reduction of fat tissue. The reduction of insulin is a fundamental, beneficial effect of fasting. IGF-1 levels are also reduced during fasting, thus slowing down the aging process.[19, 20] Valter Longo demonstrated this connection with the aid of Laron dwarf mice. These mice are dwarfed because they are genetically engineered not to react to the growth factor IGF-1. They live longer than other mice, and if they are fed a calorie-restricted diet on top of that, they live twice as long: four instead of two years.[21]

While looking for similar connections in humans, Longo happened upon a community in Ecuador that shows precisely this resistance to growth hormones. All members of the village are short because they have Laron syndrome. Longo found that despite their unhealthy diets, the people in this community rarely suffer from diabetes, cancer, or other age-related diseases.[22] Based on these discoveries, Longo began to suspect that we could slow down the aging process by avoiding the two large food groups that boost the adverse growth factors and genes responsible for premature aging: animal proteins and sugar.[23, 24] Animal proteins heighten the concentration of the growth hormone IGF-1 and mTOR, while sugar elevates RAS and PKA.[25] Many of the animal proteins we consume come from milk, which is why I constantly advise switching to plant-based milks.

Seven Truths About Fasting

Forgoing food has astonishing health-promoting effects—whether you fast for days or even just several hours. In the following pages, I have summarized the positive effects of fasting, both therapeutic and intermittent.

1) Fasting leads to fat loss and hormone changes.

Fasting of any kind will result in fat loss. In the past two years, it has been proven beyond a doubt that obesity has negative consequences—the risk of cardiovascular diseases, cancer, diabetes, and inflammatory diseases clearly increases. Fat doesn't just lie around idly in the body; it releases substances into the body that trigger inflammation and metabolic disorders. After fasting, the fat surrounding the internal organs, on the hips, on the abdomen, and in the muscle tissue is significantly reduced, and the inflammatory substances are detectable in the blood in much lower concentrations.[26]

Fasting leads to the recovery of various hormones and control systems that deal with the digestion and processing of food in the body. Eating too often and too much causes these hormones and control systems to go into overdrive, become overwhelmed, and become "resistant." In this case, fasting works like a reset button.[27, 28]

2) Fasting leads to the production of ketone bodies.

Our bodies generally rely on glucose (sugar) for energy. When we eat food—carbohydrates, specifically—we digest the carbohydrates and break them down into molecules of glucose. Any excess glucose is stored in the liver as glycogen. The amount of glycogen that can be stored in the liver, however, is limited. As soon as the storage capacity is reached (that is, when the reserve is full), the body begins to build fat reserves in other places. In other words, surplus carbohydrates are stored in the form of body fat.

It is assumed that the glycogen reserve in the liver isn't very large. It only contains roughly 700 to 900 kcal—which provides enough energy for the body for ten to sixteen hours, depending on how high the individual's basal metabolism is. When the glycogen reserve is depleted (such as during a twelve- to sixteen-hour intermittent fast), blood sugar levels fall, and the fasting metabolism is activated. Our body then turns to our fat reserve as its fuel source. In the body's process of breaking down fats for energy, ketone bodies are produced. These ketone bodies (ketones) serve as an alternate source of fuel for our brain and muscles.

Ketone bodies are beneficial for the brain, for diseased nerve cells, and for the healthy cells in cancer patients.[29] Production of ketones starts after twelve to fourteen hours of fasting, but they can also be produced when we cut sugar and carbohydrates out of our diet and instead adopt a diet rich in fat and protein (aka the keto diet).

Changing from sugar to ketones as a messenger substance for the brain and the body is believed to be beneficial for our health. Neurobiologists have suspected for quite some time that ketones can have positive effects on brain disease. Many brain diseases damage the cells to such an extent that they can no longer properly absorb and metabolize sugar. Deriving energy from ketones is easier for these damaged cells, which suggests that ketones are a good source of energy in neurological diseases such as dementia, Parkinson's disease, and multiple sclerosis.[30, 31] The glycogen in the liver, by the way, is used up quicker and the switch from sugar to ketones is made earlier if we exercise.[32, 33] You can boost the effects of intermittent fasting, therefore, by exercising in the morning after waking up or, if you skip dinner, by going for a run in the evenings.

3) Fasting activates self-healing through hormesis.

At the start of every fast, our body experiences a slight stress reaction triggered by hunger. Stress hormones are briefly produced to initiate fat breakdown and repair processes. Now, some of you might be thinking: Isn't stress a rather negative occurrence? Isn't it something we usually try to avoid? But this controlled, brief stress (eustress) is positive for the body, contrary to permanent stress (distress), over which we have no control. It enables the body to adapt to the situation better. Exercise is also a temporary stress stimulus for the body. It's not surprising, then, that fasting causes similar changes in the body in the long run as regular physical exercise: The heart beats a little slower, blood pressure normalizes, and muscle performance increases.[34, 35] The body uses this eustress to better arm itself and optimize cell functions.

The stress reaction activates genes and proteins that are responsible for cell protection and repair. In this sense, fasting is a kind of "training" for the cells' energy plants, the mitochondria, which regenerate and multiply through fasting.[36, 37]

In its initial reaction to fasting, the body releases the stress hormones adrenaline and norepinephrine as well as cortisol. Every paramedic knows that adrenaline can be used to stimulate the heart and boost blood pressure—in cases of heart attack or cardiovascular shock, for example—when the heart is beating slowly and the blood pressure is too low. But despite the increase in these hormones during fasting, the opposite happens after a few days: The blood pressure drops and the heart beats more slowly. Both are very healthy.

Using the stress hormone cortisol as an example, researchers have found that while fasting causes more cortisol to flood the brain, the receptors are reduced. This process is comparable to exercise. Initially, more adrenaline is released, but regular training leads to the development of a lower-than-normal resting heart rate, which protects the heart. The body adapts to the healthy stress. Fasting stress is the equivalent of hormesis—the idea that exposure to a low dose of something harmful can stimulate a beneficial reaction (vaccines are a great example of this concept).[38]

For this reason, a protective effect on the heart can be observed in almost all laboratory tests on fasting.[39] Mark Mattson, a passionate runner, conducted a few studies exploring whether exercise and fasting complement each other. The results show that exercise and fasting increase beneficial effects in the cells—such as the regeneration of mitochondria. This answers the question: Fasting and exercise are an effective combination.[40] Fasting, by the way, also leads to more muscle strength as we get older if it is combined with exercise.[41]

Fasting also promotes the formation of stem cells.[42] These are essential for the maintenance of the organs and for cell function. Together with the various cell repair mechanisms, fasting acts as an internal fresh cell therapy. This explains the beneficial effects of fasting on diabetes, since type 2 diabetes is an age-related illness. If muscle cells are able to regenerate through fasting, their metabolism also normalizes.[43]

4) Fasting is linked to autophagy—cell repair.

Perhaps the most surprising discovery in the latest research on fasting is that fasting actually "detoxes" and rejuvenates. Fasting periods allow the body to tend to the repair of genes, proteins, and mitochondria. The body's ability to repair itself through fasting has been confirmed by human studies. The German researcher Katja Matt and her team examined the cells' ability to repair their DNA in test subjects before and after a week of fasting according to the Mayr technique. To do so, they took blood samples and damaged the cells in those samples through UV radiation. Afterward, they measured the rate of cell repair processes in the damaged cells. They found that after the fasting period there was an increased ability to repair. This ability to repair could have positive long-term effects on other diseases, such as cancer. But so far, this is merely speculation.[44]

During fasting, it is important not to put any extra strain on the body. This includes smoking, which counteracts the "detoxification" process. Smoking also puts additional strain on the body, which becomes more sensitive due to fasting. We've noticed that patients who smoke during their fast can develop severe circulatory problems, including collapse, because blood pressure can drop or be somewhat changeable during fasting. Smoking should therefore be stopped during fasting. Fasting is the ideal time to quit smoking altogether. That would be a nice additional "side effect" of the fasting therapy!

Autophagy, the cell's self-cleaning mechanism, has been extensively researched. One of the leading researchers in this process, Frank Madeo, has been so influenced by his scientific findings that he has adopted a strict intermittent fasting regime: He only ever eats between five and eight p.m. In this short time, however, he eats whatever he wants until he is full.[45] According to Madeo, the human body activates autophagy, the process by which old and damaged cell components are removed and replaced, after fourteen to sixteen hours without food.[46]

Loosely translated, the Ancient Greek word *autophagos* means "self-devouring," which hints at the autophagy process: Over the course of our entire life, mainly influenced by our diet, a kind of "microjunk" is collected in all our cells. This consists of deformed and damaged proteins and cell components. With increasing age, the burden of these cell components rises. The process of taking care of these components is heavily supported by fasting, because when there is no supply of food, the cells start to recycle old material. For this recycling, the cell surrounds the defunct protein components within it with a membrane, and essentially deconstructs these old protein parts, using them to create new proteins. The key to autophagy can be found in insulin: High insulin levels inhibit the process. If insulin levels are low, as they are during fasting, the recycling process is activated.[47] We now know that diminished autophagy plays a role in aging processes and diseases such as dementia.[48, 49]

The process of cell cleaning seems to be essential for fighting infections and slowing down aging processes. Refraining from eating for periods of time is beneficial, while constant eating is counterproductive. Or, as Madeo puts it: "From an evolutionary standpoint, having a bite at every little sensation of hunger is nonsense."[50]

5) Fasting strengthens the immune system.

Fasting supports the body's defenses against bacteria and toxins. This is especially important when undergoing chemotherapy for cancer. When you're fasting, healthy cells enter a state of hibernation that protects them from the effects of chemotherapy, whereas cancer cells become more susceptible to the chemotherapy.

6) Fasting has a healing effect on the microbiome.

Recent studies show that various forms of fasting have a beneficial effect on the microbiome. Therapeutic and intermittent fasting allow the intestine to recover and the intestinal flora to normalize. The intestinal bacteria in particular can regenerate during this time and develop greater diversity. This has great relevance for the prevention of many diseases.

The effect of fasting on the microbiome is one of the possible explanations for why fasting has such a beneficial effect on autoimmune diseases. It is believed that these diseases often begin in the intestine.[51, 52]

The microbiome, by the way, also has a circadian rhythm. Lab experiments show that intermittent fasting can restore that rhythm.[53, 54] Interestingly, fasting can also improve an impaired permeability of the intestine, which occurs in so-called leaky gut syndrome, and thereby lower the tendency toward inflammation in the body.[55]

7) Fasting has a strong effect on the psyche.

Fasting has strong mental and emotional effects. It improves mood, promotes mental and psychological balance, and reinforces a person's confidence and trust in being able to initiate positive changes for their own health. It promotes self-efficacy and the power to overcome one's weaker self.

Neurobiologically, fasting leads to an increased availability of serotonin. Endorphins (happiness hormones) and endocannabinoids (cannabis-like substances that lift the mood) are increasingly released.[56] This explains the good mood, even euphoria, that can often be observed in fasting patients.

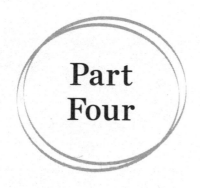

Part
Four

Healing Through Nutrition and Fasting

My Therapeutic Program for a Healthy Life

Chapter Nine

Using Nutrition and Fasting
to Cure Chronic Illness

In chapter two, I took you on a journey around the world to the Blue Zones, showing you how we can live longer, healthier lives with a traditional diet.

What Is a "Traditional Diet"?

A traditional diet consists of:

- whole foods
- vegetarian or vegan foods
- fresh foods
- lots of vegetables, legumes, and spices
- fruit, especially berries
- nuts
- eating superfoods several times a day

In chapters five through eight, I introduced the second secret to health and longevity: caloric restriction. Whether it's through hara hachi bun me (eating until you're 80 percent full) or therapeutic fasting once or twice a year, or through daily intermittent fasting, each of these methods benefits your health!

A healthy, traditional diet in combination with regular exercise, stress reduction (especially meditation), and regular fasting can have a healing and preventive effect on many diseases—including hypertension and atherosclerosis (which cause heart attack and stroke), mild forms of depression, diabetes, fatty liver disease, gout, irritable bowel syndrome, arthrosis, and gallstones and other gallbladder problems.

In this chapter you'll find treatment methods for the most common chronic diseases and my specific recommendations for a long and healthy life.

My Therapy for Obesity

Why All Diets Have Failed

The countless diet and weight loss programs, the yearly flood of self-help books, cookbooks, and television shows that are all about losing weight—they have all failed.

The diet industry is constantly developing new, supposedly effective appetite suppressants and weight loss medications. However, these often have to be taken off the market a few years later due to the severe side effects they cause. To me, the increasing number of bariatric surgeries in which obesity is surgically tackled with gastric bands, gastric balloons, or sleeve gastrectomies are a sign of medical desperation. There are indeed situations in which I recommend such procedures. But I find it alarming that medicine and nutritional science are seemingly unable to help many people lose weight with less drastic measures.

Never before have humans lived as long as they do today, and never before has obesity been such a widespread problem. Muscle burns the most calories in our body, but we tend to lose muscle mass as we get older. The average fifty-year-old possesses less muscle mass than the average thirty-year-old, which is why you generally burn fewer calories as you get older; the basal metabolism decreases. It follows, then, that if a fifty-year-old eats the same way they did when they were thirty, they are bound to put on weight.

Losing weight takes more time and patience with increasing age. I'm not saying this to dishearten you, but patience is crucial for successful weight loss. As are realistic goals.

Losing a lot of weight in a short amount of time almost always leads to a yo-yo effect. In other words, if you lose a few pounds relatively quickly with a new diet, you will likely be quite pleased. This creates—consciously or unconsciously—an expectation that you'll continue to lose weight at a similar pace. But the biological truth is that when weight is lost too quickly, alarm bells are raised in the body. The body does everything it can to prevent further weight loss. The somatic cells can't know, after all, that we have chosen to diet and are following a precise plan. If weight is lost too quickly, the body lowers energy consumption and optimizes the energy yield of food. That's why you should stay away from diets to avoid sending your body the wrong signals.

Intermittent fasting, however, is useful in cases of obesity because it raises—rather than lowers—the body's energy consumption. That's why losing weight becomes relatively easy.

How to Lose Weight

ADOPT A PLANT-BASED MEDITERRANEAN OR MEDITERRASIAN DIET

Both the Mediterranean and the MediterrAsian diets lead to weight loss as a "side effect" over a longer period of time.[1] However, you should avoid alcohol. Like sugar, alcohol is empty calories, whether you're drinking expensive Italian red wine or beer. I also recommend following a vegan or vegetarian diet (lots of fruit and vegetables, supplemented with milk and dairy products). If you follow a vegan diet, your resting metabolic rate will be a little higher.[2, 3]

If you want to lose weight, substituting chicken for pork is, unfortunately, not a successful strategy. Of all types of meat, chicken facilitates weight gain the most.[4, 5] You can blame factory farms and their methods of breeding animals with hormones and other unhealthy additives. If you don't want to give up the taste of umami, I recommend using plant-based meat options made from tofu, seitan, or mushrooms on an occasional basis.

Other diets I mentioned in previous chapters, such as Atkins, Paleo, and low-carb diets, are not healthy and I therefore don't recommend them. I would only recommend a vegetarian low-carb diet if you have elevated insulin levels, as in type 2 diabetes. If you suspect that this may apply to you, have your GP check your insulin levels to see if you may be developing a resistance to insulin.

Again, not all carbohydrates are equal. Make sure to eat whole, complex carbohydrates such as whole grains. A good way to reduce the potentially fattening quality of carbohydrates is to let potatoes, pasta, and rice cool down before you eat them. This creates a resistant starch, which leads to a lower insulin release. You can eat the potatoes, pasta, or rice cold, or you can reheat them—either way, they'll be more resistant to digestion than before.[6] Eat plenty of plant-based proteins, because proteins are very filling. Avoid animal proteins as much as possible because they boost inflammation and aging processes in the body.[7, 8]

You should also avoid chemicals that promote obesity. Environmental toxins such as persistent organic pollutants (POPs)—which include insecticides and dioxins—accumulate in the fat tissue. Since these environmental toxins accumulate across the food chain, they are mainly found in animal products, particularly in fish.[9]

SET A REALISTIC GOAL

Losing two to four pounds a month is ideal.

How to Dampen Your Appetite and Boost Your Metabolism

There are more and more grandiose advertisements for special teas, powders, and medicinal plants that are said to boost weight loss. Those promises are generally nonsense. Here is what really helps:

- **Apple cider vinegar:** In one study, the consumption of one or two tablespoons of apple cider vinegar per day was associated with weight loss of four pounds after three months. This study was financed by a vinegar manufacturer, but since the positive effects of vinegar on diabetes and blood pressure are generally known, I can recommend apple cider vinegar as a supplement for weight loss with a clear conscience. It's important to consume it regularly, and to not rely on the vinegar alone.

- **Bitter compounds:** Bitter compounds are natural fat burners. They stimulate the production of digestive enzymes in the gallbladder and pancreas very effectively and, moreover, stimulate fat digestion. Bitter flavors also make you feel full faster and are beneficial for the microbiome.[10] These days, the taste of bitterness is bred out of vegetables and salads more and more, unfortunately. I recommend having radicchio, chicory, endive, olives, cabbage, or wild plants such as dandelion and ground elder every day. If you have to have chocolate, only dark chocolate will do.

- **Nuts:** I will never tire of recommending nuts. They are just unbeatably healthy. Even though nuts are high in fat, you will still lose weight because they are very filling, so you end up eating less with your meals. Also make use of the "pistachio principle" (see page 121).

- **Drink water:** Here is a simple trick: Drink one or two glasses of water before you eat. The metabolism expert at Charité, Michael Boschmann, and his team were able to demonstrate that this facilitates weight loss. Ideally, drink the water fifteen to thirty minutes before a meal.[11] Not only does it make you feel full, it also has its own positive effects on the metabolism.

- **Exercise and stress reduction:** Both exercise and stress reduction are nearly as important as your diet. You'll manage to shed excess weight in the long run only if you exercise, reduce stress, and develop mindfulness.

INTERMITTENT FASTING AND OBESITY

According to all the data currently available, most people lose weight with intermittent fasting, especially the 16:8 method (see page 243). You can achieve a sixteen-hour break from eating by skipping dinner or by having it early. Alternatively, you can skip breakfast (or have a late breakfast) instead. In any case, you should strive to ensure that lunch is your most calorie-rich meal of the day.

For losing weight, the 5:2 method is almost as effective as intermittent fasting, but it's generally harder to maintain and therefore less sustainable. Sooner or later, most of my patients switch from this method to the more easily accomplished and effective 16:8 method of fasting.

Prolonged therapeutic fasting can be a good starting point for weight loss. However, it is extremely important to really change your diet afterward. If you are one of those people who weigh more several months after therapeutic fasting than before (this is quite rare), you should not repeat therapeutic fasting—at least not with the aim of normalizing your weight. Instead, try intermittent fasting. A good practice to incorporate into your routine after therapeutic fasting is a weekly relief day.

My Therapy for Hypertension

Around 25 million people in Germany suffer from hypertension. This is such an unimaginably high number that you almost have to ask yourself who *doesn't* have high blood pressure. There are several reasons why there are so many cases of hypertension. First, medical guidelines have lowered the threshold for high blood pressure in recent years— what may have been considered a normal blood pressure reading several years ago is now considered high. Second, our modern lifestyle facilitates this disease. We sit for too long, move too little, experience too much stress, and above all we eat too much and our diet is too unhealthy. Considering all these factors, hypertension is basically inevitable.

On our short trip to the Blue Zones I mentioned studies on people living in Uganda and Kenya that suggest, as does current research on people living in the Amazon, that people *don't* suffer from hypertension even in old age if their living conditions are "natural"—in other words, if they get enough exercise and follow a traditionally healthy diet.

A large-scale study conducted in France analyzed which risks determine whether someone will suffer from hypertension. The risk is heightened by 17 to 30 percent if a person's diet is rich in salt, meat, and animal protein. It is lowered by 15 to 30 percent if the diet mainly consists of fruit, vegetables, vegetable protein, nuts, and whole grains, as well as fiber containing potassium and magnesium.

It Is Possible to Do Without Medication

There are a lot of good medications that can be used to effectively treat hypertension. But for a lot of patients, these medications eventually stop having an effect; the patients slowly become resistant to treatment. Or the side effects are intolerable. Innovative and elaborate methods, on the other hand, interfere with the body. For example, nerves in the renal arteries that cause chronic stress and thus lead to high blood pressure can be clipped with the use of a catheter.

I strongly urge you to exhaust all possibilities of dietary change before submitting to such a procedure.

It's important to consume a lot of potassium and little sodium (salt) if you suffer from high blood pressure. Almost all plants are rich in potassium. Our ancestors probably ate two or three times as much potassium (contained in vegetables, fruit, nuts, and seeds) as we do today. Instead, we've become champions at using salt. Nowadays, salt is added to almost all food products. It is not healthy.

By the way, it's a myth that bananas contain a lot of potassium. You would have to eat more than ten bananas a day to meet the minimum daily potassium requirement. Leafy greens, sweet potatoes, legumes, and nuts are good sources of this mineral.

My Dietary Recommendations for Hypertension

- **Low salt:** If you suffer from hypertension, try to refrain from using salt for a few months. Monitor your blood pressure during this time. The major sources of salt are bread, cheese, sausage, french fries, and industrially processed meat, poultry, or fish, as well as ready-made foods. Some of the products that contain the most salt include pizza, chips, and crackers.

You can break the habit of eating dishes that are too rich in salt. Often, our desire for more salt stems from a dulled sense of taste. One of the great effects of therapeutic fasting is that you'll be able to properly taste food afterward—your sense of taste will be readjusted.

Try to avoid using salt when cooking. Instead, experiment with spices. The dishes may taste bland or different at first, but after a while you'll adjust, and when you go to restaurants you'll start thinking that the chef put too much salt in your dish.

- **No meat:** A vegetarian or vegan diet is the ideal way to begin lowering your blood pressure in the long term. A Mediterranean diet also lowers elevated blood pressure, as does the DASH diet (a diet often recommended for the prevention and control of hypertension).
- **Whole-grain products:** According to one study, three portions of whole-grain bread a day lowers the blood pressure as much as modern blood pressure medication.

What to Do If You Have High Blood Pressure

- Do not drink alcohol; it significantly raises your blood pressure.
- Eat superfoods (their antihypertensive effect has been proven in many scientific studies).
- Consume flaxseed and flaxseed oil (two tablespoons a day).
- Consume walnuts and unsalted pistachios (a handful a day).
- Drink hibiscus tea or green tea (two to three cups a day).
- Drink nonalcoholic red wine (occasionally).
- Drink beet juice (8 to 16 ounces a day).
- Eat nitrate-rich vegetables such as spinach, arugula, and Swiss chard (at least one serving a day).
- Consume plenty of olive oil daily.
- Eat dark chocolate (10 grams a day, or about 0.4 ounces).

- Eat fruits such as pomegranate and blueberries (a handful a day, fresh or frozen).
- Consume soy products such as tofu, tempeh, and soy milk (one to two servings a day).

Important: Monitor your blood pressure when you change your diet. In most cases, blood pressure medication can be reduced after a relatively short time. But only change your medication after consulting your doctor, never on your own.

Cure Hypertension Through Fasting

To prevent, treat, and cure hypertension I recommend:

THERAPEUTIC FASTING

Practicing therapeutic fasting for at least seven days at a time usually has an enormous hypotensive effect. This is due to a combination of increased secretion of antihypertensive hormones, the elimination of salt and fat, and changes to the microbiome as a result of giving the bowel some relief.

The maximum antihypertensive effect of a fasting cure is achieved after fourteen days. If you are on antihypertensive medication, the dosage must be adjusted by your doctor during and after the fast. When the fast is over, there is usually a slight rise in blood pressure, but the levels generally stay lower than they were before fasting. Therapeutic fasting is therefore a huge opportunity to strive for a sustained reduction in blood pressure supported by intermittent fasting and a healthy diet. The fasting mimicking diet (see page 179) can also be used to achieve a good reduction in blood pressure.

INTERMITTENT FASTING

For many people, intermittent fasting leads to a drop in blood pressure if it is accompanied by long-term weight loss.

RICE DAYS

Rice relief days can have a noticeable effect on lowering blood pressure. Rice days are easy to integrate into your daily routine; for example, try fitting them in once a week or just before or after the weekend. See page 246 for how to practice a rice day.

My Therapy for Type 1 Diabetes, Type 2 Diabetes, and Fatty Liver Disease

Type 1 diabetes is an autoimmune disease that often occurs in children or adolescents and is caused by the destruction of insulin-producing cells in the pancreas. It is still unclear what causes this faulty reaction of the body's own immune cells. It could be a consequence of infections, but both the role of the microbiome as well as certain dietary influences during infancy and childhood have been raised as possible causes. There's a limit to how much dietary changes can help with cases of type 1 diabetes, but often they can improve the fine-tuning of the insulin dose.

Type 2 diabetes, once considered a sign of aging, is the more common form of diabetes. Cases of type 2 diabetes are increasing rapidly around the world and causing great concern for doctors and health policy makers. The disease affects about 10 percent of Germany's population, including more and more young people. Type 2 diabetes is associated with obesity and a lack of exercise. The actual cause is insulin resistance, often a consequence of many years of nutritional deficiency and overeating.

These days, new antidiabetic drugs have become a multibillion-dollar business. These drugs effectively lower blood sugar levels, control symptoms, and protect against complications. Yet there's one major downside: They cannot cure diabetes.

By changing your diet, you can get to the root cause of type 2 diabetes. Using a combination of regular therapeutic fasting, intermittent fasting, and an optimal diet, I've seen time and again in my patients how this disease can be cured.

Chances of curing type 2 diabetes are particularly good if a patient has had the illness for less than seven years. If the disease has persisted for longer than ten years, it becomes more difficult. The ideal moment to employ diet instead of pills as treatment is when diabetes is diagnosed. There are initial convincing studies on vegan diets, but if you don't want to forgo animal products, I recommend a Mediterranean lacto-vegetarian diet—that is, a vegetarian diet with small amounts of cheese and yogurt. All dairy products should be made from organic milk.

Today we know that antidiabetic drugs not only have a direct effect on the regulation of sugar and insulin but also intervene and regulate via the intestinal bacteria.[12] This underlines the importance of a healthy diet with fiber and prebiotic vegetables for the microbiome.

Avoid Artificial Sweeteners Altogether

As a diabetic, you should stay away from artificial sweeteners completely, because some products, such as sucralose (Splenda), worsen blood sugar regulation and even promote diabetes.[13, 14, 15] If you must consume artificial sweeteners, try stevia and erythritol (I recommend them begrudgingly), since they don't affect the sugar metabolism.

My Dietary Recommendations for Type 2 Diabetes

- **Vinegar:** Balsamic vinegar and apple cider vinegar can be delicious. Patients with type 2 diabetes should use plenty of vinegar in their cooking. Numerous studies have shown that it improves blood sugar levels after meals.[16] The exact mechanism of this therapeutic effect is not yet fully understood. As with beets, arugula, and spinach—vegetables that contain nitrate—the effect seems to be the result of the production of nitric oxide. That's why vinegar also lowers blood pressure.

- **Fruit:** This might sound surprising, but I recommend fruit and berries for patients with diabetes. As sensible as it is to avoid sugar and artificial sweeteners when suffering from diabetes, it can be just as sensible to eat fruit consciously. This generally has a positive effect. Berries and apples are particularly beneficial. When eating apples, try to eat the peel as well; it's full of healthy quercetin. In one study, healthy participants ate twenty servings of fruit every day over the course of several weeks. This is an incredibly large amount of fruit, and naturally it was associated with an enormous intake of fructose. Nevertheless, the participants' metabolic sugar levels stayed within a healthy range.[17]

- **Vegetables:** An extract of broccoli has been proven to have an effect similar to that of the most important antidiabetic drug, metformin, which slows down the formation of glucose in the liver.[18] Swedish researchers found that the mustard oil sulforaphane contained in broccoli inhibits blood sugar synthesis in the liver just as effectively, albeit with a different mechanism.[19]

- **Olive oil and nuts:** Regular consumption of olive oil and 30 grams (about one ounce) of nuts a day can prevent diabetes.[20, 21] An antidiabetic effect has especially been attributed to pistachios and almonds.[22] Almonds, by the way, also lower blood fat levels.[23]

- **Ginger:** One to two cups of ginger tea or one to two teaspoons of ground ginger a day reduce appetite and improve fatty liver.[24]
- **Oats:** Oats have a proven antidiabetic effect. Oatmeal for breakfast or regular relief days with oats have a beneficial effect. The relief days are a moderate form of fasting and help the sugar metabolism.[25]
- **Flaxseed:** Flaxseed lowers cholesterol levels and blood pressure and supports an antidiabetic diet.[26]
- **Legumes:** Eating chickpeas, lentils, or beans every day improves blood sugar regulation.[27]
- **Cinnamon:** In discussions about diabetes, this spice is often mentioned as a remedy. But the devil is in the details, because there are two types of cinnamon: Ceylon and cassia. The cheaper and thus more commonly used variety, cassia, does indeed have antidiabetogenic properties. But unfortunately, it contains coumarin, a phytochemical that is harmful in large quantities. For cassia cinnamon to be effective, one would have to eat so much of it that its high content of coumarin would harm the liver. The more expensive Ceylon cinnamon is more easily tolerated and free of coumarin, but unfortunately it doesn't help against diabetes.[28]

My tip: Eating slowly helps with type 2 diabetes. If you chew your food well, starch and carbohydrates are mixed with enzymes in the saliva (mainly alpha-amylase). The amylase breaks down oligosaccharides into monosaccharides in the mouth and thus does 30 percent of the digestive work. When we eat slowly, a feeling of satiety occurs more quickly, which means that we ultimately eat less and thus less insulin is released. One study compared what happens when you wolf down a serving of ice cream in five minutes or enjoy it over the course of thirty minutes. The latter reduced unfavorable metabolic reactions by 25 percent![29] So please enjoy your food and don't gobble it up!

Cure Diabetes Through Fasting

There are several methods that can help with this disease. A combination of different methods is ideal:

THERAPEUTIC FASTING

Prolonged therapeutic fasting has a beneficial effect on type 2 diabetes, especially if you also suffer from a fatty liver. After just a week or two of therapeutic fasting, blood sugar levels and insulin resistance improve significantly, and the symptoms of a fatty liver disappear.[30, 31, 32] I recommend fasting with only vegetable juices. Fruit juices contain too much fructose and promote fatty liver.

However, if you have type 2 diabetes, therapeutic fasting should be carried out only under medical supervision. For example, it is important to stop taking the diabetes medication metformin immediately. This medication inhibits the formation of sugar in the liver; however, this process is important during fasting in order to supply the cells and the brain with sugar, in addition to ketones.

In patients with type 1 diabetes, therapeutic fasting can improve insulin effects, but due to the complex metabolic situation, side effects are more common. Therefore, medical supervision, ideally in a clinic that specializes in type 1 diabetes, is all the more advisable.

In the animal experiments conducted by Valter Longo and his research team, type 1 diabetes could be cured with a fasting mimicking diet. But these results are not yet transferrable to humans. Nevertheless, therapeutic fasting can improve the metabolism with a lower insulin requirement afterward.

INTERMITTENT FASTING

Intermittent fasting works extremely well for patients with type 2 diabetes, and it can be tested, under medical supervision, in cases of type 1 diabetes. Skipping dinner or having dinner early is advisable here. For diabetics, an intake of carbohydrates and energy in the evening leads to a higher insulin release in the morning—presumably due to an interaction with the sleep hormone melatonin.

Two meals a day is ideal—a big breakfast with oatmeal, wholegrain bread, berries, and fruit, as well as a hearty lunch (in any case, make sure you eat before five p.m.). Avoid snacks.

> Patients with type 1 diabetes must fast only under medical supervision.

Patient History: Type 1 Diabetes and Rheumatism

Lena H., age thirty-three, a product developer in the food industry, suffers from type 1 diabetes and rheumatism. She is fighting both with intermittent fasting—with great success.

"The cleansing through fasting really benefited my entire system."

I have had type 1 diabetes since I was twelve. Thanks to innovations in medical technology, I've managed well. I have an insulin pump and a blood glucose sensor that sticks on my arm and is constantly measuring my levels. Sure, I have to be careful about what I eat, but on the whole, there are very few restrictions for me. If I overdo it every now and again, I counteract that with the pump.

It's the rheumatic episodes, which started in early 2017, that have become the bigger problem. In the beginning, I only had pain in my feet, which I blamed on running or hiking too long. When the pain and severe swelling started in my hands as well, I ended up going to the doctor, who immediately referred me to a specialist and asked for a blood test. Rheumatism. At my age. The doctor suggested methotrexate as a treatment. This is a kind of "chemo light," a cytotoxin that has side effects such as nausea and headaches. This treatment also meant that I couldn't be in the sun or have any alcohol—or get pregnant. At the time, I didn't want children right away, but starting to take a drug like that at the age of thirty-two still seemed absurd to me. So instead, we tried a weaker version of a disease-modifying antirheumatic drug. But honestly it didn't work all that great, at least not all the time.

That's when my rheumatologist suggested Dr. Michalsen's clinic. Initially, I resisted. But when my symptoms kept getting worse and worse, when I could barely get out of bed for days on end, I made a decision. By then, I no longer had the strength to do anything: I got up in the mornings, went to work, came home, lay down for two hours, got up to eat, and then went back to bed. I don't know if the fatigue was caused by the rheumatism or the antirheumatic medication. But I wanted to search for alternatives.

I was a little worried about whether fasting and diabetes were compatible—and I did become hypoglycemic sometimes, usually at night. But when that happened, I just drank some apple juice and then I was fine. Just before I went to the clinic, I had to take cortisone for eight weeks, and so the cleansing through fasting really benefited my entire system. My joint pains improved significantly and didn't return for weeks after fasting. Unfortunately, they eventually did return, but they weren't as bad as they had been before.

I now fast intermittently, which means I don't eat anything for sixteen hours every day. Sometimes I skip breakfast if I'm meeting friends for dinner, for example; sometimes I leave out dinner if I want to have a leisurely breakfast on Sundays. It's easy. I also avoid meat and dairy products, because they are said to boost inflammatory processes in the body. Instead, I eat a lot of vegetables and fruit, a lot of muesli, lentils, potatoes, whole-grain bread. My boyfriend follows the same diet; luckily he isn't big on meat anyway, but he does like to have some cheese every now and then. In winter, I make a paste out of ginger, black pepper, turmeric, nutmeg, and cinnamon with a dash of oil. And then every morning, I mix a teaspoon of this paste with some boiled water and drink it. Turmeric helps against inflammation; the rest of the ingredients give me strength. In order to keep my joint pains at bay, I also plan to do therapeutic fasting twice a year.

My Therapy for Atherosclerosis, Heart Attack, and Stroke

Modern cardiology is a blessing in the treatment of acute heart attacks, dysrhythmias, and strokes. In the case of a heart attack, the affected coronary artery can be kept open with a stent through cardiac catheterization in order to restore blood flow to the heart muscle; valvular heart disease can be treated with minimal invasiveness.

In most cases, the underlying cause of a heart attack or a stroke is a long-existing chronic disease of the arterial blood vessels—atherosclerosis (a buildup of fat, cholesterol, and other substances in the walls of the arteries). This atherosclerosis is ultimately not affected by the procedures described above and can progress if the risk factors (elevated blood lipid levels, hypertension, obesity, stress, smoking) are not addressed. Unfortunately, patients often overestimate the effectiveness of drug-based therapies against a potential heart attack or stroke.

A cholesterol-lowering statin's protective effect on the heart is estimated to be twenty times more effective than it actually is.[33] This misconception can be fatal, because if you believe that taking a preventive drug makes everything okay, then your motivation and willingness to change your lifestyle will be limited. Why take on the effort of getting healthy?

My advice is: We should be grateful for the achievements of medicine and modern medications, but we should also be aware of the fact that they are not a cure-all. One pill can't fix everything. A healthy lifestyle without nicotine, with fasting, and with a corresponding diet that protects the vessels is the most important factor in cases of existing or looming cardiovascular diseases.

A Preventive and Healing Diet for the Heart and Blood Vessels

With arteriosclerosis, the best results are achieved with a vegan, low-fat diet and a Mediterranean diet. Two remarkable studies showed that the vegan diet can initiate a regression of atherosclerosis. The lead scientists in these studies, Dean Ornish and Caldwell Esselstyn, insist that the diet of patients with coronary heart disease must be very low in fat.[34, 35] On the basis of this and many more studies, I strongly recommend following a strictly plant-based diet. Your diet doesn't necessarily need to be low fat, but do make sure it contains only minimal amounts of animal fats.

Fasting for the Heart and Vessels

The risk factors that lead to coronary heart disease and stroke can be effectively treated with both intermittent fasting and periodic therapeutic fasting. Regular relief days or intermittent fasting in combination with medications that protect the vessels are also very effective.

My Dietary Recommendations
for the Heart and Blood Vessels

- **Flaxseed:** Flaxseed lowers cholesterol and blood pressure.[36]
- **Berries:** Dark berries such as blueberries and blackberries, as well as the Indian gooseberry (also known as amla), reduce the risk of heart attack.[37] I also recommend Chyawanprash, a traditional Ayurvedic product whose main components are amla and sesame oil.
- **Oils:** Olive oil, canola oil, and flaxseed oil are great for preventing heart disease.[38]
- **Garlic and red onion:** Both keep the vessels supple.[39, 40]
- **Nuts:** Walnuts, pecans, Brazil nuts, and almonds lower cholesterol and blood pressure, and reduce weight. In addition, they improve the fatty acid profile.[41]
- **Ginger:** This healthy plant lowers triglyceride levels.[42]
- **Turmeric:** This spice lowers cholesterol.[43]
- **Legumes:** Eating legumes minimizes the risk of atherosclerosis (this also applies to unsalted peanuts).[44]
- **L-arginine:** This valuable amino acid found in pumpkin seeds, almonds, pine nuts, legumes, and peanuts has an antihypertensive effect and relaxes the blood vessels.[45]
- **Beets:** This root vegetable and other vegetables containing nitrate, such as spinach, lettuce, Swiss chard, and arugula, are effective in preventing heart attack and stroke.[46]
- **Pomegranate juice:** Drinking 3.5 ounces of pomegranate juice every day improves blood flow to the coronary vessels, as a study conducted by Dean Ornish showed.[47]

You should not undergo therapeutic fasting within three months after suffering an emergency such as a heart attack or a stroke, because the heart is not yet stable enough. But you can fast even if there is an existing cardiac insufficiency, because the diuretic effect in particular is a good supplementary therapy to medication. In this situation, however, you should fast only under medical supervision in a clinic.

My Therapy for Kidney Disease

Our kidneys work hard every day: Over the course of twenty-four hours, they filter up to forty gallons of blood and produce about one to two liters of urine from blood.

Chronic kidney disease with an increasing loss of kidney function (renal insufficiency) can be caused by inflammation, autoimmune diseases, or long-term use of pain medications. The most common cause of kidney damage is existing chronic diseases such as diabetes and hypertension. Hypertension is the biggest risk factor for declining kidney function in old age. This decline can progress gradually and ultimately result in the complete loss of kidney function and thus the need for regular dialysis. But chronic kidney disease is accompanied by an increased risk of heart attack or stroke and can therefore become life-threatening much earlier.

Unfortunately, there is no cure for chronic kidney insufficiency. This is why it is so important to stop or slow down the loss of kidney function. Avoid all drugs that cause damage to the kidneys, and ensure treatment of the risk factors for kidney disease (hypertension, diabetes, high cholesterol). This is also the central goal of nutritional therapy. Therefore, the recommendations for kidney disease are the same as those for hypertension, diabetes, and atherosclerosis. In addition, there are a few particularities:

Fasting for Kidney Problems

Before there was dialysis, kidney specialists recommended fasting and thirst therapies for their patients. Many times, the condition of the

My Dietary Recommendations
for Patients with Kidney Disease

- **Low protein:** If you are suffering from chronic kidney disease, you should stop consuming animal protein. Meat, fish, and poultry put measurable stress on the kidneys; this is called hyperfiltration. Omitting animal protein is also important because the protein poses an additional strain for diseased kidneys: It adds a high acid load.[48, 49]

  If the kidney disease progresses to such an extent that dialysis becomes necessary, a larger quantity of protein might be needed again. Follow the recommendations of your nephrologist, including the amount of potassium-containing vegetables and fruits you should eat.

- **Low acid:** An alkaline diet delays the deterioration of existing kidney disease. Meat, dairy products, and fish are acidic.[50, 51]

- **Low phosphorus:** Phosphorus, like calcium, is an essential mineral. It is ingested with food in the form of phosphate and converted into phosphorus in the body. Normally, excess quantities of phosphorus are excreted in the urine. When kidney function is impaired, phosphate levels in the blood can be elevated, which is why there is danger in ingesting too much of it. Be careful: Phosphorus is much more easily absorbed from animal products, bread, grain, and soft drinks than from fruits and vegetables.

  What I consider to be particularly negative are forms of phosphate that are used as food additives. That's why you shouldn't buy any products with the phosphorus-containing additives E338, E343, E450, E452, E1410, E1412, E1413, or E1414. The acid burden created by phosphate damages not only the kidneys but also the heart.

- **Low salt and low fluid intake:** The diet of patients with kidney disease should be low in salt. Drinking large amounts of water has been shown to be surprisingly ineffective when it comes to kidney failure.[52] However, if you have kidney stones or chronic inflammation of the bladder, you should drink plenty of water. If you are on dialysis, you should follow the advice of your nephrologist.

kidneys was improved by these therapies, but the effect never lasted long. After dialysis became established, fasting was no longer recommended. Today, many doctors even say that patients with kidney disease should not fast. Their argument is that the kidneys have to play an important part in fasting as an excretory organ and therefore doctors are concerned that this would create problems in cases of impaired kidney function.

I disagree. Many patients with kidney disease have fasted successfully in our clinic without showing any particular side effects. In some patients, kidney function even improved slightly after fasting. Above all, however, blood pressure, diabetes, and hyperhydration improved. Therefore, I highly recommend fasting, but only in a clinic, where blood values can be regularly monitored.

Intermittent fasting works well for patients with kidney disease and can be practiced independently—the 16:8 method is ideal. If hypertension is also an issue, I recommend low-salt rice relief days once a week. You can try a low-calorie rice relief day once a week as recommended on page 246, or you can try the Kempner method on page 244 (which allows you to eat up to 2,000 kcal a day) for several days.

My Therapy for Arthrosis

When the skeleton of an unborn child develops in the womb, it initially consists of cartilage before it ossifies completely. Cartilage remains only at the joint surfaces as a kind of elastic shock absorber and protective layer for the bone.

The main cause of arthrosis is age. Hardly any forty-year-olds suffer from it, but it's quite common for eighty-year-olds. The layer of cartilage at the joints becomes increasingly thinner, and to compensate for that, ossification occurs at the edges of the joints. Overuse and overload are rarely the cause of arthrosis nowadays, unlike in the past, when people spent more time doing physical labor. Arthrosis from overuse and overload generally applies only to former professional athletes and people whose work is very physically demanding.

But even if arthrosis is mostly a disease of old age, there are other factors that determine how long our joints remain supple and pain-free. To name just two, there are genetic disposition (especially with arthrosis of the hands) and diet. The symptoms of arthrosis are often caused by inflammation. Commonly taken pain medications such as ibuprofen and diclofenac have an anti-inflammatory effect on the joints. Incidentally, the cartilage is not responsible for the unpleasant pain, but the structures surrounding it are (synovial membrane, articular capsule, tendons, and ligaments). It's a vicious cycle—because it is painful to move, the joint is rested too often, which in turn causes the arthrosis to progress.

In Cases of Arthrosis, It's Imperative to Lose Excess Weight

In cases of arthrosis, the first thing I recommend is to tackle any excess weight. This is not easy, especially if you can no longer walk well due to arthrosis of the knees, hips, or ankles. Exercise becomes difficult. In addition to good physiotherapy and pain therapy, it is therefore crucial to change your diet to prevent the need for surgery or an artificial joint later on. The connection between being overweight and having arthrosis, particularly of the knee and hip joints, is not only the increased weight load. The additional fat also causes the microbiome to release inflammatory metabolites that can potentially damage the articular cartilage.[53]

New materials and surgical techniques have enabled good results in joint replacement, but it is not always successful or advisable. With "simple" joints such as the hip, replacement can achieve excellent results. But the situation is different when it comes to knee, ankle, and shoulder joints. Because these joints are anatomically much more complex structures, the success rates are less optimal. In these cases, it makes sense to explore all other possibilities first.

With a combination of movement and exercise in the right dosage, warm and cold water therapies, physiotherapy, yoga, fasting, and nutritional therapy, you can ensure that you will barely or no longer feel your arthrosis—at least for some time.

During therapeutic fasting, the joints are quickly relieved due to the weight loss. In addition, the pro-inflammatory arachidonic acid is banished from the body almost completely within a few days.[54] Moreover, certain anti-inflammatory effects are initiated.[55] Depending on your initial weight, one or two weeks of therapeutic fasting is appropriate to reduce the pain as much as possible.

My Dietary Recommendations for Arthrosis

- **Vegetarian, lacto-vegetarian, or vegan diet:** Arachidonic acid is a fatty acid that occurs in notable amounts only in animal fats. If a lot of it enters the body with food, it is synthesized into pro-inflammatory semiochemicals called eicosanoids. By avoiding meat, sausage, eggs, fish, and dairy products, you can avoid the effects of arachidonic acid.[56, 57]

- **Omega-3 fatty acids:** Omega-3 fatty acids are the opponents of the pro-inflammatory eicosanoids.[58] Therefore, they should be consumed in large quantities; for example, in the form of flaxseed, flaxseed oil or canola oil, leafy greens, soy, algae, and nuts (such as walnuts).

- **Low in acid:** Too much acid weakens the bones and the cartilage and can cause inflammation in the connective tissue and around the joints.[59] When you follow a vegan or a lacto-vegetarian diet with only small amounts of dairy, you will consume more alkaline foods, which will keep your acid levels low.

- **Limited bread and cereal products:** Use them in moderation in order to slow down the intake of acid. But it is not necessary to avoid these products entirely.
- **Foods to alleviate symptoms:** Initial studies have shown that a symptom-alleviating effect was achieved in arthrosis when the following foods were eaten:

  flaxseed oil

  turmeric

  ginger

  pomegranate

  Vegetables and fruits rich in vitamin C, such as citrus, sea buckthorn, rose hip. Rose hip is effective only in the form of a pulp; heated rose hip tea has no notable affect. Rose hip also exists as a dietary supplement.

  Spice mixtures containing cumin, coriander, and nutmeg. Be sure to add turmeric and ginger, as these are more effective than the other three. Fenugreek and cardamom are also anti-inflammatory.

Wraps and Compresses

In complementary medicine, wraps are successfully used to treat arthrosis. They can be made with cabbage leaves, fenugreek, or cottage cheese.

You can make a cabbage wrap quickly: Simply roll three fresh leaves of green or savoy cabbage flat with a rolling pin. The pressure releases the effective glucosinolates. Wrap the leaves on or around the joint for at least two hours. If necessary, you can hold the leaves in place with a gauze bandage.

For arthrosis of the finger joints, you need waterproof gloves or medical gloves to create a "wrap." Prepare a small smoothie of green or savoy cabbage, then pour it into the gloves. You should wear the gloves for up to two hours.

Therapeutic Fasting for Arthrosis

During therapeutic fasting, joints are quickly relieved because of the immediate weight loss. In addition, the inflammatory arachidonic acid is almost completely eliminated from the body within a few days. Special anti-inflammatory effects are also initiated. Depending on the starting weight, one to two weeks of fasting makes sense to reduce the pain as much as possible.

Intermittent Fasting for Arthrosis

Intermittent fasting has little proven anti-inflammatory effect. However, it is ideal for further reducing weight after therapeutic fasting and in combination with a vegetarian diet.

My Therapy for Rheumatism

Rheumatoid arthritis, formerly called polyarthritis, is associated with painful joint inflammation and swelling. It leads to severe joint damage if not treated optimally.

The cause of this disease is an autoimmune reaction against your own cartilaginous tissue. It's not clear why the immune system decides to attack the body's own tissue. It's believed that genetics may be a factor, as well as the microbiome.[60, 61] Intestinal infections, stress, and possibly even diet change the composition of the intestinal flora.

Up until a few decades ago, doctors were relatively powerless when faced with rheumatoid arthritis. Now there are a few effective drugs that, while they can't cure the disease, can control the inflammation to such an extent that the damage to the joints can be well contained. However, these drugs often lose their effect after a certain amount of time, or severe side effects limit their use. When that happens, cortisol must be taken, which carries the known side effects of weight gain, increased blood pressure, increased blood sugar levels, and so on.

My Dietary Recommendations for Rheumatism

- **Plant-based food:** The low arachidonic acid content of a plant-based diet maximizes an anti-inflammatory effect.[62] The Mediterranean version of the plant-based, vegetarian diet can help especially well with the symptoms of rheumatism.
- **Elimination diet:** Many patients have discovered that certain foods can trigger a rheumatic episode. Often, the culprits are meat and dairy products. Pay attention to how your body reacts to different foods, and avoid those that aggravate your health. However, note that your reactions can change based on living conditions, age, and stress. Therefore, the suspected foods should be tested again after some time.
- **Low in acid:** Too much acid can cause inflammation in the connective tissue and around the joints.[63, 64] "Alkalize" your body by following a vegan or a lacto-vegetarian diet with only small amounts of dairy products.
- **Low in salt:** Studies at Charité showed that autoimmune processes are triggered by salt.[65]
- **Follow a diet based on the principles of Ayurveda:** The Ayurvedic diet is generally a lacto-vegetarian diet, and I have observed a lasting improvement in our patients' symptoms when they switch to this type of diet. Anti-inflammatory spices are often used, and plants of the nightshade family such as tomatoes, eggplant, bell peppers, and potatoes are avoided. The dishes are predominantly warm dishes; there are few cold dishes. I recommend following the general dietary rules of Ayurveda, such as the adherence to a certain rhythm of eating.

Individual foods that can help with rheumatism are identical to those listed under arthrosis (page 305).

Therapeutic Fasting for Rheumatism

The most effective antirheumatic method in nutritional medicine is therapeutic fasting. Otto Buchinger, the pioneer of therapeutic fasting, experienced this firsthand. His rheumatic joint inflammation improved significantly after a three-week fast. It is not known what type of rheumatic disease Buchinger was suffering from, since diagnoses were not as differentiated back then as they are today. All that is known is that the disease affected him gravely. Later on, he repeatedly treated rheumatic episodes with periods of fasting.[66]

In our clinic, we've observed that patients with rheumatoid arthritis who fast for at least seven days experience pain relief and reduced joint swelling; the inflammatory parameters in the blood also improve. Fasting according to the Buchinger method is the most effective in alleviating these symptoms.

Longer fasting periods are possible if the patient's initial weight allows it. While the antihypertensive effect of fasting sets in after only two to four days, rheumatic inflammation sometimes requires ten to twelve days of fasting before the anti inflammatory effect becomes clearly noticeable.

As good and quick as the effect of therapeutic fasting for rheumatism is, there remains the question of what diet patients should follow after fasting, so that pain relief and symptom relief last for as long as possible. If there is no change in diet, the symptoms usually return relatively quickly.

In the aforementioned study carried out by immunologist Jens Kjeldsen-Kragh (see page 164), sustainable success in treating rheumatism can be achieved with the help of an extensive dietary plan. After fasting, patients received a vegan and gluten-free diet for four months.

Moreover, a so-called elimination diet was practiced: After fasting, a new food was introduced every two days. First potatoes, then carrots two days later, apples after another two days, and so on. If the condition of the joints worsened after the addition of a new food, that food was immediately eliminated again; sometimes it was reintroduced at a later stage for testing purposes. In this way, the foods that triggered rheumatic episodes were identified and forever taken off the shopping list.[67] But as I said, this is a very complex process.

Based on further study data and my own experiences, I recommend that patients with rheumatism initially adopt a vegan diet after fasting.[68, 69] A gluten-free diet can be tried at a different time, but it's probably not as important as leaving out animal products. Ongoing studies, also conducted at Charité, will hopefully lead to more precise dietary recommendations in a few years' time.

Intermittent Fasting for Rheumatism

The anti-inflammatory effect of intermittent fasting is not noticeable enough to match the powerful effect of therapeutic fasting for rheumatism. In my experience, the fasting mimicking diet also has a weaker effect on this disease than therapeutic fasting according to the Buchinger method.

My Therapy for Irritable Bowel Syndrome (IBS) and Inflammatory Bowel Disease (IBD)

It is estimated that up to 15 percent of the population in industrialized countries suffers from irritable bowel syndrome, women more often than men.[70] Recent studies indicate a hypersensitivity of the intestinal walls and an abnormal intestinal flora or microbial imbalance as the cause.[71] Intestinal infections as well as stress are important triggers.[72]

The combination of digestive problems and a lowered pain threshold of the intestinal mucosa leads the "normal" movements of the intestine to cause pain.[73, 74] Furthermore, digestion is irregular; diarrhea, constipation, and flatulence occur more frequently.

In cases of irritable bowel syndrome, the intestinal mucosa is often easily inflamed. In cases of chronic inflammatory bowel diseases such as ulcerative colitis and Crohn's disease, the inflammation is severe. Modern medicine's only method of treating irritable bowel syndrome is the FODMAP diet (fermentable oligosaccharides, disaccharides, monosaccharides, and polyols; see page 102). This diet strictly avoids all foods that cause flatulence or are hard to digest. FODMAPs can be found in sweets, bread, and grain, as well as in cabbage plants (cabbage, broccoli, cauliflower, etc.). This diet is carried out over a period of eight weeks, during which individual foods are tested for their tolerability, just as in the elimination diet. The FODMAP principle, however, is somewhat complicated and leads to a clear restriction of nutritional diversity. Its effectiveness has been proven, but only in the medium run—not in the long run. If you decide to try it, you should ideally be supervised by a professional nutritionist.

There is a fundamental dilemma when it comes to irritable bowel syndrome: Some foods that are important and beneficial for the intestinal bacteria, such as root vegetables, legumes, and whole-grain bread, can initially aggravate the symptoms. But at the same time, these foods feed the good bacteria and cause them to multiply. Which means the benefits of these foods only become apparent in the long run. That's why I recommend eating—at least in small amounts—foods that may initially cause symptoms.

Eat high-quality foods, prepare them carefully (some spices, for example, alleviate the flatulent effect), and chew your meals slowly and thoroughly.

If your doctor diagnoses you with irritable bowel syndrome after performing a colonoscopy, you should get a breath test to check for specific intolerances such as lactose or fructose intolerance. Your pain could improve if you limit your consumption of milk and dairy products as well as fructose. For acute and severe symptoms, the FODMAP diet is a suitable start.

Basically, you should opt for a mild diet, which means as little raw food as possible. Eat steamed vegetables instead. Or fry vegetables briefly in a wok. Asian cuisine is the best example of a healthy, mild diet that can easily be digested by the intestine.

The Ayurvedic diet is also very well tolerated, especially in patients with irritable bowel syndrome. I strongly recommend it if your symptoms haven't improved enough through previously mentioned measures.

It's important to chew your food well. When properly mixed with saliva, all foods containing carbohydrates become predigested and can be tolerated much better by the intestine later on.

Don't drink anything during meals, especially cold beverages. It is believed that drinking liquids during meals dilutes the digestive enzymes and thus impairs their function. Furthermore, the addition of liquids to meals stretches the stomach walls more, which confuses the nerves and causes food to be transferred to the small intestine too early, creating digestive problems. However, this has not yet been examined in medical studies and is based on the advice of naturopathic and Ayurvedic medicine.

Don't eat when you are stressed or tired. Instead, rest first, or do a relaxation exercise. Eat only after your mind and body have calmed down, because then the intestine can do its work in peace as well.

Avoid alcohol. It's an inflammatory stimulus for the intestinal mucosa and can exacerbate leaky gut syndrome.[75, 76]

Provide your intestinal bacteria with good food: Eat prebiotics.

These should also be chewed thoroughly. If necessary, a probiotic such as sauerkraut, bread drink, or kefir can help.

If you have the impression that you cannot tolerate gluten or wheat, even though celiac disease has been ruled out, I recommend conducting a self-experiment. Omit gluten from your diet for several weeks and observe whether this has a positive effect on your gut.

My Dietary Recommendations for Irritable Bowel Syndrome

- turmeric (one to two teaspoons a day mixed with black pepper)
- ginger
- berry leaf tea (such as raspberry leaf or blackberry leaf)
- bitters (such as amara drops)
- fennel, caraway seed, or aniseed tea
- chamomile or lemon balm tea
- psyllium, flaxseed, and flaxseed gruel
- wormwood tea (very bitter)
- blueberries (dried or in the form of not-from-concentrate juice)

Fasting for Irritable Bowel Syndrome

If you have irritable bowel syndrome, I recommend therapeutic fasting for seven to ten days. This improves the composition of the microbiome. Both the Buchinger method and the F. X. Mayr method can help. You can gain a lot by chewing thoroughly and eating slowly, which is what the Mayr method teaches.

Patient History: Irritable Bowel Syndrome

Renate S., age sixty-six, a nurse from Berlin, overworked herself to such an extent that she developed irritable bowel syndrome. Switching to an Ayurvedic diet helped bring peace back to her digestive system.

"I have made peace with my gut. . . . I'm doing really well!"

As a nurse, I've worked shifts for forty-five years. In recent years, my workload became so overwhelming that I couldn't sit down and eat some proper food or even go to the bathroom during an eight-hour shift. My body responded with constipation, sometimes for a whole week, then extreme diarrhea lasting for hours. On top of that, I had intense heartburn.

When I retired, I had to take a small job to be able to afford my rent. So I didn't really rest then, either. But I felt that I needed to make a fundamental change, because my gut was torturing me, no matter how often I tried to change my diet. Then I saw Dr. Michalsen on television and realized that he was describing all the symptoms I had. I went to see my GP and asked if Dr. Michalsen's clinic could be the right fit for me—but my GP dismissed my complaints and prescribed a proton pump inhibitor. So, I called the clinic myself. There was a study that was just right for me, but there were no more spaces. Luckily, a few weeks later, the nurse called me back and told me that they could take me.

I had a consultation at admission and was weighed. The scale showed 178 pounds, which was embarrassing for me since I'm only 5'4". Then, over the course of several weeks, I had to write down everything I ate, when I ate, and how my bowel movements were doing. After that, I received nutritional counseling with a naturopathic

Ayurvedic focus, and the doctor explained to me that I could eat much better and healthier. I was, for example, eating a lot of chicken and salad, because I thought that was healthy. And it is—but not for me. I'm a fiery, so-called *pitta* type, and that would need to be dampened. I was given a meal plan. In the mornings, for example, I should have oatmeal with fruit. For lunch, couscous or bulgur with lentils, sweet potatoes, vegetables, mung beans. In the evenings, soup with hempseed, tofu, or seitan. I was to eat three warm meals a day, no salads or cold dishes, and nothing in between—no snacks. When I felt like eating something sweet, I could have steamed fruit with cinnamon and raisins after lunch. And I was to stick to eating at set times: breakfast at seven, lunch at noon, dinner at six p.m.

At first, I thought that I wouldn't be able to keep this up. I was virtually always busy cooking, but at some stage, it started to relax me. Cutting up fruit and vegetables is almost meditative. I got to know a lot of new foods, like soy protein. Spicy food is taboo, so I use a lot of spices like caraway seeds, fennel, cilantro, and turmeric instead. At some point, I was craving chicken—but I noticed how quickly the desire for it evaporated. I just don't need as much meat or fish as I did before.

I don't have scales at home, which is why I only learned at the end of the study, after three months, that I had lost more than 17 pounds! My body fat percentage fell from 44.5 percent to 35.3 percent, and my muscle mass increased from 23.9 percent to 28.5 percent thanks to the exercise in rehab. My body mass index is now 27 instead of 30, my waist shrank from 44 to 35 inches, and my belly circumference went from 46 to 42 inches. Those numbers are nothing to sneeze at! For me, though, what's more important is that I have made peace with my gut. I have hardly any symptoms now—no diarrhea, constipation, or heartburn, and I only take one of the prescribed pills a day. I'm doing really well!

But I also learned to treat myself to rest. I quit my job and moved to a different, cheaper part of the city. That took away a lot of financial pressure. I now do volunteer work, go for walks, or go shopping with elderly people. That gives me some exercise, interaction with other people, and a positive attitude, because I can help others while taking care of myself.

My Recommendations for Inflammatory Bowel Diseases

For inflammatory bowel diseases such as ulcerative colitis and Crohn's disease, my recommendations are essentially the same as for irritable bowel syndrome. IBD occurs in inflammatory episodes, and only a few, very mild foods can be tolerated during such episodes. I recommend eating only rice, potatoes, pureed soups, gruel, and white bread at first—that is, no or little fiber.

Constipation

Many people suffer from constipation and bloating if they have not had a bowel movement for several days. Regular bowel movements (once or twice a day) are undoubtedly healthy. However, constipation is much less threatening than is often assumed. As a rule of thumb, the more fiber you eat, the more regular and natural the type and number of bowel movements. Dietary fiber increases the so-called transit time, the speed at which food is metabolized and its end products are excreted as stool. A transit time of one to two days is optimal. Vegetarians have a clear advantage here, since the intestine needs much more time to digest meat.

You can find out how quickly your intestine works with a beet test: Eat beets and observe when your stool turns a reddish color. If this happens within twenty-four to forty-eight hours, your intestine works well and fast.

If you suffer from IBD and wish to try therapeutic fasting, you should go to a clinic to do so. You should also be very careful and not take any strong laxative measures.

My Therapy for Skin Diseases

In our clinic we treat many patients with skin diseases—psoriasis, neurodermatitis, and rosacea. For these patients, fasting and a change in diet always results in a significant improvement. Often, this is the beginning of the healing process.

> Fasting works for skin diseases in at least two ways: It relieves the metabolism and the liver and reduces stress. This calms the autonomic nervous system; pulse, blood pressure, and breathing rate are lowered.

Psoriasis

Psoriasis is a disease that affects the skin, nails, and often also the joints. Red, flaky inflammation and swelling are characteristic. During an episode, the regeneration of cells is sped up due to the inflammation. While the exfoliation and renewal of the skin cells can take four weeks in healthy people, the cycle is accelerated to a few days in patients with psoriasis. Although psoriasis has a strong hereditary component, most people who are afflicted with it report that triggers such as stress and the wrong diet can worsen symptoms. Excess weight, saturated fats, and alcohol are proven to trigger episodes.[77]

Alcohol, saturated fats, and foods rich in arachidonic acid (meat, sausage, eggs, and dairy products) should be avoided. Patients with celiac disease are more likely to suffer from psoriasis. That's why there are discussions on whether a gluten-free diet could also improve psoriasis. I recommend trying a gluten-free diet only when celiac antibodies in the blood are positive. Although these alone do not prove gluten intolerance, it has been shown that psoriasis patients whose antibodies test positive benefit from a gluten-free diet.

My Dietary Recommendations for Psoriasis

The following foods help with this skin disease:

- turmeric
- flaxseed oil, flaxseed, walnuts (which are rich in omega-3 fatty acids)
- algae
- green tea
- wheat germ oil, black cumin seed oil
- borage
- pomegranate
- ginger
- foods containing quercetin, such as apples, capers, red grapes, onions, broccoli, kale, berries, and sea buckthorn
- fiber (the microbiome of people with psoriasis is often out of balance; fiber helps get it back in balance)

FURTHER MEASURES

Externally, brine baths (with a salinity up to 6 percent) have a soothing effect. Run a bath and pour in some good sea salt. You can tell there's enough salt when the water tastes like seawater.

Therapeutic Fasting for Psoriasis

Therapeutic fasting for seven to ten days leads to a significant improvement for the majority of psoriasis patients with skin or joint problems. Studies show that weight loss helps with this skin disease. Therapeutic fasting, followed by intermittent fasting and a change in diet, can normalize weight in the long run.

Patient History: Psoriasis

Mona N., age forty-eight, a vehicle sales director at a large automobile company in Berlin, had suffered from psoriasis for decades—until she completely changed her diet.

"For me, it was the beginning of a new life."

I realized that I had reached rock bottom when I dropped a file on the sales floor because my hand was simply not strong enough to hold it. I have had psoriasis for thirty years. I used cortisone for years, until my skin became paper-thin. Twenty-three years ago, I was diagnosed with psoriatic arthritis. This means that I have very itchy and painful flaky skin as well as intense joint pain—my hands would get so stiff that I could barely hold anything in them.

For years, I consulted naturopaths to find ways to treat the disease without medication. I have been vegetarian since I was twelve years old, which was probably very lucky, because meat would have fueled the inflammation further. I learned about Dr. Michalsen's clinic in Berlin from a friend. For me, it was the beginning of a new life.

Fasting is an integral part of the clinic's program. I felt great while fasting. I experienced the famous fasting high, was completely euphoric, and my symptoms improved significantly. However, one of the doctors told me that I shouldn't overestimate this; there could be a setback after the stay at the hospital—and that's exactly what happened. But I used it to change my diet and work on my attitude toward the disease. Until then, it had been my enemy, something I needed to fight. Through yoga I understood that the psoriasis is part of me and that I need to treat it and myself carefully—that I don't need to fight it but treat myself well. I listened to Dr. Michalsen's recommendation and started to eat a mostly vegan diet. Instead of focusing on all the things I could no longer eat, I focused on the exciting new recipes I could try and how good they would be for me.

In addition, I followed the dietary directions of Ayurvedic medicine. I've given up snacks, for example. The fruit plate I used to make for myself in the afternoons I now have right after lunch. That way, my intestine gets some time to relax. And I'm following a third recommendation: I no longer eat any plants of the nightshade family, such as bell pepper, tomatoes, or potatoes. They contain lectins, which supposedly also boost inflammation in some people.

My husband and my seven-year-old daughter looked a little startled when I first returned from the clinic with this project, but they quickly enjoyed eating all the different dishes that I cooked. Sure, my husband likes to have a good steak when he's at a restaurant, and my daughter has yogurt and cheese from the school cafeteria, but in the evening we all eat something vegetarian and healthy together, and it gives me joy when my husband comes through the front door and says how wonderful it smells. Recently, I made a mung bean pasta and my loved ones didn't even realize that they weren't eating "real" pasta. And have you ever tried warm lentil salad with spinach? It's excellent!

The best thing for me is that not only is this new diet fun, but I also feel how good it is for me. My joint pain is almost completely gone! And the psoriasis has shrunk to a few small spots. I haven't had that happen in thirty years. I developed the courage to quit my well-paid job in order to have more time for myself and my family and to grow—I'm planning on training as a naturopath. Who better, if not someone who was afflicted herself and has found a way out of her health crisis, to motivate others to try the same? I have already started my new passion: I teach vegan cooking classes for other patients.

Neurodermatitis

Neurodermatitis is more difficult to treat than psoriasis. For many patients, the symptoms are alleviated during a seven- to fourteen-day period of therapeutic fasting, but they often return later on. That's why an individual elimination diet is recommended after fasting. Many patients report that the condition of the skin improves significantly if, for example, they largely avoid sugar and fructose.

Recent findings indicate that probiotics and prebiotics, which support the microbiome, are helpful.[78] That's why I recommend fiber and fermented foods, such as raw sauerkraut, bread drink, tempeh, and organic yogurt. In many cases, extracts of gamma linolenic acid (an unsaturated omega-6 fatty acid that occurs in evening primrose oil, black currant seeds, and borage) as well as plant-based omega-3 fatty acids (flaxseed oil) can also help.[79, 80]

The Ayurvedic dietary therapy recommends avoiding plants of the nightshade family (tomatoes, eggplant, potatoes, and bell pepper) for skin diseases such as psoriasis and neurodermatitis. Possible toxins are no longer a problem in ripe plants of the nightshade family, and these vegetables are very healthy. Nevertheless, I know some patients whose skin improved significantly when they avoided them. My recommendation: It doesn't hurt to try.

Rosacea

Rosacea, also called facial erysipelas, manifests in a reddening and breaking out of the skin. These skin irritations typically appear on the nose and cheeks like a stripe across the face. Often, the skin shows red patches and you can see delicate blood vessels. The cause is believed to be a dysfunction of the nerves in these areas. Triggers such as stress, heat, cold, sun exposure, alcohol, and spices can intensify or trigger rosacea.

There is no reliable data on nutritional therapy for rosacea. But I've observed clear success with therapeutic fasting and intermittent fasting in our patients. During therapeutic fasting the reddening of the skin usually becomes a little worse in the first days, but after the third or fourth day of fasting the skin improves. Therapeutic fasting (a week or two) should be followed by intermittent fasting and a Mediterranean or vegetarian diet.

My Therapy for Allergies and Asthma

Immune diseases such as allergies, hay fever, and allergic asthma have been increasing for years.[81] In a large-scale observational study of more than 140,000 children, an increased allergy rate correlated with the consumption of large amounts of fast food and saturated fats, while fruits and vegetables protected against allergies.[82, 83] Further studies have shown that a Mediterranean and vegetarian diet with few saturated fats can reduce the risk of allergy and asthma.[84, 85] A dysfunctional microbiome and heightened stress levels are further causal factors.[86]

We ask a lot of our immune system. On the one hand, it should quickly and actively ward off hostile attacks. On the other hand, it's not supposed to harm our own body. An allergic shock is a prime example of an overreaction in which the immune system is unable to maintain this balance and reacts too strongly to a trigger (bee venom, for example). The immune defense can then be fatal.

Only a few foods are known to both stimulate the immune system and prevent an overreaction at the same time. These include brewer's yeast and oats, which contain beta-glucans.[87, 88] Yeast or oats can be mixed into food during allergy season as a dietary supplement. Trying prebiotics and fiber can also support the microbiome. Eat less grain, particularly less bread.

Most people suffering from an allergy react to early flowering plants and trees such as birch pollen, and in summer to grass and rye pollen. If you have a pollen allergy or hay fever, watch out for a possible cross allergy. Pip fruit (such as apples and pears) and stone fruit can often cause symptoms for people who have birch pollen allergies; celery can cause symptoms for those with an existing mugwort pollen allergy. However, try not to restrict your diet too much. Especially when it comes to allergic asthma, a diverse diet with a lot of vegetables and fruits can alleviate symptoms.

One new way of looking at food allergies is interesting. Severe reactions occur most commonly to cow's milk, eggs, and peanuts. Until recently, there were only two recognized strategies: first, avoiding the allergens, and second, carrying an emergency kit. But now medical professionals recommend desensitization. Instead of avoiding it, a controlled "encounter" with the allergen is carried out as therapy. Due to the possible side effects, the desensitization should be carried out only under the supervision of an experienced allergist and never on your own.[89] Particularly when it comes to peanut allergy, this seems to be the best method of prevention.

Fasting for Allergies and Asthma

In our clinic, patients suffering from allergies have had good experiences with regular therapeutic fasting. Since the therapeutic method has a strong influence on the microbiome, this effect is not surprising.

Patients have also told me that their allergies improved with intermittent fasting (16:8). Therapeutic fasting followed by intermittent fasting has proven particularly effective in allergic asthma.

My Therapy for Migraines

Migraines are often not taken seriously enough. It is a painful and extremely torturous disease. A very effective group of drugs called triptans have made it so that those afflicted are no longer as vulnerable as they used to be. Triptans, however, do not cure migraines. On the contrary: If taken intensively for a long time (ten to twelve pills a month), they can, like other pain relievers, even worsen the disease.[90] In technical jargon this is called a medication overuse headache or a rebound headache.

There is a genetic component to migraines, as well as familial aggregation. But it is undisputed that environmental factors and lifestyle also play a crucial role as triggers. This explains why the number of migraine sufferers has risen sharply in recent decades. Important causal factors are lack of sleep, stress, hormonal factors, and diet.

Many migraine sufferers are familiar with this fact: They eat a certain food and an attack occurs immediately. Try to identify the foods that trigger a migraine. A headache diary can help. However, my advice is to not only avoid the trigger foods, but to generally choose a diet that can improve the migraines.

My Dietary Recommendations for Migraines

- Avoid foods that can trigger a migraine attack.
- Avoid histamine-containing foods such as cheese (especially hard cheese), smoked meats, canned fish, legumes, chocolate, cocoa, and red wine (or alcohol in general). The fresher a food item is, the less histamine it contains.
- Avoid foods containing tyramine. Like histamine, tyramine blocks the enzyme diamine oxidase (DAO), which is responsible for metabolizing histamine. Accordingly, the foods listed above should be avoided. If necessary, you might also want to avoid the following: citrus fruits, bananas, strawberries, avocado, nuts, yeast, condiments such as stock cubes, and soy sauce.
- Coffee can be a migraine trigger.
- Choose a plant-based diet and make sure to consume whole carbohydrates.
- Give pure sugar a wide berth; avoid sweets and white flour in general—it is believed that fluctuating sugar levels can cause a migraine attack.
- Omega-3 fatty acids have a protective effect, which is why I recommend flaxseed, canola, and soybean oil as well as walnuts.
- Magnesium can have a preventive effect; the mineral is found in legumes, nuts, sprouted grains, and magnesium-rich mineral water.
- Folic acid seems to be effective in preventing migraines; it occurs in leafy greens (the Latin *folia* means "leaves") and many other types of vegetables.
- Choose organic products wherever possible, since they contain little to no preservatives or flavor enhancers, which are also suspected of causing migraine attacks.

> ### My Recommendations for When Migraines Occur
>
> - Ginger extract can be almost as effective as triptans in a migraine attack. When migraines start, drink a strong ginger tea (slice one to two centimeters of gingerroot into thin slices, then pour hot water over them).
> - Bitter substances and bitter foods are traditionally used in naturopathy for impending migraines.
> - I also recommend a hot foot bath.

Therapeutic Fasting for Migraines

Therapeutic fasting (up to fourteen days) can significantly improve migraines by decreasing the frequency and length of attacks. There are no major studies on this, but it is the experience of almost all physicians who specialize in fasting. That said, a severe migraine attack can occur at the start of the therapeutic fasting period. Self-help measures and naturopathic remedies can help alleviate some of the pain when this occurs. It's often better for patients not to take any strong laxative measures at the beginning of the fast—don't use Glauber's salt, just a little Epsom salts. It is especially important to drink enough during the fasting period.

I recommend therapeutic fasting for migraines once or twice a year. For most patients, the intensity and frequency of attacks decrease. After that, the diet can be changed by eliminating all foods that could trigger an attack.

Intermittent Fasting for Migraines

There is no data yet on the therapy and prevention of migraines with intermittent fasting. However, our patients keep telling me that their migraines have improved ever since they started intermittent fasting.

In my experience, migraines, like chronic tension headaches, are mostly triggered by excessive stress. That is why it's imperative to pay attention to stress reduction as well as nutrition.

My Therapy for Depression

According to the Centers for Disease Control and Prevention, 12.7 percent of Americans take antidepressants.[91] Depression is on the rise in all industrialized nations. The causes are multifaceted and have not yet been sufficiently studied.[92]

In conventional medicine, depression is treated with psychotherapy and medications such as tricyclic antidepressants and selective serotonin reuptake inhibitors. Scientific studies show, however, that their effects, when compared with placebo treatments, are rather modest.[93] Of course, in cases of severe depression, drug-based therapy is indispensable.

Less severe forms of depression, on the other hand, can be treated with naturopathic remedies such as Saint-John's-wort, exercise, and thermotherapy. A common side effect of antidepressants is severe weight gain. For this reason alone, I recommend nutritional therapy as an important alternative. Indeed, diet can have a significant effect on depression.

Consuming fruits and vegetables can significantly reduce the risk of depression. Important neurotransmitters in the brain, such as serotonin and dopamine, which ensure a positive mood, are broken down by the enzyme monoamine oxidase (MAO). That's why MAO inhibitors are prescribed for depression.

These inhibitors are naturally found in fruit such as berries, grapes, and apples; vegetables such as onions; and green tea and numerous spices. Australian researchers divided patients with moderate to severe depression into two groups. One group was placed on a Mediterranean diet; the other received psychological support in the form of group sessions. Three months later, the group who followed the Mediterranean diet showed a significant improvement of symptoms, with remission in 32 percent of them, meaning the depression had regressed. In the control group, this was the case in only 8 percent of the participants.[94] Therefore, in the case of mild to moderate depression, a vegetarian or Mediterranean diet is highly recommended.

> **Important:** If you are suffering from depression, don't stop taking your medication without first consulting your doctor! Diet can complement a drug-based therapy or psychotherapy in a meaningful way.

My Dietary Recommendations for Antidepressant Effects

- **Tomatoes and tomato products:** In an observational study, the regular consumption of tomatoes halved the risk of depression.[95] This is probably due to the phytochemical lycopene, which is found in tomatoes in large quantities.
- **Saffron:** Extracts from the most expensive spice in the world seem to inhibit certain receptors in the brain that are also responsible for depression.[96]
- **Chili and ginger:** These hot spices are able to stimulate the brain's serotonin production and stimulate the body's endorphins, which also lift the mood.[97, 98]
- **Tryptophan:** Tryptophan is a precursor to serotonin, which is unable to reach the brain from food due to the blood-brain barrier (a protective barrier to ward off toxins and harmful substances). Tryptophan, on the other hand, can pass this barrier; it is found in walnuts, cocoa, soy, cashews, and milk. Incidentally, carbohydrates ease

> the move of tryptophan to the brain, which may be why we like to eat pasta, cake, and chocolate when we are stressed.
>
> In cases of depression I recommend a healthy plant-based diet including the regular consumption of superfoods, because current scientific data suggests that phytochemicals can have a positive effect on our mood and psyche.[99, 100]

Fasting for Depression

Fasting usually has a mood-lifting, sometimes even euphoric effect. This is most likely due to the increased release of serotonin and other neurotransmitters in the brain.

Depression is often a concomitant symptom in people who are suffering from pain or metabolic syndrome. In these cases, fasting relieves symptoms and improves the quality of life. And this in turn has a positive effect on the mood.

My Therapy for Neurological Diseases

Multiple Sclerosis

Multiple sclerosis (MS) is a chronic autoimmune disease that usually occurs in episodes. The symptoms are diverse and the disease is difficult to diagnose. It is also called the disease of a thousand faces. Unfortunately, the frequency of MS, like other autoimmune diseases, is on the rise in industrialized nations. The causes of this are unclear, but scientists believe a connection to diet and the microbiome is likely.[101] There has been great progress in the drug-based therapy of multiple sclerosis in recent years thanks to new antibody therapies and biologics (biotechnological drugs), but there is still no cure in sight.[102]

So far, there are only a few studies on diet and MS; most findings come from laboratory tests. Scientific data indicate an advantage of Mediterranean and plant-based nutrition. This affects prevention in particular; it has little healing effect on active MS.[103] Patients have repeatedly told me about their good experiences with a ketogenic diet. The ketogenic diet causes the body to shift to a partial fasting metabolism, while also providing it with sufficient calories. This is mainly achieved through meat and dairy products. I would rather recommend a vegetarian version, but it's not that easy to implement. In an initial study, however, we were able to show that a vegetarian ketogenic diet over the course of several months—similar to therapeutic fasting— improves the quality of life in patients with MS.[104]

Another diet that has been propagated for multiple sclerosis for years is the Evers diet. The American physician Joseph Evers blamed environmental factors for MS and developed a plant-based, raw food diet. I would like to advise against this diet. Raw foods are difficult to digest and put additional strain on the body in the event of an existing chronic illness.

My Dietary Recommendations for Multiple Sclerosis

Avoid or reduce these foods:

- saturated fats and foods rich in arachidonic acid (meat, sausage, cheese)
- milk and dairy products (because of their harmful fats; they are also suspected of being a risk factor for the development of MS)[105, 106]
- salt (One study conducted at Charité showed a connection between the consumption of salt and autoimmune processes in multiple sclerosis.[107])

If you are suffering from multiple sclerosis, you should eat more of these foods:

- fiber from whole grains and vegetables
- prebiotics such as chicory, root vegetables, sunchoke, fermented vegetables
- omega-3 fatty acids (flaxseed and canola oil, walnuts)
- longer-chain omega-3 fatty acids from algae
- turmeric
- blueberries
- yarrow (A study conducted in Iran showed surprisingly good effects from an extract containing 250 milligrams of yarrow.[108] In complementary medicine, this plant is traditionally used as an anticonvulsant for gastrointestinal problems and painful menstrual cramps. Yarrow contains flavonoids.)
- frankincense (According to results of an experiment conducted at Charité, this extract may have a supplementary effect in MS.[109])

Important: Taking extracts should always be discussed with your neurologist first.

Therapeutic Fasting for Multiple Sclerosis

The brain researcher Mark Mattson used countless animal laboratory tests to investigate the preventive effects of fasting, particularly intermittent fasting, on chronic neurological diseases. He found the same impressive effects again and again: Intermittent fasting clearly protected the animals from neurodegenerative diseases such as multiple sclerosis, Parkinson's, and dementia.[110] The problem is that these results aren't so easily transferrable to humans.

However, in our first comparative dietary study on MS, we were able to show that both the ketogenic diet and therapeutic fasting, followed by a Mediterranean diet, moderately increase the quality of life in patients after three to six months.[111]

Patients with these diseases should undergo therapeutic fasting only with medical supervision.

Intermittent Fasting for Multiple Sclerosis

Intermittent fasting seems to make sense in addition to therapeutic fasting. After twelve hours of fasting, there is an increase in ketone bodies, which presumably have a beneficial effect on diseased nerve cells. In an ongoing large-scale study, we are currently researching the effects of fasting and intermittent fasting, the Mediterranean diet, and the ketogenic diet with regard to the effects they have on MS centers in the brain.[112]

Parkinson's Disease

In Parkinson's disease there is a slow, progressive destruction of the nerve cells in one region of the midbrain, the substantia nigra, where dopamine is produced. The increasing lack of dopamine leads to movement disorders, tremors, and a general deterioration and slowing down of movement.

Changes in the intestine and environmental toxins are mainly discussed as the cause. The person after whom this disease was named, the British physician James Parkinson (1755–1824), noticed that years before the onset of the disease his patients suffered from digestive problems such as constipation.[113] It has long been suspected that the intestine and the microbiome play a role in the development of Parkinson's. Neurologists in Marburg, Germany, were able to show that ten years before the first symptoms of Parkinson's appear, the bacterial composition of patients' stool was already different from that of healthy people.[114]

Interestingly, the dopaminergic nerves responsible for the disease also exist in the gut, our so-called "stomach brain." Today, the cell disorders typical of Parkinson's disease, the so-called Lewy bodies, can also be detected in intestinal cells. It seems, therefore, that Parkinson's disease actually has its origin in the intestine and only then affects the brain. It fits that the disease occurs less often in people whose vagus nerve, which connects the brain and the gastrointestinal tract, has been severed (this happens in the context of gastric ulcer surgery).[115]

Another curiosity in Parkinson's research explains how the disease could start in the intestine: People whose appendix was removed when they were young are noticeably less likely to develop Parkinson's disease. Scientists discovered a protein called alpha-synuclein, which accumulates in the appendix as well as in the substantia nigra of patients with Parkinson's. One theory assumes that this protein migrates from the appendix to the brain and damages the nerve cells there, especially if other harmful factors such as pesticides are added to our food. This, in turn, would explain why removing the appendix protects the rural population particularly well against Parkinson's. This part of the population is increasingly exposed to pesticides, unless organic farming is practiced nearby. American researchers also found that eating more vegetable fats can reduce the negative impact of pesticides in the rural population in terms of Parkinson's disease.[116, 117] But it would be better not to use pesticides in the first place, and to practice more organic farming!

Environmental toxins such as pesticides and heavy metals are nerve toxins, or neurotoxins. These include dioxin, arsenic, lead, mercury, and many more. These are all substances that we do not want in our bodies.

If Parkinson's disease is diagnosed, I definitely recommend reducing the intake of these toxins via food. The easiest way to do this is to avoid fish, meat, eggs, and dairy products.[118] I explained the harmful substances in fish in the section "Is Fish Healthy?" (see page 57). The pollutant load of the meat of animals such as beef is elevated because they eat one to two tons of plant-based fodder in their lifetime before

they are killed. The pesticides found in the fodder accumulate in the
meat of the animals.

> ### My Dietary Recommendations for Parkinson's Disease
>
> - **Coffee:** It is well known that the caffeine in coffee can prevent Parkinson's disease, but it is not yet clear if it has a curative effect in the case of an already existing illness.[119]
> - **Plants of the nightshade family:** Consuming tomatoes, bell peppers, and eggplant has a preventive effect.[120]
> - **Berries and apples:** People who regularly eat large amounts of berries and apples are better protected against Parkinson's.[121]

Fasting with Parkinson's Disease

See my remarks on fasting with multiple sclerosis (page 331).

My Therapy for Dementia and Alzheimer's

Alzheimer's is the most common form of dementia. The world's lowest
Alzheimer's rates are found in the rural regions of India, where people
follow a predominantly lacto-vegetarian diet. Correspondingly, there is
a rapidly growing number of scientific publications that point to the
role of diet in preventing dementia.[122]

The risk of developing Alzheimer's increases significantly as the
cholesterol level rises. Another factor is alcohol. Studies show that even
small amounts (about 100 ml of wine, which is less than a glass), consumed daily, damage certain areas of the brain such as the hippocampus, where short-term knowledge is transferred to long-term memory.
These studies also observed a limitation of language competence,
which is a fine indicator of the onset of dementia.[123]

The Mediterranean diet in particular, with its high percentage of vegetables and fruits, does well in terms of dementia prevention. According to one study, the MIND-diet (Mediterranean-DASH Intervention for Neurodegenerative Delay), which was specially developed to fight dementia, is said to reduce the risk of Alzheimer's by more than 50 percent. MIND's rule of thumb is three whole-grain products plus vegetables and salad every day.[124, 125]

If you notice memory and concentration diminishing with age (scientists call this cognitive decline) in yourself, a relative, or a friend, a strict Mediterranean or vegetarian/vegan diet can lead to improvement. In studies, three servings of berries (about a handful) and a few glasses of vegetable juice on a regular basis significantly delayed further deterioration of brain performance.[126, 127]

Saffron in particular has an alleviating effect on Alzheimer's symp-

---

A Diet to Improve Cognitive Performance
(Anti-Alzheimer's Diet)

- **Apples:** The active ingredient quercetin in the peel prevents dementia and memory lapses.[128]
- **Dark chocolate:** The phytochemicals in cocoa improve cognitive abilities.[129]
- **Green tea:** The antioxidant epigallocatechin gallate seems to prevent memory loss and nerve damage.[130]
- **Walnuts:** They look like our brain, and they are beneficial for it! The antioxidants contained in walnuts are likely to prevent the protein deposits in the brain that are typical of Alzheimer's.[131, 132]
- **Blueberries:** They stimulate areas of the brain responsible for cognitive and motor skills as well as learning.[133, 134]
- **Saffron:** A plant-based remedy against forgetting.
- **Broccoli and other cruciferous vegetables:** Sulforaphane, an active ingredient found in broccoli, can assist in the treatment of Alzheimer's.[135]

toms. In a comparative study, this alleviation even equaled that of the commonly prescribed Alzheimer's drug donepezil.[136] That said, the latter's effect isn't great. But saffron at least doesn't have any known side effects.

I recommend buying organic foods when following a Mediterranean or plant-based diet. These contain no pesticides and fewer heavy metals. Both toxins are further risk factors for dementia. Also, avoid saltwater fish, as it is polluted with heavy metals.

Fasting for Alzheimer's

Fasting can be a supportive therapy for mild early stages of dementia and also has a preventive effect against Alzheimer's. A research group headed by dementia researcher Agnes Flöel at Charité was able to demonstrate in an initial small-scale human study that slight cognitive impairments in overweight people improved after a modified fast (with liquid food and weight loss).[137] It is possible that during fasting, nerve-enhancing (neurotrophic) factors are released and that the protein plaques surrounding the nerve cells, which are typical in Alzheimer's, are reduced.[138] If dementia is severe, fasting should not be done.

Prevent Cancer Through Diet and Fasting

Different types of cancer differ considerably in terms of risk factors, causes, and progression. But uncontrolled cell growth is common to all types of cancer.

Lifestyle is the cause of certain types of cancer, such as smoking and lung cancer. Other types of cancer, such as leukemia and brain tumors, occur regardless of lifestyle. A familial disposition and other genetic factors such as spontaneous mutations in the course of life are further causes. Generally, diet does play a role, but not to the same extent as for heart attack or hypertension. The degree to which diet can play a role in the development of cancer is estimated at around 30 percent for all types of cancer.[139] Of course, I believe this is something we should take seriously.

In the Blue Zones, it's primarily the Mediterranean and the MediterrAsian diets that are associated with a low risk of cancer. Clinical studies have shown a reduced frequency of cancer for the Mediterranean diet.[140, 141] This is not surprising, since animal protein promotes cancer while fruits and vegetables reduce it.[142, 143] Meat and sausage usually contain carcinogenic substances such as nitrosamines and AGEs (advanced glycation end products; they occur during grilling, for example, and increase the level of harmful substances).[144] It has been proven that milk has carcinogenic effects on prostate cancer (see page 74).[145]

The preventive effect of a healthy diet has been scientifically proven, especially for the most common types of cancer (colon, prostate, and breast cancers).[146] In addition to lots of vegetables and fruit, a low-fat diet provides preventive protection from breast cancer and prevents recurrences.[147]

To prevent colon cancer, avoid meat and eat more fiber.[148] According to recent study data, if you already have colon cancer, you can significantly reduce your risk of a relapse by eating a lot of fiber and nuts.[149, 150]

Patients with prostate cancer should ideally adopt a vegan diet. If you can't manage this, you should at least leave out eggs and poultry. According to one study, three to five servings of poultry a week quadruples the growth rate of prostate cancer tissue.[151]

Avoiding alcohol or at least limiting your intake clearly reduces the general risk of cancer.[152] Red wine seems to be the least carcinogenic alcoholic drink due to the resveratrol contained in the skin of red grapes.[153] But I recommend eating red grapes instead; those with seeds are the healthiest. Unfortunately, more and more types of seedless grapes are cultivated.

A consistent intake of anticarcinogenic substances through food strengthens the immune system and thus its ability to fight cancer cells. In their bestselling book, *Foods That Fight Cancer*, Canadian scientists Richard Béliveau and Denis Gingras compiled a list of suitable foods. That said, as tempting as it is to believe that we can protect ourselves from cancer with onions, tomatoes, and oranges, we need to caution against false hope. No food eaten in isolation is a miracle

---

Nutrition for Cancer Prevention

I can wholeheartedly recommend the following foods for cancer prevention. Thanks to their phytochemicals, they might be able to slow down or even prevent the growth of microtumors in the body.[154] Smaller cell growths occur naturally in the body all the time. It's the task of the immune system—and it usually works very well—to thwart their growth.

- Cruciferous vegetables (broccoli, broccoli sprouts, kale, brussels sprouts, cauliflower, cress, radish)
- green tea
- red grapes with seeds; grape juice
- garlic and onions (especially red onions)
- mushrooms (maitake, shiitake, oyster mushrooms, champignons)
- flaxseed
- olive oil and olives
- turmeric
- berries (blueberries, blackberries, black currants)
- soy products
- parsley
- coffee
- nuts
- whole grains
- apples and pears (not peeled)

weapon that protects against cancer. Most of the data collected so far comes from laboratory tests with cancer cells and cancer tissue. The proof of what this means for cancer prevention in real life is yet to come. But since most of the foods tested in the lab also show preventive and supportive effects on many other diseases, I definitely recommend them.

Fasting for Cancer

Therapeutic fasting and intermittent fasting are probably the only two biological ways to prolong life and prevent old-age diseases. All studies on age research have come to this result.[155] Most cancers result from the fact that the body's own defense mechanisms no longer function as seamlessly due to age.[156]

Almost all data on cancer research and fasting comes from cell and animal studies. Nevertheless, most researchers assume that regular fasting is also particularly suitable for preventing cancer in humans. Initial human studies seem to confirm this.[157, 158, 159] It has been shown that fasting reduces growth hormones and other substances that stimulate the growth of cancer cells while simultaneously promoting the secretion of important protective factors.[160]

It seems it's not important how periods of fasting are scheduled; the main thing is that the body is given the chance to fast. One initial large-scale observational study has shown that women who fasted intermittently for at least thirteen hours daily after breast cancer had a 30 percent lower risk of recurrence.[161] These relationships may not necessarily be causal, but the large amount of data derived from laboratory research strongly indicates that they are. I think it is sufficient to recommend moderate intermittent fasting (14:10) after cancer surgery. Similar effects for regular therapeutic fasting or the fasting mimicking diet are not known.

Fasting During Chemotherapy

It has not yet really been proven whether short-term fasting during chemotherapy improves the patient's well-being, reduces side effects, or even increases the success of the therapy. The results of the largest study to date, conducted by our own research group, suggest that therapeutic fasting according to the Buchinger method at least thirty-six to forty-eight hours before and up to twenty-four hours after chemotherapy can improve quality of life.[162] But it's too early to make a clear assessment, and we need to wait for the results of ongoing studies.

Supplementing chemotherapy with fasting is more difficult when the chemotherapy is administered weekly. Severe weight loss or being underweight should be avoided at all costs. That's why in our ongoing studies with weekly chemotherapy, we conduct only a twenty-four-hour fast from the evening before until the evening of chemotherapy.

I also recommend the fasting mimicking diet during traditional chemotherapy. It starts forty-eight hours before chemotherapy and ends twenty-four hours after; it's a calorie-reduced (700 to 1,100 kcal), vegan, and sugar-free diet. This means that sucrose, added fructose, and artificially sweetened products are avoided; fruit is allowed. But why should the diet be maintained during those twenty-four hours after chemotherapy? This prevents healthy cells from becoming active again while the chemotherapeutic agent is still in the blood, and thus damage to the healthy cells is avoided.

Many patients ask me about the ketogenic diet, since there are indications that it could have a beneficial effect on brain diseases and tumors. Most scientists, however, doubt that it is as powerful as fasting, because it only makes up part of the fasting effect. If you would like to try it, you should make sure to avoid (or only have very little) animal products. This version is harder to do, but it prevents animal proteins from promoting the growth of the cancer cells.

New Knowledge from Age Research

In his painting *The Fountain of Youth*, Lucas Cranach the Elder captured man's eternal longing for everlasting youth, beauty, and immortality. Roughly five hundred years later—in 2013, to be precise—Google founded the biotechnology company Calico (California Life Company), designed to research and stop the aging process. Almost one billion dollars was invested; together with "big data," its research is meant to one day find the magic formula. As commercially successful as Google is, I don't believe the "fountain of youth" can be found this way.

The body is a highly complex system. Billions of signals are sent back and forth from cell to cell in a fraction of a second. Aging processes take place within this constantly communicating marvel of biology—and they have done so since birth. I think the idea of finding eternal life through a supermolecule is naive. We can achieve a life that is as long and as healthy as possible only if we get in sync with our body and its programs. And the best way to do this is to maintain our health through diet and fasting. Because health is a guarantee of autonomy and mobility in old age, and thus of a higher quality of life and more joy in that phase of life.

Spermidine

Healthy centenarians have remarkably high concentrations of spermidine in their blood. It regenerates the DNA, the mitochondria (the power plants of our cells), and various tissues (see page 269). It has anti-inflammatory and anticarcinogenic properties and promotes autophagy.[163] A preliminary observational study and a clinical trial have now shown spermidine's positive effect on life expectancy and cognitive performance.[164, 165, 166]

Many superfoods contain spermidine, and even though I advocate healthy eating as a whole and not individual substances, I would like to recommend a few foods that are rich in spermidine. These include:

- amaranth
- apple
- broccoli and cauliflower
- ripened, sharp cheese
- mushrooms (shiitake)
- salad
- soy and soy products
- whole-grain products
- wheat germ

Our intestinal bacteria, by the way, produce spermidine when they are fed a lot of fiber and prebiotics.

Green and Yellow Vegetables Keep You Young

Scientists have observed that eating green and yellow vegetables is associated with less pronounced wrinkling around the eyes (crow's feet).[167, 168] Lactic acid bacteria (lactobacilli) in yogurt have a similar effect.[169, 170]

Fruit and vegetables with plenty of beta-carotene such as carrots, tomatoes, and sweet potatoes ensure a healthier and fresher complexion.[171] This, while not a direct medical anti-aging effect, is certainly a pleasant side effect.

Sirtfood Diet

Sirt is the abbreviation for "sirtuins." These are proteins that slow down the cell metabolism and thus create an antiaging effect.[172] Fasting increases the production of sirtuins in the body.[173, 174]

Foods containing sirtuins are said to imitate the effect of fasting without your having to fast. In this book, you have met them many times: green tea, kale, apples, citrus fruits, capers, berries, turmeric, chili, dark chocolate, red grapes. So you don't need to spend money on a special sirtuin diet. But these foods do not replace the extensive effects of fasting on the body.

COVID-19

With the coronavirus pandemic, humanity is facing a health threat for which no specific therapy is scientifically established yet. Such a global crisis makes one thing abundantly clear: Our health needs to be a priority. Not someday, but right now.

COVID-19 is not the first new virus that has challenged the world. In the past two decades, we have seen the emergence of other viral diseases such as SARS, MERS, Ebola, and H1N1. It's fair to assume that viruses will continue to challenge health care systems, societies, and economies worldwide in the future. The coronavirus pandemic has shown us that sustainable food production, climate change mitigation, and nature and biodiversity protection cannot be regarded as topics in isolation—they are inextricably linked to one another.

There is clear evidence that the increase in virus transmission from animals to humans is a consequence of the destructive way we humans exploit and interact with nature. Around 70 percent of the newly emerging infectious diseases, and almost all recent pandemics, have originated from animals.[175] Disease emergence correlates with human population density and wildlife diversity; it is driven by deforestation, expansion of land used for livestock production, and increased hunting.[176, 177, 178] Thus, the coronavirus pandemic tells us one important thing: The sooner we adopt a more plant-based diet with less demand for animal products, land, and agricultural intensification and fewer CO_2 emissions, the better the world will be for nature, for animals and—because this is all interconnected—for us humans. Perhaps this can motivate us all to adopt plant-based diets—our health and the health of our planet depend on it!

But can we also protect ourselves individually against viral diseases through nutrition? Yes, we can. Of course, the most urgent medical actions during a pandemic are disinfection, social distancing, protection through personal protective equipment (such as masks and gloves), and medical treatment for those who are ill. However, let's consider disease even more closely. There is the virus, and there is the host. There are two main factors in any infection: first, the pathogenic potency of the microbes, and second, the resilience and autonomy of the host, with the immune system at the forefront. Our immune systems have coexisted with viruses for hundreds of thousands of years over the course of human evolution. Our bodies are well equipped with immune cells and functions to combat viruses, even new ones. And, importantly, we can support and even boost our immune system with our lifestyle and the food we eat. Research so far tells us that the majority of the COVID-19 deaths are linked to age and underlying chronic health conditions. Besides age, the most important risk factors are obesity, followed by heart disease, type 2 diabetes, kidney disease, and cancer. As I've previously mentioned in this book, the number one key to the prevention of these chronic diseases is the food on our plate. A whole-food, plant-based, Mediterranean diet can drastically reduce your risk for these dangerous COVID-19 risk factors and other chronic diseases.

Obesity has been identified in recent studies as a very important risk factor for severe COVID-19 infections.[179, 180, 181] Obesity weakens the body and its immune system through metabolic and inflammatory signals produced by the fat tissue, especially abdominal fat.[182] Moreover, breathing is much more difficult in the case of obesity.[183] Weight normalization, therefore, offers us protection from a severe infection with the coronavirus.

Even age should not be considered a non-modifiable risk factor. Obviously we cannot change our numeric age, but we can influence our biological age. One reason the elderly are at increased risk for COVID-19 is the gradual deterioration of the immune system due to age. Researchers call it "immunosenescence." But as we've learned from the abundant research, with a combination of fasting, lifestyle, exercise, and sufficient sleep, we can influence parts of biological aging to a certain degree. We cannot stop it, but we can decelerate it. Therapeutic fasting, intermittent fasting, fasting mimicking diets, and low-sugar, low-animal-protein diets may impact immunosenescence by stimulating the replacement of old and damaged cells with young and functional cells.[184] Diets that are rich in antioxidants, phytochemicals, and anti-inflammatory nutrients can have a significant impact with regard to chronic diseases, aging, and longevity.[185, 186, 187]

Nutrition plays a major role both in individual susceptibility to infective agents and, if infected, in the outcome of the infectious disease.[188] Hopefully, a vaccination against the coronavirus will soon be available. But even then, food matters. In the Ageing and Dietary Intervention Trial, researchers found 83 healthy volunteers aged 65 to 85 who normally had a low fruit and vegetable intake (2 portions per day or less). The participants were divided into two groups: Those in one group were asked to continue their normal diets; those in the other group were asked to consume at least five servings of fruit and vegetables per day for four months. At the beginning of the study, the participants received a vaccination against pneumococcus, and the antibody response to this vaccination was measured. The results showed that the group that ate five or more servings of fruit and vegetables a day had a much better response to the vaccination. That means the function of our immune system and the quantity of antibody production also depends on our nutrition.[189] We should not forget, a vaccination doesn't work 100 percent. For example, on average, the seasonal flu vaccine has a response rate of slightly above 50 percent, meaning almost half of vaccine recipients don't make enough antibodies to successfully fight the virus. This could also happen with the coronavirus vaccine. So we should make use of the benefits of good nutrition before and after a vaccination is available against COVID-19.

Specific Nutrients and Superfoods

There are a number of superfoods I recommend specifically to strengthen the immune system and our defenses against viruses. We know that many spices and herbs have antimicrobial and antiviral effects.[190, 191] With evolution, nature provided plants with phytochemicals, especially in the outer layers and the peel, to protect them against microbes. When we eat plants, these phytochemicals, with their antimicrobial and antiviral activity, are transferred to us. German researchers have found that many spices and herbs have antiviral effects. Among them are oregano, thyme, pepper, ginger, rosemary, eucalyptus, cinnamon, and lemon peel. At the time the research was conducted, the antiviral effect was mostly measured against herpes, HIV, and influenza. Some spices were also tested against the precursor of COVID-19, the SARS virus, and here, for example, bay leaves showed antiviral activity.[192] Other research has found that numerous aromatic plant oils (specifically found in spices) show antiviral activity against the SARS virus.[193] That plant compounds may act against viruses has been known for many years. For example, the influenza remedy Tamiflu was developed from specific compounds of star anise.

Other research has focused on single substances within plants that may inhibit inflammation and trigger antimicrobial and antiviral activity. These include:

Vitamin C: Found in parsley, peppers, cauliflower, turnips, broccoli, cress, lemons, oranges, brussels sprouts, chives, etc.[194]

Epigallocatechin gallate: Green tea contains catechins, a type of flavonoid and antioxidant, which includes epigallocatechin gallate. Green tea showed antiviral effects in different viral infections from the common cold to influenza to dengue fever.[195, 196, 197]

Quercetin: Found in onions, apples, oregano, chili peppers, and dill. Quercetin has proven antiviral activity in numerous lab studies. It has been tested and documented to have an effect against Zika and Ebola. Interestingly, quercetin also enhances the effect of zinc in the body, and we know that zinc has a beneficial effect on respiratory viral infections.[198, 199, 200]

Myricetin: Found in tomatoes, oranges, garlic, and berries (e.g., cranberries).

Apigenin: Found in chamomile, parsley, goji berries, star fruit, and celery.[201]

Mustard oils: Such as sulforaphane, found in garlic, leeks, onion, green onion, broccoli, kale, and cabbage.[202]

Since the coronavirus is a new virus, we don't know if these nutrients and foods also have antiviral activity against COVID-19, but some new research gives promising hints that this might be the case.

Researchers from Indonesia and Thailand investigated the potential of certain plant compounds to inhibit the ability of COVID-19 to invade the cells.[203] In their study, they found the following plant substances to be effective:

Quercetin: See page 347.

Luteolin: Found in olives, star fruit, chili pepper, leeks.

Demethoxycurcumin: Found in turmeric.

Naringenin: Found in citrus fruits such as lemon, orange, and grapefruit, especially in the peel.

Apigenin: See page 347.

Oleuropein: Found in olives.

Curcumin: Found in turmeric.

Epigallocatechin gallate: See page 347.

Zingerol and gingerol: Found in ginger.

A Vietnamese research group used the same study method for investigating the potential antiviral activity of garlic. Several of the compounds in garlic showed an inhibitory effect on the ACE receptors of somatic cells, which are also used as receptors for the COVID-19 virus.[204]

Probiotics may also have a beneficial influence on defense against COVID-19. In three out of four studies on common cold and respiratory infections of viral origin, the intake of common probiotic lactobacillus and bifidobacterium strains reduced the severity and led to a shorter duration of viral respiratory infections.[205]

Finally, there is one berry that appears to have promising potential, the elderberry.[206] A study of sixteen people with influenza found that those who took 15 ml of elderberry syrup four times a day showed symptom improvement in two to four days, whereas the control group took seven to eight days to improve.[207] Another study of sixty-four people found that taking 175 mg elderberry extract lozenges for two days resulted in significant improvement in flu symptoms, including fever, headache, muscle aches, and nasal congestion after just twenty-four hours.[208] In the lab, elderberry extract was able to inhibit a previous form of coronavirus, different from SARS-COV-2 but still belonging to the same coronavirus family.[209] But note that the bark, unripe berries, and seeds of elderberries contain small amounts of lectins, which can cause stomach problems if too much is eaten. Elderberry is not recommended for children or for pregnant or lactating women. I like to eat it in the form of a syrup or jam—this reduces the amount of beneficial antioxidants but it's very tasty. Or I add fresh elderberries to salad.

Can Fasting Help Prevent or Treat COVID-19?

In several studies, Valter Longo and his team have demonstrated that cycles of fasting or a fasting mimicking diet, followed by a normal diet, are beneficial to stem cells and rejuvenate the immune system in mice. Early clinical trials confirmed that this process of cleaning up older white blood cells during short periods of fasting, then spurring the restoration of the normal levels of the infection-fighting cells when fasting stops may also happen in humans, providing potential health benefits.[210, 211, 212] With its effect on stem cells and its promotion of autophagy, fasting may allow the body to get rid of damaged cells and replace them with younger and more effective immune cells.[213] This is what we know from experiments with mice.

However, there is also some concern about fasting and viral infections. In a 2016 study, researchers at Yale published the results of their experiments with mice. One group of mice fasted, and the other group was fed with glucose. The fasting group had improved defense and survival in the case of bacterial infection with leptospirosis, compared to the group that was fed. But the fasting group had a worse reaction in the case of viral infection with influenza, compared to the group that was fed.[214] But I think it's important to point out that the experiments were done with rather small numbers and a test protocol that does not necessarily reflect the human situation of a natural viral infection with respiratory disease. In the meantime, further research results shed more light on this issue: Another study from Yale found that mice fed a ketogenic diet and infected with the influenza virus had a higher survival rate than mice on a high-carb normal diet. This means that ketones might have a role in infection defense.[215] Furthermore, a recent study on the H1N1 virus found that calorie restriction improved the outcome for this infection.[216]

What we know for sure is that an intermittent or therapeutic fasting routine may better prepare the body for any infectious attack. However, when acutely infected with a virus, one should not start a very strict fast, since for virus defense a certain amount of nutritional energy and glucose are needed. Here, the best guide is the body itself. For centuries, doctors have known about the loss of appetite during an infection. If this is the case, I would not force the body to eat, but give the body what it desires—a (moderate) fast. If the appetite is very pronounced during an infection, or when you or your doctors notice too much weight loss, you should feed the body adequately.

Further recent research points to another aspect of fasting that may be advantageous in viral infections, namely autophagy. In 2020 the German scientist Nils Gassen and his team published an intriguing paper elucidating that autophagy is not only key for prevention of chronic diseases and aging but is also an essential cellular process affecting viral infections.[217] They found that a relative of COVID-19, the Middle East respiratory syndrome coronavirus (MERS), inhibits autophagy and that in turn, enhancers of autophagy fight the replication of the MERS coronavirus. As fasting is one of the strongest inductors of autophagy, this may be a hint for rather beneficial effects of fasting in viral infections.

Gassen's research team, together with the renowned German virologist Christian Drosten, went one step further and looked at the effects of a well-known autophagy enhancer, spermidine.[218] I've already mentioned spermidine several times in this book because of its important function as an elixir that mimics some effects of fasting. In this study, researchers found that the SARS virus limits autophagy. In turn, exogenous administration of spermidine inhibited SARS propagation by 85 percent. However, the high concentrations of spermidine used in the study are not really achievable by simply eating spermidine-rich food. Still, I think considering this, along with all of spermidine's wonderful effects on aging and chronic diseases, we should not miss the opportunity to regularly eat spermidine-rich foods such as wheat germ, apples, pears, mushrooms, soy, and legumes.

When describing the potential benefits of intermittent fasting in viral infection, another substance comes into play—melatonin. This hormone has inhibitory effects on infections, especially on lung injury and inflammation during viral infections.[219] Unfortunately, there is an age-related decline in melatonin production in the body.[220] Supplementing appears not to be so useful, as this does not take into account the complex rhythm of melatonin secretion in the body. The best way to optimize melatonin function and availability in the body is to get enough sleep, to sleep in a dark environment, and to avoid metabolic jet lag by adhering to a regular eating rhythm.

Three Recommendations for Improving Your Defense System Against COVID-19

1) Adopt a plant-based diet with lots of fresh fruit (particularly berries), vegetables, legumes, spices, and nuts.

2) Integrate superfoods into your everyday meals; among them are ginger, turmeric, onions, garlic, celery, broccoli, arugula, cabbage, wheat germ, green tea, elderberries, and cranberries.

3) Practice intermittent fasting with an individual rhythm adapted to your preferences. Once or twice a year, a five- to seven-day therapeutic fasting period will rejuvenate your immune system. For COVID-19, a fasting mimicking diet, which provides some energy and glucose, is especially beneficial.

Clearly, we do not yet know if all the measures I've described here definitely work against COVID-19. And none of this advice should replace social distancing, protection with masks, and (hopefully) a soon-to-be-developed vaccine. Only more clinical trials will bring the necessary evidence, and it's possible not all my suggestions will be confirmed by future science. However, there is one important thing to remember: All of this advice on fasting and nutrition will certainly help your body in the prevention of chronic diseases and decelerating biological aging. And above all, it will enhance your well-being and quality of life.

Epilogue

We know more about nutrition today than ever before. If we eat well—eat better and simply fast—we have done the most important thing we can to keep ourselves healthy, and we will be able to counteract a wide variety of diseases and their progression with great effectiveness.

Of course, a certain incalculability remains, because not everything in life is in our hands alone—as American baseball legend Lawrence Peter "Yogi" Berra once said, "Predictions are difficult, especially about the future."

But if you implement the latest study results and recommendations from my naturopathic experience for yourself, change your diet and tailor it to your individual needs, and start fasting, you have done the most important thing for the protection and maintenance of your health. And you'll learn how much diet can contribute to health.

Because fasting and diet complement each other so ideally, they are the key to our health and to a longer life. Therefore, I would like to answer the question of whether we can live longer through a combination of a healthy diet and regular fasting with a wholehearted yes!

Acknowledgments

My first thank-you goes to my wife, Ileni, who, in the midst of our busy family life, gave me the support and the space I needed to write this book.

The entire team of physicians and therapists of complementary medicine at Immanuel Hospital Berlin and especially the management team of Dr. Ursula Hackermeier, Dr. Christian Kessler, Dr. Barbara Koch, Dr. Susanne Frank, and Dipl.-Psych. Chris von Scheidt for the cooperative work on the subject of healthy nutrition and therapeutic fasting.

The research team on fasting and diet with Dr. Daniel Liebscher, Dr. Michael Jeitler, Dr. Nico Steckhan, and other colleagues for the wonderful cooperation on research projects; special thanks to Alexandra Prus for the compilation of the fasting schedules as well as the critical reading of the manuscript.

The Buchinger Wilhelmi clinics and Françoise Wilhelmi de Toledo in particular for the decades of pioneering work in the field of fasting therapy.

The Medical Association for Fasting and Nutrition (AGHE) for the decades of commitment to fasting therapy, even when it was rejected by many.

Scientists Valter Longo, Frank Madeo, Satchin Panda, Rafael de Cabo, Michael Boschmann, Michelle Harvie, and Krista Varady for their research work, scientific exchange, and the many inspiring conversations on the topic of fasting.

The executive board of Immanuel Hospital Berlin and the Immanuel Albertinen Diakonie for the continuing support of the Department and the Center for Complementary Medicine.

The many clinics and colleagues at Charité Berlin and many other hospitals in Berlin who cooperate in our research on fasting and nutrition.

The donors and foundations for their generous funding, which made possible the research into fasting and plant-based diets.

Professor Claus Leitzmann for his decades of pioneering work in the field of a plant-based whole-food nutrition.

The initiators, organizers, and supporters of the scientific conference VegMed, particularly Dr. Christian Kessler and Elmar Stapelfeldt, the organization ProVeg Germany, as well as Rainer Plum (Reformhaus Akademie Foundation). The conference is an ongoing inspiration for healthy nutrition!

My patients, who inspire me every day with their therapeutic successes thanks to fasting and dietary changes, and who are the most important resource for research into fasting and nutrition.

And last but not least, I would like to thank my editorial publisher, Friedrich-Karl Sandmann, who conceptualized this book and directed its realization with the utmost commitment, and his team: Dr. Suzann Kirschner-Brouns, Eva Römer, Regina Carstensen, Florian Frohnholzer, and Viktoria Kaiser.

Notes

Introduction

1. Luigi Fontana and Samuel Klein, "Aging, Adiposity, and Calorie Restriction," *Journal of the American Medical Association* 297, no. 9 (2007): 986–94, https://doi .org/10.1001/jama.297.9.986.
2. Mark P. Mattson, Valter D. Longo, and Michelle Harvie, "Impact of Intermittent Fasting on Health and Disease Processes," *Ageing Research Reviews* 39 (2017): 46–58, https://doi.org/10.1016/j.arr.2016.10.005.
3. Andreas Michalsen and Chenying Li, "Fasting Therapy for Treating and Preventing Disease—Current State of Evidence," *Forschende Komplementärmedizin Research in Complementary Medicine* 20, no. 6 (2013): 444–53, https://doi.org /10.1159/000357765.
4. World Health Organization, *Diet, Nutrition and the Prevention of Chronic Diseases* (Geneva: 2003), https://www.who.int/dietphysicalactivity/publications/trs916/en.
5. "Global, Regional, and National Life Expectancy, All-Cause Mortality, and Cause-Specific Mortality for 249 Causes of Death, 1980–2015: A Systematic Analysis for the Global Burden of Disease Study 2015," *Lancet* 388, no. 10053 (2016): 1459–1544, https://doi.org/10.1016/S0140-6736(16)31012-1.

Chapter One: Rediscovering the Natural and Healthy Rhythm of Eating

1. World Health Organization, *Diet, Nutrition and the Prevention of Chronic Diseases*.
2. Patrice D. Cani, "Human Gut Microbiome: Hopes, Threats and Promises," *Gut* 67, no. 9 (2018): 1716–25, https://doi.org/10.1136/gutjnl-2018-316723.

3. Alex R. DeCasien, Scott A. Williams, and James P. Higham, "Primate Brain Size Is Predicted by Diet but Not Sociality," *Nature Ecology and Evolution* 1, no. 5 (2017), https://doi.org/10.1038/s41559-017-0112.

4. Detlev Ganten, Thilo Spahl, and Thomas Deichmann, *Die Steinzeit Steckt Uns in Den Knochen: Gesundheit Als Erbe Der Evolution* (Munich: Piper, 2009).

5. Jared Diamond, *The Third Chimpanzee: The Evolution and Future of the Human Animal* (New York: HarperCollins, 1992).

6. David J. A. Jenkins et al., "The Garden of Eden—Plant Based Diets, the Genetic Drive to Conserve Cholesterol and Its Implications for Heart Disease in the 21st Century," *Comparative Biochemistry and Physiology Part A: Molecular and Integrative Physiology* 136, no. 1 (2003): 141–51, https://doi.org/10.1016/s1095 -6433(02)00345-8.

7. Bethany L. Turner and Amanda L Thompson, "Beyond the Paleolithic Prescription: Incorporating Diversity and Flexibility in the Study of Human Diet Evolution," *Nutrition Reviews* 71, no. 8 (2013): 501–10, https://doi.org/10.1111/nure.12039.

8. Valter D. Longo and Mark P. Mattson, "Fasting: Molecular Mechanisms and Clinical Applications," *Cell Metabolism* 19, no. 2 (2014): 181–92, https://doi.org /10.1016/j.cmet.2013.12.008.

9. Hans Konrad Biesalski, Susanne Warmuth, and Oliver Domzalski, *Unsere Ernährungsbiografie Wer Sie Kennt, Lebt Gesünder* (Munich: Knaus, 2017).

10. Nissim Silanikove, Gabriel Leitner, and Uzi Merin, "The Interrelationships Between Lactose Intolerance and the Modern Dairy Industry: Global Perspectives in Evolutional and Historical Backgrounds," *Nutrients* 7, no. 9 (2015): 7312–31, https://doi.org/10.3390/nu7095340.

11. Biesalski, Warmuth, and Domzalski, *Unsere Ernährungsbiografie Wer Sie Kennt, Lebt Gesünder.*

12. "Global, Regional, and National Life Expectancy."

13. Chelsea E. Hawley et al., "Statins for Primary Prevention in Those Aged 70 Years and Older: A Critical Review of Recent Cholesterol Guidelines," *Drugs and Aging* 36, no. 8 (2019): 687–99, https://doi.org/10.1007/s40266-019-00673-w.

14. J. Casale and M. R. Huecker, "Fasting," in *StatPearls* (Treasure Island, FL: StatPearls, 2020).

15. Daniela Artemis Tahère Liebscher, *Religiöses Fasten im Medizinischen Kontext Auswirkungen auf Anthropometrische Parameter, Blutfettwerte und Hämodynamik* (Essen, Germany: KVC Verlag, 2013).

16. Otto Buchinger, *Das Heilfasten und Seine Hilfsmethoden Als Biologischer Weg* (Stuttgart, Germany: Georg Thieme Verlag, 2005).

17. Buchinger, *Das Heilfasten und Seine Hilfsmethoden Als Biologischer Weg.*

18. Mark Twain, *Following the Equator: A Journey Around the World* (Hartford, CT: American Pub. Co., 1899).

19. Upton Sinclair, *The Fasting Cure* (Scholar Select, 2015).

20. Robert A. Gunn, *Forty Days Without Food! A Biography of Henry S. Tanner, M.D., Including a Complete and Accurate History of His Wonderful Fasts, Viz.: 42 Days in Minneapolis, Minn., and 40 Days in New York City, with Valuable Deductions* (New York: A. Metz, 1880).

21. Edward Hooker Dewey, *The No-Breakfast Plan and the Fasting-Cure* (Meadville, PA: 1900).

22. Mandy Oaklander, "Valter Longo: The Fasting Evangelist," *Time*, October 18, 2018, https://time.com/collection/health-care-50/5425015/valter-longo.

23. Valter D. Longo and Satchidananda Panda, "Fasting, Circadian Rhythms, and Time-Restricted Feeding in Healthy Lifespan," *Cell Metabolism* 23, no. 6 (2016): 1048–59, https://doi.org/10.1016/j.cmet.2016.06.001.

24. Samuel M. Flaxman and Paul W. Sherman, "Morning Sickness: A Mechanism for Protecting Mother and Embryo," *Quarterly Review of Biology* 75, no. 2 (2000): 113–48, https://doi.org/10.1086/393377.

25. Flaxman and Sherman, "Morning Sickness."

26. Jean-Jacques Hublin, *The Evolution of Hominin Diets: Integrating Approaches to the Study of Paleolithic Subsistence* (Dordrecht, Netherlands: Springer, 2009).

27. Rob Dunn, "Human Ancestors Were Nearly All Vegetarians," *Guest Blog, Scientific American*, July 23, 2012, https://blogs.scientificamerican.com/guest-blog/human-ancestors-were-nearly-all-vegetarians.

28. Lucy J. E. Cramp et al., "Immediate Replacement of Fishing with Dairying by the Earliest Farmers of the Northeast Atlantic Archipelagos," *Proceedings of the Royal Society B: Biological Sciences* 281, no. 1780 (2014), https://doi.org/10.1098/rspb.2013.2372.

29. Ursula E. Bauer et al., "Prevention of Chronic Disease in the 21st Century: Elimination of the Leading Preventable Causes of Premature Death and Disability in the USA," *Lancet* 384, no. 9937 (2014): 45–52, https://doi.org/10.1016/s0140-6736(14)60648-6.

30. Hashem B. El-Serag et al., "Update on the Epidemiology of Gastro-Oesophageal Reflux Disease: A Systematic Review," *Gut* 63, no. 6 (2013): 871–80, https://doi.org/10.1136/gutjnl-2012-304269.

31. Human Microbiome Jumpstart Reference Strains Consortium, "A Catalog of Reference Genomes from the Human Microbiome," *Science* 328, no. 5981 (2010): 994–9, doi:10.1126/science.1183605.

32. Cani, "Human Gut Microbiome."

33. Mi Young Lim et al., "The Effect of Heritability and Host Genetics on the Gut Microbiota and Metabolic Syndrome," *Gut* 66, no. 6 (2016): 1031–8, https://doi.org/10.1136/gutjnl-2015-311326.

34. Susan V. Lynch and Oluf Pedersen, "The Human Intestinal Microbiome in Health and Disease," *New England Journal of Medicine* 375, no. 24 (2016): 2369–79, https://doi.org/10.1056/nejmra1600266.

35. Vinod K. Gupta, Sandip Paul, and Chitra Dutta, "Geography, Ethnicity or Subsistence-Specific Variations in Human Microbiome Composition and Diversity," *Frontiers in Microbiology* 8 (2017): 1162, https://doi.org/10.3389/fmicb.2017.01162.

36. Jose C. Clemente et al., "The Microbiome of Uncontacted Amerindians," *Science Advances* 1, no. 3 (2015), https://advances.sciencemag.org/content/1/3/e1500183.

37. Lawrence A. David et al., "Diet Rapidly and Reproducibly Alters the Human Gut Microbiome," *Nature* 505, no. 7484 (2014): 559–63, https://doi.org/10.1038/nature12820.

38. Marlene Remely et al., "Increased Gut Microbiota Diversity and Abundance of Faecalibacterium Prausnitzii and Akkermansia after Fasting: A Pilot Study," *Wiener Klinische Wochenschrift* 127, no. 9–10 (2015): 394–8, https://doi.org/10.1007/s00508-015-0755-1.

39. Xinpu Chen and Sridevi Devaraj, "Gut Microbiome in Obesity, Metabolic Syndrome, and Diabetes," *Current Diabetes Reports* 18, no. 12 (2018), https://doi.org/10.1007/s11892-018-1104-3.

40. Christoph A. Thaiss et al., "A Day in the Life of the Meta-Organism: Diurnal Rhythms of the Intestinal Microbiome and Its Host," *Gut Microbes* 6, no. 2 (2015): 137–42, https://doi.org/10.1080/19490976.2015.1016690.

41. Mairi H. McLean et al., "Does the Microbiota Play a Role in the Pathogenesis of Autoimmune Diseases?" *Gut* 64, no. 2 (2014): 332–41, https://doi.org/10.1136/gutjnl-2014-308514.

42. J. S. Bell et al., "Invited Review: From Nose to Gut—The Role of the Microbiome in Neurological Disease," *Neuropathology and Applied Neurobiology* 45, no. 3 (2019): 195–215, https://doi.org/10.1111/nan.12520.

43. Jimmy Moore and Jason Fung, *Fasten—Das Große Handbuch Heilen Sie Ihren Körper mit Kurzem, Langem und Intermittierendem Fasten* (Munich: Riva, 2017).

44. Suzanne Floyd et al., "The Insulin-like Growth Factor-I–mTOR Signaling Pathway Induces the Mitochondrial Pyrimidine Nucleotide Carrier to Promote Cell Growth," *Molecular Biology of the Cell* 18, no. 9 (2007): 3545–55, https://doi.org/10.1091/mbc.e06-12-1109.

Chapter Two: The Healthiest Places in the World

1. Dan Buettner, *The Blue Zones: Lessons for Living Longer from the People Who've Lived the Longest* (Washington, DC: National Geographic Books, 2008).

2. S. Miyagi et al., "Longevity and Diet in Okinawa, Japan: The Past, Present and Future," *Asia Pacific Journal of Public Health* 15, no. 1_suppl (2003): S3–9, https://doi.org/10.1177/101053950301500s03.

3. David G. Le Couteur et al., "New Horizons: Dietary Protein, Ageing and the Okinawan Ratio," *Age and Ageing* 45, no. 4 (2016): 443–7, https://doi.org/10.1093/ageing/afw069.

4. Tyler Garner et al., "Sweet Potato (Ipomoea Batatas) Attenuates Diet-Induced Aortic Stiffening Independent of Changes in Body Composition," *Applied Physiology, Nutrition, and Metabolism* 42, no. 8 (2017): 802–9, https://doi.org/10.1139/apnm-2016-0571.

5. Kayo Kurotani et al., "Quality of Diet and Mortality Among Japanese Men and Women: Japan Public Health Center Based Prospective Study," *BMJ* 352:i1209 (2016), https://doi.org/10.1136/bmj.i1209.

6. "Rekord: Mehr Als 70.000 Hundertjährige in Japan—Doch Es Gibt ein Problem," Watson.de, September 13, 2019, https://www.watson.de/international/japan/412822759-rekord-mehr-als-70-000-hundertjaehrige-in-japan-doch-es-gibt-ein-problem.

7. Buettner, *The Blue Zones.*

8. Marc Luy, "Causes of Male Excess Mortality: Insights from Cloistered Populations," *Population and Development Review* 29, no. 4 (2003): 647–76, https://doi .org/10.1111/j.1728-4457.2003.00647.x.

9. G. M. Pes et al., "Male Longevity in Sardinia, a Review of Historical Sources Supporting a Causal Link with Dietary Factors," *European Journal of Clinical Nutrition* 69, no. 4 (2015): 411–8, https://doi.org/10.1038/ejcn.2014.230.

10. Androniki Naska et al., "Siesta in Healthy Adults and Coronary Mortality in the General Population," *Archives of Internal Medicine* 167, no. 3 (2007): 296–301, https://doi.org/10.1001/archinte.167.3.296.

11. Basil H. Aboul-Enein, William C. Puddy, and Joshua Bernstein, "Ancel Benjamin Keys (1904–2004): His Early Works and the Legacy of the Modern Mediterranean Diet," *Journal of Medical Biography* (2017), 096777201772769, https://doi .org/10.1177/0967772017727696.

12. C. Michael Wright, "Biographical Notes on Ancel Keys and Salim Yusuf: Origins and Significance of the Seven Countries Study and the INTERHEART Study," *Journal of Clinical Lipidology* 5, no. 6 (2011): 434–40, https://doi.org/10.1016/j .jacl.2011.09.003.

13. Leah M. Kalm and Richard D. Semba, "They Starved So That Others Be Better Fed: Remembering Ancel Keys and the Minnesota Experiment," *Journal of Nutrition* 135, no. 6 (2005): 1347–52, https://doi.org/10.1093/jn/135.6.1347.

14. Ancel Keys, *Seven Countries: A Multivariate Analysis of Death and Coronary Heart Disease* (Cambridge, MA: Harvard University Press, 1980).

15. Keys, *Seven Countries.*

16. Keys, *Seven Countries.*

17. Antonia Trichopoulou et al., "Definitions and Potential Health Benefits of the Mediterranean Diet: Views from Experts Around the World," *BMC Medicine* 12, no. 1 (2014): 112, https://doi.org/10.1186/1741-7015-12-112.

18. H. E. Bloomfield et al., *Benefits and Harms of the Mediterranean Diet Compared to Other Diets* (Washington, DC: Department of Veterans Affairs, 2015), https:// www.ncbi.nlm.nih.gov/books/NBK379574.

19. Trichopoulou et al., "Definitions and Potential Health Benefits of the Mediterranean Diet."

20. Susana Casal et al., "Olive Oil Stability Under Deep-Frying Conditions," *Food and Chemical Toxicology* 48, no. 10 (2010): 2972–9, https://doi.org/10.1016/j .fct.2010.07.036.

21. David S. Ludwig et al., "Dietary Fat: From Foe to Friend?" *Science* 362, no. 6416 (2018): 764–70, https://doi.org/10.1126/science.aau2096.

22. Matthew L. Lindberg and Ezra A. Amsterdam, "Alcohol, Wine, and Cardiovascular Health," *Clinical Cardiology* 31, no. 8 (2008): 347–51, https://doi.org /10.1002/clc.20263.

23. Anya Topiwala et al., "Moderate Alcohol Consumption as Risk Factor for Adverse Brain Outcomes and Cognitive Decline: Longitudinal Cohort Study," *BMJ* 357 (2017), https://doi.org/10.1136/bmj.j2353.

24. Max G. Griswold et al., "Alcohol Use and Burden for 195 Countries and Territories, 1990–2016: A Systematic Analysis for the Global Burden of Disease Study 2016," *Lancet* 392, no. 10152 (2018): 1015–35, https://doi.org/10.1016/s0140 -6736(18)31310-2.

25. "Alcohol and Cancer," *Lancet* 390, no. 10109 (2017): 2215, https://doi.org/10.1016 /s0140-6736(17)32868-4.

26. Trichopoulou et al., "Definitions and Potential Health Benefits of the Mediterranean Diet."

27. Kathrin Pallauf et al., "Nutrition and Healthy Ageing: Calorie Restriction or Polyphenol-Rich 'MediterrAsian' Diet?" *Oxidative Medicine and Cellular Longevity* 2013 no. 1 (2013): 1–14, https://doi.org/10.1155/2013/707421.

28. Shino Oba et al., "Diet Based on the Japanese Food Guide Spinning Top and Subsequent Mortality Among Men and Women in a General Japanese Population," *Journal of the American Dietetic Association* 109, no. 9 (2009): 1540–7, https://doi.org/10.1016/j.jada.2009.06.367.

29. Kayo Kurotani et al., "Quality of Diet and Mortality Among Japanese Men and Women."

30. T. Colin Campbell and Thomas M. Campbell II, *China Study: Revised and Expanded Edition: The Most Comprehensive Study of Nutrition Ever Conducted and the Startling Implications for Diet, Weight Loss, and Long-Term Health* (Dallas: BenBella Books, 2017).

31. "22. Christlicher Lebensstil," Freikirche der Siebenten-Tags-Adventisten, https:// nib.adventisten.de/utility/ueber-uns/unsere-glaubensueberzeugungen/22 -christlicher-lebensstil.

32. Gary E. Fraser and David J. Shavlik, "Ten Years of Life: Is It a Matter of Choice?" *Archives of Internal Medicine* 161, no. 13 (2001): 1645–52, https://doi.org/10.1001 /archinte.161.13.1645.

33. Fatemeh Kiani et al., "Dietary Risk Factors for Ovarian Cancer: The Adventist Health Study (United States)," *Cancer Causes and Control* 17, no. 2 (2006): 137–46, https://doi.org/10.1007/s10552-005-5383-z.

34. J. Chan et al., "Water, Other Fluids, and Fatal Coronary Heart Disease: The Adventist Health Study," *American Journal of Epidemiology* 155, no. 9 (2002): 827–33, https://doi.org/10.1093/aje/155.9.827.

35. Buettner, *The Blue Zones.*

36. A. G. Shaper and K. W. Jones, "Serum-Cholesterol, Diet, and Coronary Heart-Disease in Africans and Asians in Uganda," *Lancet* 274, no. 7102 (1959): 534–7, https://doi.org/10.1016/s0140-6736(59)91777-5.

37. Wilbur A. Thomas et al., "Incidence of Myocardial Infarction Correlated with Venous and Pulmonary Thrombosis and Embolism," *American Journal of Cardiology* 5, no. 1 (1960): 41–7, https://doi.org/10.1016/0002-9149(60)90007-2.

38. D. P. Burkitt, "Western Diseases and Their Emergence Related to Diet," *South African Medical Journal* 61, no. 26 (1982): 1013–5.

39. C. Donnison, "Blood Pressure in the African Native. Its Bearing upon the Ætiology of Hyperpiesia and Arterio-sclerosis," *Lancet* 213, no. 5497 (1929): 6–7, https://doi.org/10.1016/s0140-6736(00)49248-2.

40. Hillard Kaplan et al., "Coronary Atherosclerosis in Indigenous South American Tsimane: A Cross-Sectional Cohort Study," *Lancet* 389, no. 10080 (2017): 1730–9, https://doi.org/10.1016/s0140-6736(17)30752-3.

41. Hilary J. Bethancourt et al., "Longitudinal Changes in Measures of Body Fat and Diet Among Adult Tsimane' Forager-Horticulturalists of Bolivia, 2002–2010," *Obesity* 27, no. 8 (2019): 1347–59, https://doi.org/10.1002/oby.22556.

42. Buettner, *The Blue Zones*.

Chapter Three: Essential Nutrients and Where They Are Found

1. Abdollah Ghavami, W. Andy Coward, and Les J. C. Bluck, "The Effect of Food Preparation on the Bioavailability of Carotenoids from Carrots Using Intrinsic Labelling," *British Journal of Nutrition* 107, no. 9 (2012): 1350–66, https://doi.org /10.1017/s000711451100451x.

2. W. C. Willett, "Dietary Fats and Coronary Heart Disease," *Journal of Internal Medicine* 272, no. 1 (2012): 13–24, https://doi.org/10.1111/j.1365-2796.2012.02553.x.

3. Ludwig et al., "Dietary Fat: From Foe to Friend?"

4. Mahshid Dehghan et al., "Association of Dairy Intake with Cardiovascular Disease and Mortality in 21 Countries from Five Continents (PURE): A Prospective Cohort Study," *Lancet* 392, no. 10161 (2018): 2288–97, https://doi.org/10.1016 /s0140-6736(18)31812-9.

5. Dean Ornish et al., "Intensive Lifestyle Changes for Reversal of Coronary Heart Disease," *Journal of the American Medical Association* 280, no. 23 (1998): 2001–7, https://doi.org/10.1001/jama.280.23.2001.

6. Michel de Lorgeril, "Mediterranean Diet and Cardiovascular Disease: Historical Perspective and Latest Evidence," *Current Atherosclerosis Reports* 15, no. 12 (2013), https://doi.org/10.1007/s11883-013-0370-4.

7. Sabri Rial et al., "Gut Microbiota and Metabolic Health: The Potential Beneficial Effects of a Medium Chain Triglyceride Diet in Obese Individuals." *Nutrients* 8, no. 5 (2016): 281, https://doi.org/10.3390/nu8050281.

8. F. Visioli et al., "Olive Oil and Prevention of Chronic Diseases: Summary of an International Conference," *Nutrition, Metabolism and Cardiovascular Diseases* 28, no. 7 (2018): 649–56, https://doi.org/10.1016/j.numecd.2018.04.004.

9. Ramón Estruch et al., "Primary Prevention of Cardiovascular Disease with a Mediterranean Diet," *New England Journal of Medicine* 368 (2014): 1279–90, https://doi.org/10.1056/NEJMoa1200303.

10. Delfin Rodriguez-Leyva et al., "Potent Antihypertensive Action of Dietary Flaxseed in Hypertensive Patients," *Hypertension* 62, no. 6 (2013): 1081–9, https://doi .org/10.1161/hypertensionaha.113.02094.

11. Aiguo Wu et al., "Curcumin Boosts DHA in the Brain: Implications for the Prevention of Anxiety Disorders," *Biochimica et Biophysica Acta (BBA)—Molecular Basis of Disease* 1852, no. 5 (2015): 951–61, https://doi.org/10.1016/j.bbadis.2014.12.005.

12. Akshay Goel et al., "Fish, Fish Oils and Cardioprotection: Promise or Fish Tale?" *International Journal of Molecular Sciences* 19, no. 12 (2018): 3703, https://doi.org /10.3390/ijms19123703.

13. O. Adam, "Dietary Fatty Acids and Immune Reactions in Synovial Tissue," *European Journal of Medical Research* 8, no. 8 (2003): 381–7.

14. Asmaa S. Abdelhamid et al., "Omega-3 Fatty Acids for the Primary and Secondary Prevention of Cardiovascular Disease," *Cochrane Database of Systematic Reviews* 7, no. 7 (2018), https://doi.org/10.1002/14651858.cd003177.pub4.

15. Mingyang Song et al., "Association of Animal and Plant Protein Intake with All-Cause and Cause-Specific Mortality," *JAMA Internal Medicine* 176, no. 10 (2016): 1453–63, https://doi.org/10.1001/jamainternmed.2016.4182.

16. J. Dyerberg et al., "Eicosapentaenoic Acid and Prevention of Thrombosis and Atherosclerosis?" *Lancet* 312, no. 8081 (1978): 117–9, https://doi.org/10.1016/s0140-6736(78)91505-2.

17. J. George Fodor et al., "'Fishing' for the Origins of the 'Eskimos and Heart Disease' Story: Facts or Wishful Thinking?" *Canadian Journal of Cardiology* 30, no. 8 (2014): 864–8, https://doi.org/10.1016/j.cjca.2014.04.007.

18. Sven O. E. Ebbesson et al., "Eskimos Have CHD Despite High Consumption of Omega-3 Fatty Acids: The Alaska Siberia Project," *International Journal of Circumpolar Health* 64, no. 4 (2005): 387–95, https://doi.org/10.3402/ijch.v64i4.18015.

19. Fodor et al., "'Fishing' for the Origins of the 'Eskimos and Heart Disease' Story."

20. M. L. Burr, F. D. J. Dunstan, and C. H. George, "Is Fish Oil Good or Bad for Heart Disease? Two Trials with Apparently Conflicting Results," *Journal of Membrane Biology* 206, no. 2 (2005): 155–63, https://doi.org/10.1007/s00232-005-0784-1.

21. Burr, Dunstan, and George, "Is Fish Oil Good or Bad for Heart Disease?"

22. Ahmad Jayedi, Mahdieh Sadat Zargar, and Sakineh Shab-Bidar, "Fish Consumption and Risk of Myocardial Infarction: A Systematic Review and Dose-Response Meta-Analysis Suggests a Regional Difference," *Nutrition Research* 62 (2019): 1–12, https://doi.org/10.1016/j.nutres.2018.10.009.

23. José G. Dórea, "Studies of Fish Consumption as Source of Methylmercury Should Consider Fish-Meal-Fed Farmed Fish and Other Animal Foods," *Environmental Research* 109, no. 1 (2009): 131–2, https://doi.org/10.1016/j.envres.2008.10.004.

24. Ryozo Nakagawa, "Concentration of Mercury in Hair of Diseased People in Japan," *Chemosphere* 30, no. 1 (1995): 135–40, https://doi.org/10.1016/0045-6535(94)00383-6.

25. Christoph D. Rummel et al., "Plastic Ingestion by Pelagic and Demersal Fish from the North Sea and Baltic Sea," *Marine Pollution Bulletin* 102, no. 1 (2016): 134–41, https://doi.org/10.1016/j.marpolbul.2015.11.043.

26. "Fischbestände Weltweit Gefährdet," NABU, https://www.nabu.de/natur-und-landschaft/meere/fischerei/index.html.

27. "International Symposium on Fisheries Sustainability," Food and Agriculture Organization of the United Nations, http://www.fao.org/about/meetings/sustainable-fisheries-symposium/en.

28. "International Symposium on Fisheries Sustainability."

29. Tizra Meyer, "Giftige Fischsuppe," *Frankfurter Allgemeine Zeitung*, March 29, 2018: https://www.faz.net/aktuell/race-to-feed-the-world/norwegischer-lachs-fuer-die-welt-giftige-fischsuppe-15499637.html.

30. Md Ashraful Islam et al., "Trans Fatty Acids and Lipid Profile: A Serious Risk Factor to Cardiovascular Disease, Cancer and Diabetes," *Diabetes and Metabolic Syndrome* 13, no. 2 (2019): 1643–7, https://doi.org/10.1016/j.dsx.2019.03.033.

31. "Trans Fat," US Food and Drug Administration, https://www.fda.gov/food/food-additives-petitions/trans-fat.

32. Ornish et al., "Intensive Lifestyle Changes for Reversal of Coronary Heart Disease."

33. C. B. Esselstyn Jr. et al., "A Way to Reverse CAD?" *Journal of Family Practice* 63, no. 7 (2014): 356–64b.

34. Esselstyn et al., "A Way to Reverse CAD?"

35. O. Adam, "Dietary Fatty Acids and Immune Reactions in Synovial Tissue."

36. "Cardiovascular Risk Reduction with Icosapent Ethyl," *New England Journal of Medicine* 380, no. 17 (2019): 1677–8, https://doi.org/10.1056/nejmc1902165.

37. John McDougall, "Plant Foods Have a Complete Amino Acid Composition," *Circulation* 105, no. 25 (2002): e197, https://doi.org/10.1161/01.cir.0000018905.97677.1f.

38. Paul J. Moughan et al., "Food-Derived Bioactive Peptides—A New Paradigm," *Nutrition Research Reviews* 27, no. 1 (2013): 16–20, https://doi.org/10.1017/s0954422413000206.

39. Selene Yeager and Emilia Benton, "Everything to Know About Eating a High-Protein Diet for Weight Loss," *Women's Health*, May 22, 2020, https://www.womenshealthmag.com/weight-loss/a19907503/protein-weight-loss.

40. Marianne Wellershoff, "Die Effekte Sind Enorm," *Der Spiegel*, August 4, 2018, https://www.spiegel.de/wissenschaft/fasten-und-kalorienreduzierte-ernaehrung-die-effekte-sind-enorm-a-557a03a0-046b-4e87-ba71-94d8e528072b.

41. Jie Yin et al., "Protein Restriction and Cancer," *Biochimica et Biophysica Acta (BBA)—Reviews on Cancer* 1869, no. 2 (2018): 256–62, https://doi.org/10.1016/j.bbcan.2018.03.004.

42. Yin et al., "Protein Restriction and Cancer."

43. Le Couteur et al., "New Horizons."

44. Katy McLaughlin and Ron Winslow, "Report Details Dr. Atkins's Health Problems," *Wall Street Journal*, February 10, 2004, https://www.wsj.com/articles/SB107637899384525268.

45. A. Bierhaus et al., "AGEs and Their Interaction with AGE-Receptors in Vascular Disease and Diabetes Mellitus. I. The AGE Concept," *Cardiovascular Research* 37, no. 3 (1998): 586–600, https://doi.org/10.1016/s0008-6363(97)00233-2.

46. A. Michalsen et al.,"Glykotoxine Und Zellaktivierung," *Bundesgesundheitsblatt Gesundheitsforschung Gesundheitsschutz* 49, no. 8 (2006): 773–9, https://doi.org/10.1007/s00103-006-0007-7.

47. Morgan E. Levine et al., "Low Protein Intake Is Associated with a Major Reduction in IGF-1, Cancer, and Overall Mortality in the 65 and Younger but Not Older Population," *Cell Metabolism* 19, no. 3 (2014): 407–17, https://doi.org/10.1016/j.cmet.2014.02.006.

48. Teresa A. Davis et al., "Amino Acid Composition of Human Milk Is Not Unique," *Journal of Nutrition* 124, no. 7 (1994): 1126–32, https://doi.org/10.1093/jn/124.7.1126.

49. Ekhard E. Ziegler, "Adverse Effects of Cow's Milk in Infants," *Issues in Complementary Feeding: Nestlé Nutrition Workshop Series: Pediatric Program* 60 (2007): 185–99, https://doi.org/10.1159/000106369.

50. Hamed Mirzaei, Rachel R. Raynes, and Valter D. Longo, "The Conserved Role of Protein Restriction in Aging and Disease," *Current Opinion in Clinical Nutrition and Metabolic Care* 19, no. 1 (2016): 74–9, https://doi.org/10.1097/mco.0000000000000239.

51. Albano Beja-Pereira et al., "Gene-Culture Coevolution Between Cattle Milk Protein Genes and Human Lactase Genes," *Nature Genetics* 35, no. 4 (2003): 311–3, https://doi.org/10.1038/ng1263.

52. Christian Løvold Storhaug, Svein Kjetil Fosse, and Lars T. Fadnes, "Country, Regional, and Global Estimates for Lactose Malabsorption in Adults: A Systematic Review and Meta-Analysis," *Lancet Gastroenterology and Hepatology* 2, no. 10 (2017): 738–46, https://doi.org/10.1016/s2468-1253(17)30154-1.

53. Priya Balasubramanian and Valter D. Longo, "Growth Factors, Aging and Age-Related Diseases," *Growth Hormone and IGF Research* 28 (2016): 66–8, https://doi.org/10.1016/j.ghir.2016.01.001.

54. Hong Seok Shim and Valter D. Longo, "A Protein Restriction-Dependent Sulfur Code for Longevity," *Cell* 160, no. 1–2 (2015): 15–7, https://doi.org/10.1016/j.cell.2014.12.027.

55. Mirzaei, Raynes, and Longo, "The Conserved Role of Protein Restriction in Aging and Disease."

56. Vahid Shaygannejad et al., "The Environmental Risk Factors in Multiple Sclerosis Susceptibility: A Case-Control Study," *Advanced Biomedical Research* 5, no. 1 (2016): 98, https://doi.org/10.4103/2277-9175.183665.

57. Christian R. Juhl et al., "Dairy Intake and Acne Vulgaris: A Systematic Review and Meta-Analysis of 78,529 Children, Adolescents, and Young Adults," *Nutrients* 10, no. 8 (2018): 1049, https://doi.org/10.3390/nu10081049.

58. Walter C. Willett and David S. Ludwig, "Milk and Health," *New England Journal of Medicine* 382, no. 7 (2020): 644–54, https://doi.org/10.1056/nejmra1903547.

59. Willett and Ludwig, "Milk and Health."

60. Mu Chen et al., "Dairy Fat and Risk of Cardiovascular Disease in 3 Cohorts of US Adults," *American Journal of Clinical Nutrition* 104, no. 5 (2016): 1209–17, https://doi.org/10.3945/ajcn.116.134460.

61. D. Iggman et al., "Replacing Dairy Fat with Rapeseed Oil Causes Rapid Improvement of Hyperlipidaemia: A Randomized Controlled Study," *Journal of Internal Medicine* 270, no. 4 (2011): 356–64, https://doi.org/10.1111/j.1365-2796.2011.02383.x.

62. K. Michaelsson et al., "Milk Intake and Risk of Mortality and Fractures in Women and Men: Cohort Studies," *BMJ* 349 (2014): g6015, https://doi.org/10.1136/bmj.g6015.

63. Khairunnuur Fairuz Azman and Rahimah Zakaria, "D-Galactose-Induced Accelerated Aging Model: an Overview," *Biogerontology* 20, no. 6 (2019): 763–82, https://doi.org/10.1007/s10522-019-09837-y.

64. Walter Willett et al., "Food in the Anthropocene: The EAT–Lancet Commission on Healthy Diets from Sustainable Food Systems," *Lancet* 393, no. 10170 (2019): 447–92, https://doi.org/10.1016/s0140-6736(18)31788-4.

65. Claus Leitzmann, "Nutrition Ecology: The Contribution of Vegetarian Diets," *American Journal of Clinical Nutrition* 78, no. 3 Suppl (2003): 657S–9S, https://doi.org/10.1093/ajcn/78.3.657s.

66. Claus Leitzmann, "Wholesome Nutrition: A Suitable Diet for the New Nutrition Science Project," *Public Health Nutrition* 8, no. 6a (2005): 753–9, https://doi.org/10.1079/phn2005781.

67. Willett et al., "Food in the Anthropocene."

68. Alon Shepon et al., "The Opportunity Cost of Animal Based Diets Exceeds All Food Losses," *Proceedings of the National Academy of Sciences* 115, no. 15 (2018): 3804–9, https://doi.org/10.1073/pnas.1713820115.

69. Shepon et al., "The Opportunity Cost of Animal Based Diets Exceeds All Food Losses."

70. Evelyne Battaglia Richi et al., "Health Risks Associated with Meat Consumption: A Review of Epidemiological Studies," *International Journal for Vitamin and Nutrition Research* 85, no. 1–2 (2015): 70–8, https://doi.org/10.1024/0300-9831/a000224.

71. IARC Working Group on the Evaluation of Carcinogenic Risk to Humans, *Red Meat and Processed Meat* (Lyon, France: International Agency for Research on Cancer, 2018).

72. Andrea Bellavia, Frej Stilling, and Alicja Wolk, "High Red Meat Intake and All Cause Cardiovascular and Cancer Mortality: Is the Risk Modified by Fruit and Vegetable Intake?" *American Journal of Clinical Nutrition* 104, no. 4 (2016): 1137–43, https://doi.org/10.3945/ajcn.116.135335.

73. C. S. C. Yip, W. Lam, and R. Fielding, "A Summary of Meat Intakes and Health Burdens," *European Journal of Clinical Nutrition* 72, no. 1 (2018): 18–29, https://doi.org/10.1038/ejcn.2017.117.

74. Itziar Abete et al., "Association Between Total, Processed, Red and White Meat Consumption and All-Cause, CVD and IHD Mortality: A Meta-Analysis of Cohort Studies," *British Journal of Nutrition* 112, no. 5 (2014): 762–75, https://doi.org/10.1017/s000711451400124x.

75. Hamish J. Love and Danielle Sulikowski, "Of Meat and Men: Sex Differences in Implicit and Explicit Attitudes Toward Meat," *Frontiers in Psychology* 9 (2018): 559, https://doi.org/10.3389/fpsyg.2018.00559.

76. N. E. Allen et al., "Hormones and Diet: Low Insulin-like Growth Factor-I but Normal Bioavailable Androgens in Vegan Men," *British Journal of Cancer* 83, no. 1 (2000): 95–7, https://doi.org/10.1054/bjoc.2000.1152.

77. Karl E. Anderson et al., "Diet-Hormone Interactions: Protein/Carbohydrate Ratio Alters Reciprocally the Plasma Levels of Testosterone and Cortisol and Their Respective Binding Globulins in Man," *Life Sciences* 40, no. 18 (1987): 1761–8, https://doi.org/10.1016/0024-3205(87)90086-5.

78. Paul Enck et al., *Darm an Hirn! Der Geheime Dialog Unserer Beiden Nervensysteme und Sein Einfluss auf Unser Leben* (Freiburg im Breisgau, Germany: Herder, 2017).

79. Enck et al., *Darm an Hirn!*.
80. Elisabeth Krafft, "Hack Aus der Petrischale: Kunst-Fleisch Gilt Als Alternative, doch Was Kann Es Wirklich?" Focus Online, August 13, 2018, https://www .focus.de/gesundheit/ernaehrung/wissen-der-stall-der-zukunft_id_9362620.html.
81. Andrés González and Silke Koltrowitz, "The $280,000 Lab-Grown Burger Could Be a More Palatable $10 in Two Years," Reuters, July 9, 2019, https://www.reuters .com/article/us-food-tech-labmeat/the-280000-lab-grown-burger-could -be-a-more-palatable-10-in-two-years-idUSKCN1U41W8.
82. "On a Mission to Create Slaughter-Free Meat: Prof. Dr. Mark Post on Food Grown From Cells," *Vegconomist*, February 22, 2019, https://vegconomist.com /interviews/on-a-mission-to-create-slaughter-free-meat-prof-dr-mark-post -on-food-grown-from-cells.
83. Dagfinn Aune et al., "Whole Grain Consumption and Risk of Cardiovascular Disease, Cancer, and All Cause and Cause Specific Mortality: Systematic Review and Dose-Response Meta-Analysis of Prospective Studies," *BMJ* 353 (2016): i2716, https://doi.org/10.1136/bmj.i2716.
84. Cecilie Kyrø et al., "Higher Whole-Grain Intake Is Associated with Lower Risk of Type 2 Diabetes Among Middle-Aged Men and Women: The Danish Diet, Cancer, and Health Cohort," *Journal of Nutrition* 148, no. 9 (2018): 1434–44, https://doi.org/10.1093/jn/nxy112.
85. A. R. Vieira et al., "Foods and Beverages and Colorectal Cancer Risk: A Systematic Review and Meta-Analysis of Cohort Studies, an Update of the Evidence of the WCRF-AICR Continuous Update Project," *Annals of Oncology* 28, no. 8 (2017): 1788–802, https://doi.org/10.1093/annonc/mdx171.
86. Aune et al., "Whole Grain Consumption and Risk of Cardiovascular Disease."
87. Hongyu Wu et al., "Association Between Dietary Whole Grain Intake and Risk of Mortality," *JAMA Internal Medicine* 175, no. 3 (2015): 373–84, https://doi.org /10.1001/jamainternmed.2014.6283.
88. Michael Winterdahl et al., "Sucrose Intake Lowers µ-Opioid and Dopamine D⅔ Receptor Availability in Porcine Brain," *Scientific Reports* 9, no. 1 (2019): 16918, https://doi.org/10.1038/s41598-019-53430-9.
89. Ludwig et al., "Dietary Fat: From Foe to Friend?"
90. Lewis C. Cantley, "Cancer, Metabolism, Fructose, Artificial Sweeteners, and Going Cold Turkey on Sugar," *BMC Biology* 12, no. 8 (2014), https://doi.org/10.1186 /1741-7007-12-8.
91. N. Rafie et al., "Dietary Patterns, Food Groups and Telomere Length: A Systematic Review of Current Studies," *European Journal of Clinical Nutrition* 71, no. 2 (2017): 151–8, https://doi.org/10.1038/ejcn.2016.149.
92. Amy Mullee et al., "Association Between Soft Drink Consumption and Mortality in 10 European Countries," *JAMA Internal Medicine* 179, no. 11 (2019): 1479–90, https://doi.org/10.1001/jamainternmed.2019.2478.
93. Biesalski, Warmuth, and Domzalski, *Unsere Ernährungsbiografie Wer Sie Kennt, Lebt Gesünder*.
94. Robert Lustig, *Fat Chance: The Bitter Truth About Sugar* (London, UK: Fourth Estate, 2012).

95. Quanhe Yang et al., "Added Sugar Intake and Cardiovascular Diseases Mortality Among US Adults," *JAMA Internal Medicine* 174, no. 4 (2014): 516–24, https://doi.org/10.1001/jamainternmed.2013.13563.

96. Gary Taubes, *Good Calories, Bad Calories* (New York: Anchor Books, 2008).

97. Cantley, "Cancer, Metabolism, Fructose, Artificial Sweeteners, and Going Cold Turkey on Sugar."

98. Lustig, *Fat Chance.*

99. E. Zomer et al., "The Effectiveness and Cost Effectiveness of Dark Chocolate Consumption as Prevention Therapy in People at High Risk of Cardiovascular Disease: Best Case Scenario Analysis Using a Markov Model," *BMJ* 344: e3657 (2012), https://doi.org/10.1136/bmj.e3657.

100. Alonso Romo-Romo et al., "Sucralose Decreases Insulin Sensitivity in Healthy Subjects: A Randomized Controlled Trial," *American Journal of Clinical Nutrition* 108, no. 3 (2018): 485–91, https://doi.org/10.1093/ajcn/nqy152.

101. Yasmin Mossavar-Rahmani et al., "Artificially Sweetened Beverages and Stroke, Coronary Heart Disease, and All-Cause Mortality in the Women's Health Initiative," *Stroke* 50, no. 3 (2019): 555–62, https://doi.org/10.1161/strokeaha.118.023100.

102. Samir Softic, David E. Cohen, and C. Ronald Kahn, "Role of Dietary Fructose and Hepatic De Novo Lipogenesis in Fatty Liver Disease," *Digestive Diseases and Sciences* 61, no. 5 (2016): 1282–93, https://doi.org/10.1007/s10620-016-4054-0.

103. George A. Bray, "Energy and Fructose from Beverages Sweetened with Sugar or High-Fructose Corn Syrup Pose a Health Risk for Some People," *Advances in Nutrition* 4, no. 2 (2013): 220–5, https://doi.org/10.3945/an.112.002816.

104. Lindsay J. Collin et al., "Association of Sugary Beverage Consumption with Mortality Risk in US Adults," *JAMA Network Open* 2, no. 5 (2019): e193121, https://doi.org/10.1001/jamanetworkopen.2019.3121.

105. Eloi Chazelas et al., "Sugary Drink Consumption and Risk of Cancer: Results from NutriNet-Santé Prospective Cohort," *BMJ* 366 (2019): l2408, https://doi.org/10.1136/bmj.l2408.

106. Kassem Makki et al., "The Impact of Dietary Fiber on Gut Microbiota in Host Health and Disease," *Cell Host and Microbe* 23, no. 6 (2018): 705–15, https://doi.org/10.1016/j.chom.2018.05.012.

107. Lynch and Pedersen, "The Human Intestinal Microbiome in Health and Disease."

108. Michael J. Keenan et al., "Role of Resistant Starch in Improving Gut Health, Adiposity, and Insulin Resistance," *Advances in Nutrition* 6, no. 2 (2015): 198–205, https://doi.org/10.3945/an.114.007419.

109. Keenan et al, "Role of Resistant Starch in Improving Gut Health."

110. Ganten, Spahl, and Deichmann, *Die Steinzeit Steckt Uns in Den Knochen.*

111. Ganten, Spahl, and Deichmann, *Die Steinzeit Steckt Uns in Den Knochen.*

112. Rebecca Riffkin, "One in Five Americans Include Gluten-Free Foods in Diet," Gallup, https://news.gallup.com/poll/184307/one-five-americans-include-gluten-free-foods-diet.aspx.

113. Luana Colloca and Franklin G. Miller, "The Nocebo Effect and Its Relevance for Clinical Practice," *Psychosomatic Medicine* 73, no. 7 (2011): 598–603, https://doi.org/10.1097/psy.0b013e3182294a50.

114. Yolanda Reig-Otero, Jordi Mañes, and Lara Manyes, "Amylase–Trypsin Inhibitors in Wheat and Other Cereals as Potential Activators of the Effects of Nonceliac Gluten Sensitivity," *Journal of Medicinal Food* 21, no. 3 (2018): 207–14, https://doi.org/10.1089/jmf.2017.0018.

115. P. R. Shewry and S. J. Hey, "Do We Need to Worry About Eating Wheat?" *Nutrition Bulletin* 41, no. 1 (2016): 6–13, https://doi.org/10.1111/nbu.12186.

116. Sara B. Seidelmann et al., "Dietary Carbohydrate Intake and Mortality: A Prospective Cohort Study and Meta-Analysis," *Lancet Public Health* 3, no. 9 (2018): e419–28, https://doi.org/10.1016/s2468-2667(18)30135-x.

Chapter Four: Food as a Remedy and My Superfoods

1. Mark P. Mattson, "Hormesis Defined," *Ageing Research Reviews* 7, no. 1 (2008): 1–7, https://doi.org/10.1016/j.arr.2007.08.007.

2. Rehab A. Hussein and Amira A. El-Anssary, "Plants Secondary Metabolites: The Key Drivers of the Pharmacological Actions of Medicinal Plants," IntechOpen, https://www.intechopen.com/books/herbal-medicine/plants-secondary-metabolites-the-key-drivers-of-the-pharmacological-actions-of-medicinal-plants.

3. Paula Pinto and Cláudia N. Santos, "Worldwide (Poly)Phenol Intake: Assessment Methods and Identified Gaps," *European Journal of Nutrition* 56, no. 4 (2017): 1393–1408, https://doi.org/10.1007/s00394-016-1354-2.

4. Julia Baudry et al., "Association of Frequency of Organic Food Consumption with Cancer Risk," *JAMA Internal Medicine* 178, no. 12 (2018): 1597–606, https://doi.org/10.1001/jamainternmed.2018.4357.

5. Thibault Fiolet et al., "Consumption of Ultra-Processed Foods and Cancer Risk: Results from NutriNet-Santé Prospective Cohort," *BMJ* 360 (2018): k322, https://doi.org/10.1136/bmj.k322.

6. Palanisamy Bruntha Devi et al., "Health Benefits of Finger Millet (Eleusine Coracana L.) Polyphenols and Dietary Fiber: A Review," *Journal of Food Science and Technology* 51, no. 6 (2014): 1021–40, https://doi.org/10.1007/s13197-011-0584-9.

7. Rajinder Singh, Subrata De, and Asma Belkheir, "Avena Sativa (Oat), a Potential Neutraceutical and Therapeutic Agent: An Overview," *Critical Reviews in Food Science and Nutrition* 53, no. 2 (2013): 126–44, https://doi.org/10.1080/10408398.2010.526725.

8. Pei Wang et al., "Oat Avenanthramide-C (2c) Is Biotransformed by Mice and the Human Microbiota into Bioactive Metabolites," *Journal of Nutrition* 145, no. 2 (2015): 239–45, https://doi.org/10.3945/jn.114.206508.

9. Xiao Shen et al., "Effect of Oat β-Glucan Intake on Glycaemic Control and Insulin Sensitivity of Diabetic Patients: A Meta-Analysis of Randomized Controlled Trials," *Nutrients* 8, no. 1 (2016): 39, https://doi.org/10.3390/nu8010039.

10. Xue Li et al., "Short- and Long-Term Effects of Wholegrain Oat Intake on Weight Management and Glucolipid Metabolism in Overweight Type-2 Diabetics: A Randomized Control Trial," *Nutrients* 8, no. 9 (2016): 549, https://doi.org/10.3390/nu8090549.

11. Li et al., "Short- and Long-Term Effects of Wholegrain Oat Intake."

12. C. J. Fabian et al., "Reduction in Ki-67 in Benign Breast Tissue of High-Risk Women with the Lignan Secoisolariciresinol Diglycoside," *Cancer Prevention Research* 3, no. 10 (2010): 1342–50, https://doi.org/10.1158/1940-6207.capr-10-0022.

13. X. J. Xiong et al., "Garlic for Hypertension: A Systematic Review and Meta-Analysis of Randomized Controlled Trials," *Phytomedicine* 22, no. 3 (2015): 352–61, https://doi.org/10.1016/j.phymed.2014.12.013.

14. Marjan Mahdavi-Roshan, et al., "Effect of Garlic Powder Tablet on Carotid Intima-Media Thickness in Patients with Coronary Artery Disease," *Nutrition and Health* 22, no. 2 (2013): 143–55, https://doi.org/10.1177/0260106014563446.

15. Michael K. Ang-Lee, Jonathan Moss, and Chun-Su Yuan, "Herbal Medicines and Perioperative Care," *Journal of the American Medical Association* 286, no. 2 (2001): 208–16, https://doi.org/10.1001/jama.286.2.208.

16. H. L. Nicastro, S. A. Ross, and J. A. Milner, "Garlic and Onions: Their Cancer Prevention Properties," *Cancer Prevention Research* 8, no. 3 (2015): 181–9, https://doi.org/10.1158/1940-6207.capr-14-0172.

17. S. V. Rana et al., "Garlic in Health and Disease," *Nutrition Research Reviews* 24, no. 1 (2011): 60–71, https://doi.org/10.1017/s0954422410000338.

18. Vasanthi Siruguri and Ramesh V. Bhat, "Assessing Intake of Spices by Pattern of Spice Use, Frequency of Consumption and Portion Size of Spices Consumed from Routinely Prepared Dishes in Southern India," *Nutrition Journal* 14, no. 1 (2015): 7, https://doi.org/10.1186/1475-2891-14-7.

19. Michael Greger, *How Not to Die: Discover the Foods Scientifically Proven to Prevent and Reverse Disease* (New York: Flatiron Books, 2015).

20. Jie Zheng et al., "Spices for Prevention and Treatment of Cancers," *Nutrients* 8, no. 8 (2016): 495, https://doi.org/10.3390/nu8080495.

21. Marcia Cruz-Correa et al., "Combination Treatment with Curcumin and Quercetin of Adenomas in Familial Adenomatous Polyposis," *Clinical Gastroenterology and Hepatology* 4, no. 8 (2006): 1035–8, https://doi.org/10.1016/j.cgh.2006.03.020.

22. Betül Kocaadam and Nevin Şanlier, "Curcumin, an Active Component of Turmeric (Curcuma Longa), and Its Effects on Health," *Critical Reviews in Food Science and Nutrition* 57, no. 13 (2015): 2889–95, https://doi.org/10.1080/10408398.2015.1077195.

23. Susan Hewlings and Douglas Kalman, "Curcumin: A Review of Its Effects on Human Health," *Foods* 6, no. 10 (2017): 92, https://doi.org/10.3390/foods6100092.

24. Nita G. Forouhi, "Consumption of Hot Spicy Foods and Mortality—Is Chilli Good for Your Health?" *BMJ* 351 (2015): h4141, https://doi.org/10.1136/bmj.h4141.

25. Sharon Varghese et al., "Chili Pepper as a Body Weight-Loss Food," *International Journal of Food Sciences and Nutrition* 68, no. 4 (2016): 392–401, https://doi.org/10.1080/09637486.2016.1258044.

26. Nicholas Eriksson et al., "A Genetic Variant near Olfactory Receptor Genes Influences Cilantro Preference," *Flavour* 1 (2012): 22, https://doi.org/10.1186/2044-7248-1-22.

27. Najla Gooda Sahib et al., "Coriander (Coriandrum Sativum L.): A Potential Source of High-Value Components for Functional Foods and Nutraceuticals—A Review," *Phytotherapy Research* 27, no. 10 (2012), https://doi.org/10.1002/ptr.4897.

28. Mehdi Maghbooli et al., "Comparison Between the Efficacy of Ginger and Su-
    matriptan in the Ablative Treatment of the Common Migraine," *Phytotherapy
    Research* 28, no. 3 (2013): 412–15, https://doi.org/10.1002/ptr.4996.
29. Muhammad Shoaib Akhtar et al., "Effect of Amla Fruit (Emblica Officinalis
    Gaertn.) on Blood Glucose and Lipid Profile of Normal Subjects and Type 2
    Diabetic Patients," *International Journal of Food Sciences and Nutrition* 62, no. 6
    (2011): 609–16, https://doi.org/10.3109/09637486.2011.560565.
30. Monica H. Carlsen et al., "The Total Antioxidant Content of More than 3100
    Foods, Beverages, Spices, Herbs and Supplements Used Worldwide," *Nutrition
    Journal* 9 (2010): 3, https://doi.org/10.1186/1475-2891-9-3.
31. Nikolaj Travica et al., "The Effect of Blueberry Interventions on Cognitive Per-
    formance and Mood: A Systematic Review of Randomized Controlled Trials,"
    Brain, Behavior, and Immunity 85 (2020): 96–105, https://doi.org/10.1016/j.bbi
    .2019.04.001.
32. Marshall G. Miller et al., "Dietary Blueberry Improves Cognition Among Older
    Adults in a Randomized, Double-Blind, Placebo-Controlled Trial," *European
    Journal of Nutrition* 57, no. 3 (2017): 1169–80, https://doi.org/10.1007/s00394
    -017-1400-8.
33. Adrian R. Whyte, Graham Schafer, and Claire M. Williams, "Cognitive Effects
    Following Acute Wild Blueberry Supplementation in 7- to 10-Year-Old Chil-
    dren," *European Journal of Nutrition* 55, no. 6 (2015): 2151–62, https://doi.org
    /10.1007/s00394-015-1029-4.
34. Robert Krikorian et al., "Blueberry Supplementation Improves Memory in Older
    Adults," *Journal of Agricultural and Food Chemistry* 58, no. 7 (2010): 3996–4000,
    https://doi.org/10.1021/jf9029332.
35. Travica et al., "The Effect of Blueberry Interventions on Cognitive Performance
    and Mood."
36. Ana Rodriguez-Mateos et al., "Intake and Time Dependence of Blueberry
    Flavonoid–Induced Improvements in Vascular Function: A Randomized, Con-
    trolled, Double-Blind, Crossover Intervention Study with Mechanistic Insights
    into Biological Activity," *American Journal of Clinical Nutrition* 98, no. 5 (2013):
    1179–91, https://doi.org/10.3945/ajcn.113.066639.
37. Mauro Serafini et al., "Antioxidant Activity of Blueberry Fruit Is Impaired by
    Association with Milk," *Free Radical Biology and Medicine* 46, no. 6 (2009): 769–74,
    https://doi.org/10.1016/j.freeradbiomed.2008.11.023.
38. Ana Rodriguez-Mateos et al., "Impact of Processing on the Bioavailability and
    Vascular Effects of Blueberry (Poly)Phenols," *Molecular Nutrition and Food Re-
    search* 58, no. 10 (2014): 1952–61, https://doi.org/10.1002/mnfr.201400231.
39. Riitta Törrönen et al., "Postprandial Glucose, Insulin and Glucagon-like Peptide 1
    Responses to Sucrose Ingested with Berries in Healthy Subjects," *British Journal of
    Nutrition* 107, no. 10 (2012): 1445–51, https://doi.org/10.1017/s0007114511004557.
40. L. Ryan et al., "Micellarisation of Carotenoids from Raw and Cooked Vegeta-
    bles," *Plant Foods for Human Nutrition* 63, no. 3 (2008): 127–33, https://doi.org
    /10.1007/s11130-008-0081-0.

41. Ping Chen et al., "Lycopene and Risk of Prostate Cancer: A Systematic Review and Meta-Analysis," *Medicine* 94, no. 33 (2015), https://doi.org/10.1097/md.0000000000001260.

42. Ho M. Cheng et al., "Lycopene and Tomato and Risk of Cardiovascular Diseases: A Systematic Review and Meta-Analysis of Epidemiological Evidence," *Critical Reviews in Food Science and Nutrition* 59, no. 1 (2019): 141–58, https://doi.org/10.1080/10408398.2017.1362630.

43. Lee Hooper et al., "Effects of Chocolate, Cocoa, and Flavan-3-Ols on Cardiovascular Health: A Systematic Review and Meta-Analysis of Randomized Trials," *American Journal of Clinical Nutrition* 95, no. 3 (2012): 740–51, https://doi.org/10.3945/ajcn.111.023457.

44. Hooper et al., "Effects of Chocolate."

45. Greger, *How Not to Die.*

46. Maria Ukhanova et al., "Effects of Almond and Pistachio Consumption on Gut Microbiota Composition in a Randomised Cross-over Human Feeding Study," *British Journal of Nutrition* 111, no. 12 (2014): 2146–52, https://doi.org/10.1017/s0007114514000385.

47. Emilio Ros, "Health Benefits of Nut Consumption," *Nutrients* 2, no. 7 (2010): 652–82, https://doi.org/10.3390/nu2070652.

48. Dagfinn Aune et al., "Nut Consumption and Risk of Cardiovascular Disease, Total Cancer, All-Cause and Cause-Specific Mortality: A Systematic Review and Dose-Response Meta-Analysis of Prospective Studies," *BMC Medicine* 14 (2016): 207, https://doi.org/10.1186/s12916-016-0730-3.

49. J. A. Meyerhardt et al., "The Impact of Dietary Patterns on Cancer Recurrence and Survival in Patients with Stage III Colon Cancer: Findings from CALGB 89803," *Journal of Clinical Oncology* 25, no. 18_suppl (2007): 4019, https://doi.org/10.1200/jco.2007.25.18_suppl.4019.

50. Ukhanova et al., "Effects of Almond and Pistachio Consumption on Gut Microbiota Composition."

51. Katherine A. Sauder et al., "Pistachio Nut Consumption Modifies Systemic Hemodynamics, Increases Heart Rate Variability, and Reduces Ambulatory Blood Pressure in Well-Controlled Type 2 Diabetes: A Randomized Trial," *Journal of the American Heart Association* 3, no. 4 (2014): e000873, https://doi.org/10.1161/jaha.114.000873.

52. Diane McKay et al., "A Pecan-Rich Diet Improves Cardiometabolic Risk Factors in Overweight and Obese Adults: A Randomized Controlled Trial," *Nutrients* 10, no. 3 (2018): 339, https://doi.org/10.3390/nu10030339.

53. Tricia Y. Li et al., "Regular Consumption of Nuts Is Associated with a Lower Risk of Cardiovascular Disease in Women with Type 2 Diabetes," *Journal of Nutrition* 139, no. 7 (2009): 1333–8, https://doi.org/10.3945/jn.108.103622.

54. Eunyoung Park, Indika Edirisinghe, and Britt Burton-Freeman, "Avocado Fruit on Postprandial Markers of Cardio-Metabolic Risk: A Randomized Controlled Dose Response Trial in Overweight and Obese Men and Women," *Nutrients* 10, no. 9 (2018): 1287, https://doi.org/10.3390/nu10091287.

55. R. Ozolua et al., "Acute and Sub-Acute Toxicological Assessment of the Aqueous Seed Extract of *Persea Americana* Mill (Lauraceae) in Rats," *African Journal of Traditional, Complementary and Alternative Medicines* 6, no. 4 (2009): 573–8, https://doi.org/10.4314/ajtcam.v6i4.57214.

56. A. J. Butt et al., "A Novel Plant Toxin, Persin, with in Vivo Activity in the Mammary Gland, Induces Bim-Dependent Apoptosis in Human Breast Cancer Cells," *Molecular Cancer Therapeutics* 5, no. 9 (2006): 2300–9, https://doi.org/10.1158/1535-7163.mct-06-0170.

57. H. Ding et al., "Chemopreventive Characteristics of Avocado Fruit," *Seminars in Cancer Biology* 17, no. 5 (2007): 386–94, https://doi.org/10.1016/j.semcancer.2007.04.003.

58. Maria D. Jackson et al., "Associations of Whole-Blood Fatty Acids and Dietary Intakes with Prostate Cancer in Jamaica," *Cancer Causes and Control* 23, no. 1 (2012): 23–33, https://doi.org/10.1007/s10552-011-9850-4.

59. Tom Philpott, "We Have Some Bad News for You About Avocados," *Mother Jones*, October 1, 2014, https://www.motherjones.com/food/2014/10/avocado-drought-chile-california.

60. Alexis Soyer, *Food, Cookery, and Dining in Ancient Times: Alexis Soyer's Pantropheon* (Mineola, NY: Dover Publications, 2004).

61. Alena Vanduchova, Pavel Anzenbacher, and Eva Anzenbacherova. "Isothiocyanate from Broccoli, Sulforaphane, and Its Properties," *Journal of Medicinal Food* 22, no. 2 (2019): 121–6, https://doi.org/10.1089/jmf.2018.0024.

62. Anika Eva Wagner, Anna Maria Terschluesen, and Gerald Rimbach, "Health Promoting Effects of Brassica-Derived Phytochemicals: From Chemopreventive and Anti-Inflammatory Activities to Epigenetic Regulation," *Oxidative Medicine and Cellular Longevity* 2013 (2013): 1–12, https://doi.org/10.1155/2013/964539.

63. Yoko Yagishita et al., "Broccoli or Sulforaphane: Is It the Source or Dose That Matters?" *Molecules* 24, no. 19 (2019): 3593, https://doi.org/10.3390/molecules24193593.

64. Akinori Yanaka, "Role of Sulforaphane in Protection of Gastrointestinal Tract Against H. Pylori and NSAID-Induced Oxidative Stress," *Current Pharmaceutical Design* 23, no. 27 (2017): 4066–75, https://doi.org/10.2174/1381612823666170207103943.

65. Greger, *How Not to Die*.

66. Dunja Šamec, Branimir Urlić, and Branka Salopek-Sondi, "Kale (Brassica Oleracea Var. Acephala) as a Superfood: Review of the Scientific Evidence Behind the Statement," *Critical Reviews in Food Science and Nutrition* 59, no. 15 (2019): 2411–22, https://doi.org/10.1080/10408398.2018.1454400.

67. Bryan Lufkin, "How Avocados and Kale Became so Popular," BBC, https://www.bbc.com/worklife/article/20190304-how-avocados-and-kale-became-so-popular.

68. Jose Medina-Inojosa et al., "The Hispanic Paradox in Cardiovascular Disease and Total Mortality," *Progress in Cardiovascular Diseases* 57, no. 3 (2014): 286–92, https://doi.org/10.1016/j.pcad.2014.09.001.

69. Francisco Lopez-Jimenez and Carl J. Lavie, "Hispanics and Cardiovascular Health and the 'Hispanic Paradox': What Is Known and What Needs to Be Discovered?" *Progress in Cardiovascular Diseases* 57, no. 3 (2014): 227–9, https://doi.org/10.1016/j.pcad.2014.09.007.

70. "Eat a Diet Rich in Whole Grains, Vegetables, Fruits, and Beans," American Institute for Cancer Research, https://www.aicr.org/cancer-prevention/recommendations/eat-a-diet-rich-in-whole-grains-vegetables-fruits-and-beans.

71. Yuxia Wei et al., "Soy Intake and Breast Cancer Risk: A Prospective Study of 300,000 Chinese Women and a Dose–Response Meta-Analysis," *European Journal of Epidemiology* (2019), https://doi.org/10.1007/s10654-019-00585-4.

72. Qianghui Wang, Xingming Liu, and Shengqiang Ren, "Tofu Intake Is Inversely Associated with Risk of Breast Cancer: A Meta-Analysis of Observational Studies," *PLoS One* 15, no. 1 (2020): e0226745, https://doi.org/10.1371/journal.pone.0226745.

73. Yan Zhao et al., "In Vitro Antioxidant Activity of Extracts from Common Legumes," *Food Chemistry* 152 (2014): 462–6, https://doi.org/10.1016/j.foodchem.2013.12.006.

74. Dita Moravek et al., "Carbohydrate Replacement of Rice or Potato with Lentils Reduces the Postprandial Glycemic Response in Healthy Adults in an Acute, Randomized, Crossover Trial," *Journal of Nutrition* 148, no. 4 (2018): 535–41, https://doi.org/10.1093/jn/nxy018.

75. Adriana N. Mudryj, Nancy Yu, and Harold M. Aukema, "Nutritional and Health Benefits of Pulses," *Applied Physiology, Nutrition, and Metabolism* 39, no. 11 (2014): 1197–204, https://doi.org/10.1139/apnm-2013-0557.

76. T. M. Wolever et al., "Second-Meal Effect: Low-Glycemic-Index Foods Eaten at Dinner Improve Subsequent Breakfast Glycemic Response," *American Journal of Clinical Nutrition* 48, no. 4 (1988): 1041–7, https://doi.org/10.1093/ajcn/48.4.1041.

77. Mario Siervo et al., "Inorganic Nitrate and Beetroot Juice Supplementation Reduces Blood Pressure in Adults: A Systematic Review and Meta-Analysis," *Journal of Nutrition* 143, no. 6 (2013): 818–26, https://doi.org/10.3945/jn.112.170233.

78. Stephen J. Bailey et al., "Dietary Nitrate Supplementation Reduces the O2 Cost of Low-Intensity Exercise and Enhances Tolerance to High-Intensity Exercise in Humans," *Journal of Applied Physiology* 107, no. 4 (2009): 1144–55, https://doi.org/10.1152/japplphysiol.00722.2009.

79. Barbara Hohensinn et al., "Sustaining Elevated Levels of Nitrite in the Oral Cavity Through Consumption of Nitrate-Rich Beetroot Juice in Young Healthy Adults Reduces Salivary PH," *Nitric Oxide* 60 (2016): 10–5, https://doi.org/10.1016/j.niox.2016.08.006.

80. Dyah Setyorini, Yani C. Rahayu, and Tita Sistyaningrum, "The Effects of Rinsing Red Beet Root (Beta Vulgaris L.) Juice on Streptococcus Sp. Dental Plaque," *Journal of Dentomaxillofacial Science* 2, no. 1 (2017): 18–22, https://doi.org/10.15562/jdmfs.v2i1.460.

81. H.-C. Hung et al., "Fruit and Vegetable Intake and Risk of Major Chronic Disease," *JNCI: Journal of the National Cancer Institute* 96, no. 21 (2004): 1577–84, https://doi.org/10.1093/jnci/djh296.

82. C. Jubert et al., "Effects of Chlorophyll and Chlorophyllin on Low-Dose Aflatoxin B1 Pharmacokinetics in Human Volunteers," *Cancer Prevention Research* 2, no. 12 (2009): 1015–22, https://doi.org/10.1158/1940-6207.capr-09-0099.

83. Dalia Akramienė et al., "Effects of ß-Glucans on the Immune System," *Medicina* 43, no. 8 (2007): 597, https://doi.org/10.3390/medicina43080076.

84. Tongtong Xu, Robert B. Beelman, and Joshua D. Lambert, "The Cancer Preventive Effects of Edible Mushrooms," *Anti-Cancer Agents in Medicinal Chemistry* 12, no. 10 (2012): 1255–63, https://doi.org/10.2174/187152012803833017.

85. Şeyda Karaman et al., "Comparison of Antioxidant Capacity and Phenolic Composition of Peel and Flesh of Some Apple Varieties," *Journal of the Science of Food and Agriculture* 93, no. 4 (2013): 867–75, https://doi.org/10.1002/jsfa.5810.

86. Athanasios Koutsos et al., "Two Apples a Day Lower Serum Cholesterol and Improve Cardiometabolic Biomarkers in Mildly Hypercholesterolemic Adults: A Randomized, Controlled, Crossover Trial," *American Journal of Clinical Nutrition* 111, no. 2 (2019): 307–18, https://doi.org/10.1093/ajcn/nqz282.

87. Roberta Fadda et al., "Effects of Drinking Supplementary Water at School on Cognitive Performance in Children," *Appetite* 59, no. 3 (2012): 730–7, https://doi.org/10.1016/j.appet.2012.07.005.

88. Chan et al., "Water, Other Fluids, and Fatal Coronary Heart Disease."

89. Dominique S. Michaud et al., "Fluid Intake and the Risk of Bladder Cancer in Men," *New England Journal of Medicine* 340, no. 18 (1999): 1390–7, https://doi.org/10.1056/nejm199905063401803.

90. Thomas M. Hooton et al., "Effect of Increased Daily Water Intake in Premenopausal Women with Recurrent Urinary Tract Infections," *JAMA Internal Medicine* 178, no. 11 (2018): 1509–15, https://doi.org/10.1001/jamainternmed.2018.4204.

91. William F. Clark et al., "Effect of Coaching to Increase Water Intake on Kidney Function Decline in Adults with Chronic Kidney Disease," *Journal of the American Medical Association* 319, no. 18 (2018): 1870–9, https://doi.org/10.1001/jama.2018.4930.

92. O. De Giglio et al., "Mineral Water or Tap Water? An Endless Debate," *Annali di Igiene* 27, no. 1 (2015): 58–65, doi:10.7416/ai.2015.2023.

93. Vera Zylka-Menhorn, "Arzneimittelrückstände im Wasser: Vermeidung und Elimination," Aktion Deutschland Hilft, https://www.aerzteblatt.de/archiv/198237/Arzneimittelrueckstaende-im-Wasser-Vermeidung-und-Elimination.

94. F. D. Daschner et al., "Microbiological Contamination of Drinking Water in a Commercial Household Water Filter System," *European Journal of Clinical Microbiology and Infectious Diseases* 15, no. 3 (1996): 233–7, https://doi.org/10.1007/bf01591360.

95. Eddo J. Hoekstra and Catherine Simoneau, "Release of Bisphenol A from Polycarbonate—A Review," *Critical Reviews in Food Science and Nutrition* 53, no. 4 (2011): 386–402, https://doi.org/10.1080/10408398.2010.536919.

96. Beverly S. Rubin, "Bisphenol A: An Endocrine Disruptor with Widespread Exposure and Multiple Effects," *Journal of Steroid Biochemistry and Molecular Biology* 127, no. 1–2 (2011): 27–34, https://doi.org/10.1016/j.jsbmb.2011.05.002.

97. Robin Poole et al., "Coffee Consumption and Health: Umbrella Review of Meta-Analyses of Multiple Health Outcomes," *BMJ* 359 (2017): j5024, https://doi.org/10.1136/bmj.j5024.

98. Adela M. Navarro et al., "Coffee Consumption and Total Mortality in a Mediterranean Prospective Cohort," *American Journal of Clinical Nutrition* 108, no. 5 (2018): 1113–20, https://doi.org/10.1093/ajcn/nqy198.

99. Erikka Loftfield et al., "Association of Coffee Drinking with Mortality by Genetic Variation in Caffeine Metabolism," *JAMA Internal Medicine* 178, no. 8 (2018): 1086–97, https://doi.org/10.1001/jamainternmed.2018.2425.

100. Poole et al., "Coffee Consumption and Health."

101. Loftfield et al., "Association of Coffee Drinking with Mortality."

102. Loftfield et al., "Association of Coffee Drinking with Mortality."

103. Thomas Remer and Friedrich Manz, "Potential Renal Acid Load of Foods and Its Influence on Urine pH," *Journal of the American Dietetic Association* 95, no. 7 (1995): 791–7, https://doi.org/10.1016/s0002-8223(95)00219-7.

104. B. Wendl et al., "Effect of Decaffeination of Coffee or Tea on Gastro-Oesophageal Reflux," *Alimentary Pharmacology and Therapeutics* 8, no. 3 (1994): 283–7, https://doi.org/10.1111/j.1365-2036.1994.tb00289.x.

105. Gang Liu et al., "Effects of Tea Intake on Blood Pressure: A Meta-Analysis of Randomised Controlled Trials," *British Journal of Nutrition* 112, no. 7 (2014): 1043–54, https://doi.org/10.1017/s0007114514001731.

106. Anja Mähler et al., "Metabolic Response to Epigallocatechin-3-Gallate in Relapsing-Remitting Multiple Sclerosis: A Randomized Clinical Trial," *American Journal of Clinical Nutrition* 101, no. 3 (2015): 487–95, https://doi.org/10.3945/ajcn.113.075309.

107. Yohei Shirakami and Masahito Shimizu, "Possible Mechanisms of Green Tea and Its Constituents against Cancer," *Molecules* 23, no. 9 (2018): 2284, https://doi.org/10.3390/molecules23092284.

108. Anna H. Wu and Lesley M. Butler, "Green Tea and Breast Cancer," *Molecular Nutrition and Food Research* 55, no. 6 (2011): 921–30, https://doi.org/10.1002/mnfr.201100006.

109. Sawako Masuda et al., "'Benifuuki' Green Tea Containing O-Methylated Catechin Reduces Symptoms of Japanese Cedar Pollinosis: A Randomized, Double-Blind, Placebo-Controlled Trial," *Allergology International* 63, no. 2 (2014): 211–7, https://doi.org/10.2332/allergolint.13-oa-0620.

110. A. C. Nobre, A. Rao, and G. N. Owen, "L-theanine, a Natural Constituent in Tea, and Its Effect on Mental State," *Asia Pacific Journal of Clinical Nutrition* 17, suppl. 1 (2008): 167–8.

111. Terry Lopez et al., "Green Tea Polyphenols Extend the Lifespan of Male Drosophila Melanogaster While Impairing Reproductive Fitness," *Journal of Medicinal Food* 17, no. 12 (2014): 1314–21, https://doi.org/10.1089/jmf.2013.0190.

112. S. Pérez-Burillo et al., "Effect of Brewing Time and Temperature on Antioxidant Capacity and Phenols of White Tea: Relationship with Sensory Properties," *Food Chemistry* 248 (2018): 111–8, https://doi.org/10.1016/j.foodchem.2017.12.056.

113. Erica Sharpe et al., "Effects of Brewing Conditions on the Antioxidant Capacity of Twenty-Four Commercial Green Tea Varieties," *Food Chemistry* 192 (2016): 380–7, https://doi.org/10.1016/j.foodchem.2015.07.005.

114. Griswold et al., "Alcohol Use and Burden for 195 Countries and Territories, 1990–2016."

115. Griswold et al., "Alcohol Use and Burden for 195 Countries and Territories, 1990–2016."

116. "Alcohol and Cancer."
117. Angela M. Wood et al., "Risk Thresholds for Alcohol Consumption: Combined Analysis of Individual-Participant Data for 599 912 Current Drinkers in 83 Prospective Studies," *Lancet* 391, no. 10129 (2018): 1513–23, https://doi.org/10.1016 /s0140-6736(18)30134-x.
118. Sarah Boseley, "Extra Glass of Wine a Day 'Will Shorten Your Life by 30 Minutes.'" *Guardian*, April 13, 2018, https://www.theguardian.com/science/2018 /apr/12/one-extra-glass-of-wine-will-shorten-your-life-by-30-minutes.
119. Griswold et al., "Alcohol Use and Burden for 195 Countries and Territories, 1990– 2016."

Chapter Five: Why Fasting Is So Important for Us

1. World Health Organization, *Diet, Nutrition and the Prevention of Chronic Diseases*.
2. Luigi Fontana and Linda Partridge, "Promoting Health and Longevity Through Diet: From Model Organisms to Humans," *Cell* 161, no. 1 (2015): 106–18, https://doi.org/10.1016/j.cell.2015.02.020.
3. Longo and Mattson, "Fasting: Molecular Mechanisms and Clinical Applications."
4. Michalsen and Li, "Fasting Therapy for Treating and Preventing Disease."
5. Michalsen and Li, "Fasting Therapy for Treating and Preventing Disease."
6. Hamed Mirzaei, Stefano Di Biase, and Valter D. Longo, "Dietary Interventions, Cardiovascular Aging, and Disease," *Circulation Research* 118, no. 10 (2016): 1612–25, https://doi.org/10.1161/circresaha.116.307473.
7. Longo and Mattson, "Fasting: Molecular Mechanisms and Clinical Applications."
8. Buchinger, *Das Heilfasten und Seine Hilfsmethoden Als Biologischer Weg*.
9. Buchinger, *Das Heilfasten und Seine Hilfsmethoden Als Biologischer Weg*.
10. Andreas Michalsen et al., "Incorporation of Fasting Therapy in an Integrative Medicine Ward: Evaluation of Outcome, Safety, and Effects on Lifestyle Adherence in a Large Prospective Cohort Study," *Journal of Alternative and Complementary Medicine* 11, no. 4 (2005): 601–7, https://doi.org/10.1089/acm.2005.11.601.
11. Shubhroz Gill and Satchidananda Panda, "A Smartphone App Reveals Erratic Diurnal Eating Patterns in Humans That Can Be Modulated for Health Benefits," *Cell Metabolism* 22, no. 5 (2015): 789–98, https://doi.org/10.1016/j.cmet.2015.09.005.
12. G. F. Cahill, O. E. Owen, and A. P. Morgan, "The Consumption of Fuels During Prolonged Starvation," *Advances in Enzyme Regulation* 6 (1968): 143–50, https:// doi.org/10.1016/0065-2571(68)90011-3.
13. Philip Felig et al., "Amino Acid Metabolism During Prolonged Starvation," *Journal of Clinical Investigation* 48, no. 3 (1969): 584–94, https://doi.org/10.1172 /jci106017.
14. Leonie K. Heilbronn et al., "Alternate-Day Fasting in Nonobese Subjects: Effects on Body Weight, Body Composition, and Energy Metabolism," *American Journal of Clinical Nutrition* 81, no. 1 (2005): 69–73, https://doi.org/10.1093/ajcn/81.1.69.
15. Stephen D. Anton et al., "Flipping the Metabolic Switch: Understanding and Applying the Health Benefits of Fasting," *Obesity* 26, no. 2 (2017): 254–68, https://doi.org/10.1002/oby.22065.

16. Mark P. Mattson et al., "Intermittent Metabolic Switching, Neuroplasticity and Brain Health," *Nature Reviews Neuroscience* 19, no. 2 (2018): 63–80, https://doi.org/10.1038/nrn.2017.156.

17. Buchinger, *Das Heilfasten und Seine Hilfsmethoden Als Biologischer Weg.*

18. Buchinger, *Das Heilfasten und Seine Hilfsmethoden Als Biologischer Weg.*

19. Roman Huber, Sven Weisser, and Rainer Luedtke, "Effects of Abdominal Hot Compresses on Indocyanine Green Elimination—A Randomized Cross Over Study in Healthy Subjects," *BMC Gastroenterology* 7, no. 1 (2007): 27, https://doi.org/10.1186/1471-230x-7-27.

20. Alex Witasek, *Lehrbuch der F.X. Mayr-Medizin: Grundlagen, Diagnostik und Therapie* (Berlin: Springer, 2019).

21. A. G. Christen and J. A. Christen, "Horace Fletcher (1849–1919): 'The Great Masticator,'" *Journal of the History of Dentistry* 45, no 3 (1997): 95–100.

22. Hendrik Jan Smit et al., "Does Prolonged Chewing Reduce Food Intake? Fletcherism Revisited," *Appetite* 57, no. 1 (2011): 295–8, https://doi.org/10.1016/j.appet.2011.02.003.

23. Alan Goldhamer et al., "Medically Supervised Water-Only Fasting in the Treatment of Hypertension," *Journal of Manipulative and Physiological Therapeutics* 24, no. 5 (2001): 335–9, https://doi.org/10.1067/mmt.2001.115263.

24. J. Kjeldsen-Kragh et al., "Controlled Trial of Fasting and One-Year Vegetarian Diet in Rheumatoid Arthritis," *Lancet* 338, no. 8772 (1991): 899–902, https://doi.org/10.1016/0140-6736(91)91770-u.

25. H. Müller, F. Wilhelmi de Toledo, and K.-L. Resch, "Fasting Followed by Vegetarian Diet in Patients with Rheumatoid Arthritis: A Systematic Review," *Scandinavian Journal of Rheumatology* 30, no. 1 (2001): 1–10, https://doi.org/10.1080/030097401750065256.

26. Rainer Stange et al., "Therapeutic Fasting in Patients with Metabolic Syndrome and Impaired Insulin Resistance," *Forschende Komplementärmedizin/Research in Complementary Medicine* 20, no. 6 (2013): 421–6, https://doi.org/10.1159/000357875.

27. Chenying Li et al., "Effects of a One-Week Fasting Therapy in Patients with Type-2 Diabetes Mellitus and Metabolic Syndrome—A Randomized Controlled Explorative Study," *Experimental and Clinical Endocrinology and Diabetes* 125, no. 09 (2017): 618–24, https://doi.org/10.1055/s-0043-101700.

28. Chenying Li et al., "Metabolic and Psychological Response to 7-Day Fasting in Obese Patients with and Without Metabolic Syndrome," *Forschende Komplementärmedizin/Research in Complementary Medicine* 20, no. 6 (2013): 413–20, https://doi.org/10.1159/000353672.

29. Chia-Wei Cheng et al., "Fasting-Mimicking Diet Promotes Ngn3-Driven β-Cell Regeneration to Reverse Diabetes," *Cell* 168, no. 5 (2017): 775–88, https://doi.org/10.1016/j.cell.2017.01.040.

30. J. Hermanides et al., "Lagere Incidentie van Diabetes Mellitus Type 2 bij Verandering van Leefstijl: Aanwijzingen uit de Tweede Wereldoorlog" ["Lower Incidence of Type 2 Diabetes Mellitus with Changes in Lifestyle: Clues from World War II"]. *Nederlands Tijdschrift voor Geneeskunde* 152, no. 44 (2008): 2415–7.

31. M. L. Roditis et al., "Epidemiology and Predisposing Factors of Obesity in Greece: From the Second World War Until Today," *Journal of Pediatric Endocrinology and Metabolism* 22, no. 5 (2009): 389–405, https://doi.org/10.1515/jpem.2009.22.5.389.

32. Claire Saraux et al., "Plasticity in Foraging Strategies of Inshore Birds: How Little Penguins Maintain Body Reserves While Feeding Offspring," *Ecology* 92, no. 10 (2011): 1909–16, https://doi.org/10.1890/11-0407.1.

33. C. Habold et al., "Effects of Fasting and Refeeding on Jejunal Morphology and Cellular Activity in Rats in Relation to Depletion of Body Stores," *Scandinavian Journal of Gastroenterology* 39, no. 6 (2004): 531–9, https://doi.org/10.1080/00365520410004514.

34. Suzanne Dunel-Erb et al., "Restoration of the Jejunal Mucosa in Rats Refed After Prolonged Fasting," *Comparative Biochemistry and Physiology Part A: Molecular and Integrative Physiology* 129, no. 4 (2001): 933–47, https://doi.org/10.1016/s1095-6433(01)00360-9.

35. Alexis M. Stranahan et al., "Diet-Induced Insulin Resistance Impairs Hippocampal Synaptic Plasticity and Cognition in Middle-Aged Rats," *Hippocampus* 18, no. 11 (2008): 1085–8, https://doi.org/10.1002/hipo.20470.

36. Mark P. Mattson, "Energy Intake, Meal Frequency, and Health: A Neurobiological Perspective," *Annual Review of Nutrition* 25 (2005): 237–60, https://doi.org/10.1146/annurev.nutr.25.050304.092526.

37. Mark P. Mattson, "Gene-Diet Interactions in Brain Aging and Neurodegenerative Disorders," *Annals of Internal Medicine* 139, no. 5, part 2 (2003): 441–4, https://doi.org/10.7326/0003-4819-139-5_part_2-200309021-00012.

38. S. M. Rothman and M. P. Mattson, "Activity-Dependent, Stress-Responsive BDNF Signaling and the Quest for Optimal Brain Health and Resilience Throughout the Lifespan," *Neuroscience* 239 (2013): 228–40, https://doi.org/10.1016/j.neuroscience.2012.10.014.

39. Mattson et al., "Intermittent Metabolic Switching, Neuroplasticity and Brain Health."

40. Jo Sourbron et al., "Ketogenic Diet for the Treatment of Pediatric Epilepsy: Review and Meta-Analysis," *Child's Nervous System* 36, no. 6 (2020): 1099–109, https://doi.org/10.1007/s00381-020-04578-7.

41. In Young Choi et al., "A Diet Mimicking Fasting Promotes Regeneration and Reduces Autoimmunity and Multiple Sclerosis Symptoms," *Cell Reports* 15, no. 10 (2016): 2136–46, https://doi.org/10.1016/j.celrep.2016.05.009.

42. Andreas Michalsen et al., "In-Patient Treatment of Fibromyalgia: A Controlled Nonrandomized Comparison of Conventional Medicine Versus Integrative Medicine Including Fasting Therapy," *Evidence-Based Complementary and Alternative Medicine* 2013 (2013): 1–7, https://doi.org/10.1155/2013/908610.

43. Alessio Nencioni et al., "Fasting and Cancer: Molecular Mechanisms and Clinical Application," *Nature Reviews Cancer* 18, no. 11 (2018): 707–19, https://doi.org/10.1038/s41568-018-0061-0.

44. Stephan P. Bauersfeld et al., "The Effects of Short-Term Fasting on Quality of Life and Tolerance to Chemotherapy in Patients with Breast and Ovarian Cancer: A

Randomized Cross-over Pilot Study," *BMC Cancer* 18, no. 1 (2018): 476, https://doi.org/10.1186/s12885-018-4353-2.

45. Yan-Bo Zhang et al., "Combined Lifestyle Factors, Incident Cancer, and Cancer Mortality: A Systematic Review and Meta-Analysis of Prospective Cohort Studies," *British Journal of Cancer* 122, no. 7 (2020): 1085–93, https://doi.org/10.1038/s41416-020-0741-x.

46. Sebastian Brandhorst and Valter D. Longo, "Protein Quantity and Source, Fasting-Mimicking Diets, and Longevity," *Advances in Nutrition* 10, suppl. 4 (2019), https://doi.org/10.1093/advances/nmz079.

47. Roberta Buono and Valter D. Longo, "Starvation, Stress Resistance, and Cancer," *Trends in Endocrinology and Metabolism* 29, no. 4 (2018): 271–80, https://doi.org/10.1016/j.tem.2018.01.008.

48. Valter Longo, *The Longevity Diet: Discover the New Science Behind Stem Cell Activation and Regeneration to Slow Aging, Fight Disease, and Optimize Weight* (New York: Avery, 2018).

49. Fondazione Valter Longo Onlus, https://www.fondazionevalterlongo.org.

50. Min Wei et al., "Fasting-Mimicking Diet and Markers/Risk Factors for Aging, Diabetes, Cancer, and Cardiovascular Disease," *Science Translational Medicine* 9, no. 377 (2017): eaai8700, https://doi.org/10.1126/scitranslmed.aai8700.

51. Sebastian Brandhorst et al., "A Periodic Diet That Mimics Fasting Promotes Multi-System Regeneration, Enhanced Cognitive Performance, and Healthspan," *Cell Metabolism* 22, no. 1 (2015): 86–99, https://doi.org/10.1016/j.cmet.2015.05.012.

52. Christoph A. Thaiss et al., "The Microbiome and Innate Immunity," *Nature* 535, no. 7610 (2016): 65–74, https://doi.org/10.1038/nature18847.

53. Marlene Remely et al., "Increased Gut Microbiota Diversity and Abundance of Faecalibacterium Prausnitzii and Akkermansia after Fasting: A Pilot Study," *Wiener Klinische Wochenschrift* 127, no. 9–10 (2015): 394–8, https://doi.org/10.1007/s00508-015-0755-1.

54. In Young Choi, Changhan Lee, and Valter D. Longo, "Nutrition and Fasting Mimicking Diets in the Prevention and Treatment of Autoimmune Diseases and Immunosenescence," *Molecular and Cellular Endocrinology* 455 (2017): 4–12, https://doi.org/10.1016/j.mce.2017.01.042.

55. Choi et al., "A Diet Mimicking Fasting Promotes Regeneration."

56. Gerald Huether et al., "Long-Term Food Restriction Down-Regulates the Density of Serotonin Transporters in the Rat Frontal Cortex," *Biological Psychiatry* 41, no. 12 (1997): 1174–80, https://doi.org/10.1016/s0006-3223(96)00265-x.

57. Li et al., "Metabolic and Psychological Response to 7-Day Fasting."

58. Chrysoula Boutari et al., "The Effect of Underweight on Female and Male Reproduction," *Metabolism* 107 (2020): 154229, https://doi.org/10.1016/j.metabol.2020.154229.

59. Li et al., "Metabolic and Psychological Response to 7-Day Fasting."

60. Stefan Drinda et al., "Effects of Periodic Fasting on Fatty Liver Index—A Prospective Observational Study," *Nutrients* 11, no. 11 (2019): 2601, https://doi.org/10.3390/nu11112601.

61. Rinella, Mary E. "Nonalcoholic Fatty Liver Disease: A Systematic Review," *Journal of the American Medical Association* 313, no. 22 (2015): 2263–73, https://doi.org/10.1001/jama.2015.5370.
62. Amedeo Lonardo et al., "Hypertension, Diabetes, Atherosclerosis and NASH: Cause or Consequence?" *Journal of Hepatology* 68, no. 2 (2018): 335–52, https://doi.org/10.1016/j.jhep.2017.09.021.
63. Chenying et al., "Effects of a One-Week Fasting Therapy in Patients with Type-2 Diabetes Mellitus."
64. Stange et al., "Therapeutic Fasting in Patients with Metabolic Syndrome and Impaired Insulin Resistance."
65. Drinda et al., "Effects of Periodic Fasting on Fatty Liver Index."
66. Michalsen and Li, "Fasting Therapy for Treating and Preventing Disease."

Chapter Six: Therapeutic Fasting—The Practical Program

1. Tatiana Moro et al., "Effects of Eight Weeks of Time-Restricted Feeding (16/8) on Basal Metabolism, Maximal Strength, Body Composition, Inflammation, and Cardiovascular Risk Factors in Resistance-Trained Males," *Journal of Translational Medicine* 14, no. 1 (2016): 290, https://doi.org/10.1186/s12967-016-1044-0.
2. Heilbronn et al., "Alternate-Day Fasting in Nonobese Subjects."

Chapter Seven: Intermittent Fasting—The Brilliant New Discovery Suitable for Everyday Life

1. Buchinger, *Das Heilfasten und Seine Hilfsmethoden Als Biologischer Weg.*
2. Satchin Panda, *The Circadian Code: Lose Weight, Supercharge Your Energy, and Transform Your Health from Morning to Midnight* (New York: Rodale Books, 2018).
3. Daniela Artemis Tahère Liebscher, *Religiöses Fasten im Medizinischen Kontext Auswirkungen auf Anthropometrische Parameter, Blutfettwerte und Hämodynamik* (Essen, Germany: KVC Verlag, 2013).
4. Nader Lessan and Tomader Ali, "Energy Metabolism and Intermittent Fasting: The Ramadan Perspective," *Nutrients* 11, no. 5 (2019): 1192, https://doi.org/10.3390/nu11051192.
5. Lessan and Ali, "Energy Metabolism and Intermittent Fasting."
6. Fraser and Shavlik, "Ten Years of Life."
7. Buettner, *The Blue Zones.*
8. Grant M. Tinsley and Benjamin D. Horne, "Intermittent Fasting and Cardiovascular Disease: Current Evidence and Unresolved Questions," *Future Cardiology* 14, no. 1 (2018): 47–54, https://doi.org/10.2217/fca-2017-0038.
9. Benjamin D. Horne et al., "Usefulness of Routine Periodic Fasting to Lower Risk of Coronary Artery Disease in Patients Undergoing Coronary Angiography," *American Journal of Cardiology* 102, no. 7 (2008): 814–9, https://doi.org/10.1016/j.amjcard.2008.05.021.
10. Benjamin D. Horne et al., "Relation of Routine, Periodic Fasting to Risk of Diabetes Mellitus, and Coronary Artery Disease in Patients Undergoing Coronary

Angiography," *American Journal of Cardiology* 109, no. 11 (2012): 1558–62, https://doi.org/10.1016/j.amjcard.2012.01.379.

11. C. M. McCay, Mary F. Crowell, and L. A. Maynard, "The Effect of Retarded Growth upon the Length of Life Span and upon the Ultimate Body Size," *Journal of Nutrition* 10, no. 1 (1935): 63–79, https://doi.org/10.1093/jn/10.1.63.

12. Fontana and Partridge, "Promoting Health and Longevity Through Diet."

13. Wanda Rizza, Nicola Veronese, and Luigi Fontana, "What Are the Roles of Calorie Restriction and Diet Quality in Promoting Healthy Longevity?" *Ageing Research Reviews* 13 (2014): 38–45, https://doi.org/10.1016/j.arr.2013.11.002.

14. R. L. Walford, L. Weber, and S. Panov, "Caloric Restriction and Aging As Viewed from Biosphere 2," *Receptor* 5, no 1 (1995): 29–33.

15. Roy Walford, *Beyond the 120 Year Diet: How to Double Your Vital Years* (New York: Four Walls Eight Windows, 2000).

16. Longo, *The Longevity Diet.*

17. Megumi Hatori et al., "Time-Restricted Feeding Without Reducing Caloric Intake Prevents Metabolic Diseases in Mice Fed a High-Fat Diet," *Cell Metabolism* 15, no. 6 (2012): 848–60, https://doi.org/10.1016/j.cmet.2012.04.019.

18. Longo and Panda, "Fasting, Circadian Rhythms, and Time Restricted Feeding in Healthy Lifespan."

19. Amandine Chaix et al., "Time-Restricted Feeding Is a Preventative and Therapeutic Intervention Against Diverse Nutritional Challenges," *Cell Metabolism* 20, no. 6 (2014): 991–1005, https://doi.org/10.1016/j.cmet.2014.11.001.

20. John F. Trepanowski et al., "Effect of Alternate-Day Fasting on Weight Loss, Weight Maintenance, and Cardioprotection Among Metabolically Healthy Obese Adults," *JAMA Internal Medicine* 177, no. 7 (2017): 930–8, https://doi.org/10.1001/jamain ternmed.2017.0936.

21. Krista A. Varady et al., "Alternate Day Fasting for Weight Loss in Normal Weight and Overweight Subjects: A Randomized Controlled Trial," *Nutrition Journal* 12, no. 1 (2013), https://doi.org/10.1186/1475-2891-12-146.

22. Trepanowski et al., "Effect of Alternate-Day Fasting on Weight Loss."

23. Slaven Stekovic et al., "Alternate Day Fasting Improves Physiological and Molecular Markers of Aging in Healthy, Non-Obese Humans," *Cell Metabolism* 30, no. 3 (2019): 462–76, https://doi.org/10.1016/j.cmet.2019.07.016.

24. M. N. Harvie et al., "The Effects of Intermittent or Continuous Energy Restriction on Weight Loss and Metabolic Disease Risk Markers: A Randomized Trial in Young Overweight Women," *International Journal of Obesity* 35, no. 5 (2011): 714–27, https://doi.org/10.1038/ijo.2010.171.

25. Mattson, Longo, and Harvie, "Impact of Intermittent Fasting on Health and Disease Processes."

26. Mattson, Longo, and Harvie, "Impact of Intermittent Fasting on Health and Disease Processes."

27. Ruth E. Patterson and Dorothy D. Sears, "Metabolic Effects of Intermittent Fasting," *Annual Review of Nutrition* 37 (2017): 371–93, https://doi.org/10.1146/annurev -nutr-071816-064634.

28. Michalsen and Li, "Fasting Therapy for Treating and Preventing Disease."

29. A. Ziv et al., "Comprehensive Approach to Lower Blood Pressure (CALM-BP): A Randomized Controlled Trial of a Multifactorial Lifestyle Intervention," *Journal of Human Hypertension* 27 (2013): 594–600, https://doi.org/10.1038/jhh.2013.29.

30. Shigenobu Ina et al., "Bioactive Ingredients in Rice (Oryza Sativa L.) Function in the Prevention of Type 2 Diabetes," *Journal of Nutritional Science and Vitaminology* 65, suppl. (2019): S113–6, https://doi.org/10.3177/jnsv.65.s113.

31. Yue Gao et al., "Whole Grain Brown Rice Extrudate Ameliorates the Symptoms of Diabetes by Activating the IRS1/PI3K/AKT Insulin Pathway in Db/Db Mice," *Journal of Agricultural and Food Chemistry* 67, no. 42 (2019): 11657–64, https://doi.org/10.1021/acs.jafc.9b04684.

32. Philip Klemmer, Clarence E. Grim, and Friedrich C. Luft, "Who and What Drove Walter Kempner? The Rice Diet Revisited," *Hypertension* 64, no. 4 (2014): 684–8, https://doi.org/10.1161/hypertensionaha.114.03946.

33. Neus González et al., "Dietary Exposure to Total and Inorganic Arsenic via Rice and Rice-Based Products Consumption," *Food and Chemical Toxicology* 141 (2020): 111420, https://doi.org/10.1016/j.fct.2020.111420.

34. Fang-Jie Zhao, Steve P. McGrath, and Andrew A. Meharg, "Arsenic as a Food Chain Contaminant: Mechanisms of Plant Uptake and Metabolism and Mitigation Strategies," *Annual Review of Plant Biology* 61 (2010): 535–59, https://doi.org/10.1146/annurev-arplant-042809-112152.

35. Trepanowski et al., "Effect of Alternate-Day Fasting on Weight Loss."

36. Girish C. Melkani and Satchidananda Panda, "Time-Restricted Feeding for Prevention and Treatment of Cardiometabolic Disorders," *Journal of Physiology* 595, no. 12 (2017): 3691–700, https://doi.org/10.1113/jp273094.

37. Amandine Chaix et al., "Time-Restricted Eating to Prevent and Manage Chronic Metabolic Diseases," *Annual Review of Nutrition* 39 (2019): 291–315, https://doi.org/10.1146/annurev-nutr-082018-124320.

38. Longo and Panda, "Fasting, Circadian Rhythms, and Time-Restricted Feeding in Healthy Lifespan."

39. Mattson, Longo, and Harvie, "Impact of Intermittent Fasting on Health and Disease Processes."

40. Hana Kahleova et al., "Meal Frequency and Timing Are Associated with Changes in Body Mass Index in Adventist Health Study 2," *Journal of Nutrition* 147, no. 9 (2017): 1722–8, https://doi.org/10.3945/jn.116.244749.

41. Jesus Lopez-Minguez, Purificación Gómez-Abellán, and Marta Garaulet, "Timing of Breakfast, Lunch, and Dinner. Effects on Obesity and Metabolic Risk," *Nutrients* 11, no. 11 (2019): 2624, https://doi.org/10.3390/nu11112624.

42. Hana Kahleova et al., "Eating Two Larger Meals a Day (Breakfast and Lunch) Is More Effective Than Six Smaller Meals in a Reduced-Energy Regimen for Patients with Type 2 Diabetes: A Randomised Crossover Study," *Diabetologia* 57, no. 8 (2014): 1552–60, https://doi.org/10.1007/s00125-014-3253-5.

43. M. Garaulet et al., "Timing of Food Intake Predicts Weight Loss Effectiveness," *International Journal of Obesity* 37, no. 4 (2013): 604–11, https://doi.org/10.1038/ijo.2012.229.

44. Lopez-Minguez, Gómez-Abellán, and Garaulet, "Timing of Breakfast, Lunch, and Dinner."

45. Irina Uzhova et al., "The Importance of Breakfast in Atherosclerosis Disease," *Journal of the American College of Cardiology* 70, no. 15 (2017): 1833–42, https://doi.org/10.1016/j.jacc.2017.08.027.

46. Barbara V. Howard et al., "Low-Fat Dietary Pattern and Risk of Cardiovascular Disease," *Journal of the American Medical Association* 295, no. 6 (2006): 655–66, https://doi.org/10.1001/jama.295.6.655.

47. Kahleova et al., "Eating Two Larger Meals a Day (Breakfast and Lunch) Is More Effective."

48. "Intermittent Fasting: Fad or Factual?" Catalyst Coaching Institute, https://www.catalystcoachinginstitute.com/podcast/intermittent-fasting-fad-or-factual.

49. Panda, *The Circadian Code.*

50. Manuel Calcagno et al., "The Thermic Effect of Food: A Review," *Journal of the American College of Nutrition* 38, no. 6 (2019): 547–51, https://doi.org/10.1080/07315724.2018.1552544.

51. Katharina Kessler et al., "The Effect of Diurnal Distribution of Carbohydrates and Fat on Glycaemic Control in Humans: A Randomized Controlled Trial," *Scientific Reports* 7 (2017): 44170, https://doi.org/10.1038/srep44170.

52. Gregg E. Dinse et al., "Increasing Prevalence of Antinuclear Antibodies in the United States," *Arthritis and Rheumatology* 72, no. 6 (2020): 1026–35, https://doi.org/10.1002/art.41214.

53. M. Firoze Khan and Hui Wang, "Environmental Exposures and Autoimmune Diseases: Contribution of Gut Microbiome," *Frontiers in Immunology* 10 (2020), https://doi.org/10.3389/fimmu.2019.03094.

54. Hedda L. Köhling et al., "The Microbiota and Autoimmunity: Their Role in Thyroid Autoimmune Diseases," *Clinical Immunology* 183 (2017): 63–74, https://doi.org/10.1016/j.clim.2017.07.001.

55. A. J. Richard et al., "Adipose Tissue: Physiology to Metabolic Dysfunction," in *Endotext*, ed. K. R. Feingold et al. (South Dartmouth, MA: MDText.com, 2000).

56. Joachim R. Kalden and Hendrik Schulze-Koops, "Immunogenicity and Loss of Response to TNF Inhibitors: Implications for Rheumatoid Arthritis Treatment," *Nature Reviews Rheumatology* 13, no. 12 (2017): 707–18, https://doi.org/10.1038/nrrheum.2017.187.

57. Nicola Wilck et al., "The Role of Sodium in Modulating Immune Cell Function," *Nature Reviews Nephrology* 15, no. 9 (2019): 546–58, https://doi.org/10.1038/s41581-019-0167-y.

58. Mirzaei, Di Biase, and Longo, "Dietary Interventions, Cardiovascular Aging, and Disease."

Chapter Eight: Intermittent Fasting—The Practical Program

1. Angela Relógio et al., "Tuning the Mammalian Circadian Clock: Robust Synergy of Two Loops," *PLoS Computational Biology* 7, no. 12 (2011): e1002309, https://doi.org/10.1371/journal.pcbi.1002309.

2. Satchidananda Panda, "The Arrival of Circadian Medicine," *Nature Reviews Endocrinology* 15, no. 2 (2019): 67–9, https://doi.org/10.1038/s41574-018-0142-x.

3. Emily N. C. Manoogian and Satchidananda Panda, "Circadian Rhythms, Time-Restricted Feeding, and Healthy Aging," *Ageing Research Reviews* 39 (2017): 59–67, https://doi.org/10.1016/j.arr.2016.12.006.

4. Katharina Kessler et al., "Saliva Samples as a Tool to Study the Effect of Meal Timing on Metabolic and Inflammatory Biomarkers," *Nutrients* 12, no. 2 (2020): 340, https://doi.org/10.3390/nu12020340.

5. Eva Wolf and Achim Kramer, "Circadian Regulation: From Molecules to Physiology," *Journal of Molecular Biology* 432, no. 12 (2020): 3423–5, https://doi.org/10.1016/j.jmb.2020.05.004.

6. H. van Praag et al., "Exercise, Energy Intake, Glucose Homeostasis, and the Brain," *Journal of Neuroscience* 34, no. 46 (2014): 15139–49, https://doi.org/10.1523/jneurosci.2814-14.2014.

7. Mark P. Mattson, "Challenging Oneself Intermittently to Improve Health," *Dose-Response* 12, no. 4 (2014): 600–18, https://doi.org/10.2203/dose-response.14-028.mattson.

8. Frank Madeo et al., "Spermidine in Health and Disease," *Science* 359, no. 6374 (2018): eaan2788, https://doi.org/10.1126/science.aan2788.

9. Madeo et al., "Spermidine in Health and Disease."

10. Frank Madeo et al., "Caloric Restriction Mimetics Against Age-Associated Disease: Targets, Mechanisms, and Therapeutic Potential," *Cell Metabolism* 29, no. 3 (2019): 592–610, https://doi.org/10.1016/j.cmet.2019.01.018.

11. Frank Madeo et al., "Spermidine Delays Aging in Humans," *Aging* 10, no. 8 (2018): 2209–11, https://doi.org/10.18632/aging.101517.

12. Madeo et al., "Spermidine in Health and Disease."

13. Madeo et al., "Caloric Restriction Mimetics Against Age-Associated Disease."

14. Stefan Kiechl et al., "Higher Spermidine Intake Is Linked to Lower Mortality: A Prospective Population-Based Study," *American Journal of Clinical Nutrition* 108, no. 2 (2018): 371–80, https://doi.org/10.1093/ajcn/nqy102.

15. R. Walford et al., "Physiologic Changes in Humans Subjected to Severe, Selective Calorie Restriction for Two Years in Biosphere 2: Health, Aging, and Toxicological Perspectives," *Toxicological Sciences* 52, no. 2 suppl. (1999): 61–5.

16. L. Fontana, L. Partridge, and V. D. Longo, "Extending Healthy Life Span—From Yeast to Humans," *Science* 328, no. 5976 (2010): 321–6, https://doi.org/10.1126/science.1172539.

17. Longo, *The Longevity Diet.*

18. V. D. Longo and C. E. Finch, "Evolutionary Medicine: From Dwarf Model Systems to Healthy Centenarians?" *Science* 299, no. 5611 (2003): 1342–6, https://doi.org/10.1126/science.1077991.

19. Longo and Finch, "Evolutionary Medicine."

20. V. D. Longo and P. Fabrizio, "Regulation of Longevity and Stress Resistance: A Molecular Strategy Conserved from Yeast to Humans?" *Cellular and Molecular Life Sciences* 59, no. 6 (2002): 903–8, https://doi.org/10.1007/s00018-002-8477-8.

21. Longo, *The Longevity Diet.*

22. Jaime Guevara-Aguirre et al., "GH Receptor Deficiency in Ecuadorian Adults Is Associated with Obesity and Enhanced Insulin Sensitivity," *Journal of Clinical Endocrinology and Metabolism* 100, no. 7 (2015): 2589–96, https://doi.org/10.1210/jc.2015-1678.

23. Shim and Longo, "A Protein Restriction-Dependent Sulfur Code for Longevity."

24. Min Wei et al., "Life Span Extension by Calorie Restriction Depends on Rim15 and Transcription Factors Downstream of Ras/PKA, Tor, and Sch9," *PLoS Genetics* 4, no. 1 (2008): e13, https://doi.org/10.1371/journal.pgen.0040013.

25. Min et al., "Life Span Extension by Calorie Restriction."

26. Mattson, Longo, and Harvie, "Impact of Intermittent Fasting on Health and Disease Processes."

27. Françoise Wilhelmi de Toledo et al., "Safety, Health Improvement and Well-Being During a 4 to 21-Day Fasting Period in an Observational Study Including 1422 Subjects," *Plos One* 14, no. 1 (2019): e0209353, https://doi.org/10.1371/journal.pone.0209353.

28. Michalsen and Li, "Fasting Therapy for Treating and Preventing Disease—Current State of Evidence."

29. Mattson, Longo, and Harvie, "Impact of Intermittent Fasting on Health and Disease Processes."

30. Huajun Yang et al., "Ketone Bodies in Neurological Diseases: Focus on Neuroprotection and Underlying Mechanisms," *Frontiers in Neurology* 10 (2019): 585, https://doi.org/10.3389/fneur.2019.00585.

31. Simonetta Camandola and Mark P Mattson, "Brain Metabolism in Health, Aging, and Neurodegeneration," *EMBO Journal* 36, no. 11 (2017): 1474–92, https://doi.org/10.15252/embj.201695810.

32. Robert M. Edinburgh et al., "Lipid Metabolism Links Nutrient-Exercise Timing to Insulin Sensitivity in Men Classified as Overweight or Obese," *Journal of Clinical Endocrinology and Metabolism* 105, no. 3 (2020): 660–76, https://doi.org/10.1210/clinem/dgz104.

33. Mark Hopkins, "Does Hepatic Carbohydrate Availability Influence Postexercise Compensation in Energy Intake?" *Journal of Nutrition* 149, no. 8 (2019): 1305–6, https://doi.org/10.1093/jn/nxz131.

34. Françoise Wilhelmi de Toledo et al., "Fasting Therapy—an Expert Panel Update of the 2002 Consensus Guidelines" *Forschende Komplementärmedizin/Research in Complementary Medicine* 20, no. 6 (2013): 434–43, https://doi.org/10.1159/000357602.

35. De Toledo et al., "Safety, Health Improvement and Well-Being During a 4 to 21-Day Fasting Period."

36. Edward J. Calabrese and Mark P. Mattson, "How Does Hormesis Impact Biology, Toxicology, and Medicine?" *NPJ Aging and Mechanisms of Disease* 3 (2017): 13, https://doi.org/10.1038/s41514-017-0013-z.

37. Mattson, "Hormesis Defined."

38. Mattson, "Hormesis Defined."

39. Mirzaei, Di Biase, and Longo, "Dietary Interventions, Cardiovascular Aging, and Disease."

40. Krisztina Marosi et al., "Metabolic and Molecular Framework for the Enhancement of Endurance by Intermittent Food Deprivation," *FASEB Journal* 32, no. 7 (2018): 3844–58, https://doi.org/10.1096/fj.201701378rr.

41. Marosi et al., "Metabolic and Molecular Framework."

42. C.-W. Cheng et al., "Prolonged Fasting Reduces IGF-1/PKA to Promote Hematopoietic-Stem-Cell-Based Regeneration and Reverse Immunosuppression," *Cell Stem Cell* 14, no. 6 (2014): 810–23, https://doi.org/10.1016/j.stem.2014.04.014.

43. Aman Rajpal and Faramarz Ismail-Beigi, "Intermittent Fasting and 'Metabolic Switch': Effects on Metabolic Syndrome, Prediabetes and Type 2 Diabetes," *Diabetes, Obesity and Metabolism* 22 (2020), https://doi.org/10.1111/dom.14080.

44. Katja Matt et al., "Influence of Calorie Reduction on DNA Repair Capacity of Human Peripheral Blood Mononuclear Cells," *Mechanisms of Ageing and Development* 154 (2016): 24–9, https://doi.org/10.1016/j.mad.2016.02.008.

45. Bas Kast, "Gesundes Fasten: 'Begrüße den Hunger Wie Einen Freund,'" *Stern*, December 27, 2019, https://www.stern.de/gesundheit/ernaehrung/fasten-experte -frank-madeo—-begruesse-den-hunger-wie-einen-freund—8588810.html.

46. Rafael de Cabo et al., "The Search for Antiaging Interventions: From Elixirs to Fasting Regimens," *Cell* 157, no. 7 (2014): 1515–26, https://doi.org/10.1016/j.cell.2014.05.031.

47. Frank Madeo, Nektarios Tavernarakis, and Guido Kroemer, "Can Autophagy Promote Longevity?" *Nature Cell Biology* 12, no. 9 (2010): 842–6, https://doi.org/10.1038/ncb0910-842.

48. Didac Carmona-Gutierrez et al., "The Crucial Impact of Lysosomes in Aging and Longevity," *Ageing Research Reviews* 32 (2016): 2–12, https://doi.org/10.1016/j.arr.2016.04.009.

49. Qian Cai and Yu Young Jeong, "Mitophagy in Alzheimer's Disease and Other Age-Related Neurodegenerative Diseases," *Cells* 9, no. 1 (2020): 150, https://doi.org/10.3390/cells9010150.

50. Kast, "Gesundes Fasten."

51. McLean et al., "Does the Microbiota Play a Role in the Pathogenesis of Autoimmune Diseases?"

52. Joel T. Haas and Bart Staels, "Fasting the Microbiota to Improve Metabolism?" *Cell Metabolism* 26, no. 4 (2017): 584–5, https://doi.org/10.1016/j.cmet.2017.09.013.

53. Xue Liang and Garret A. FitzGerald, "Timing the Microbes: The Circadian Rhythm of the Gut Microbiome," *Journal of Biological Rhythms* 32, no. 6 (2017): 505–15, https://doi.org/10.1177/0748730417729066.

54. Francesca Cignarella et al., "Intermittent Fasting Confers Protection in CNS Autoimmunity by Altering the Gut Microbiota," *Cell Metabolism* 27, no. 6 (2018): 1222–35, https://doi.org/10.1016/j.cmet.2018.05.006.

55. Priya Rangan et al., "Fasting-Mimicking Diet Modulates Microbiota and Promotes Intestinal Regeneration to Reduce Inflammatory Bowel Disease Pathology," *Cell Reports* 26, no. 10 (2019): 2704–19, https://doi.org/10.1016/j.celrep.2019.02.019.

56. Guillaume Fond et al., "Fasting in Mood Disorders: Neurobiology and Effectiveness. A Review of the Literature," *Psychiatry Research* 209, no. 3 (2013): 253–8, https://doi.org/10.1016/j.psychres.2012.12.018.

Chapter Nine: Using Nutrition and Fasting to Cure Chronic Illness

1. Iris Shai et al., "Weight Loss with a Low-Carbohydrate, Mediterranean, or Low-Fat Diet," *New England Journal of Medicine* 359, no. 3 (2008): 229–41, https://doi.org/10.1056/nejmoa0708681.
2. Calcagno et al., "The Thermic Effect of Food."
3. Neal D. Barnard et al., "The Effects of a Low-Fat, Plant-Based Dietary Intervention on Body Weight, Metabolism, and Insulin Sensitivity," *American Journal of Medicine* 118, no. 9 (2005): 991–7, https://doi.org/10.1016/j.amjmed.2005.03.039.
4. Anne-Claire Vergnaud et al., "Meat Consumption and Prospective Weight Change in Participants of the EPIC-PANACEA Study," *American Journal of Clinical Nutrition* 92, no. 2 (2010): 398–407, https://doi.org/10.3945/ajcn.2009.28713.
5. Anne M. J. Gilsing et al., "Longitudinal Changes in BMI in Older Adults Are Associated with Meat Consumption Differentially, by Type of Meat Consumed," *Journal of Nutrition* 142, no. 2 (2012): 340–9, https://doi.org/10.3945/jn.111.146258.
6. Pinky Raigond, Rajarathnam Ezekiel, and Baswaraj Raigond, "Resistant Starch in Food: A Review," *Journal of the Science of Food and Agriculture* 95, no. 10 (2015): 1968–78, https://doi.org/10.1002/jsfa.6966.
7. Hamed Mirzaei, Jorge A. Suarez, and Valter D. Longo, "Protein and Amino Acid Restriction, Aging and Disease: From Yeast to Humans," *Trends in Endocrinology and Metabolism* 25, no. 11 (2014): 558–66, https://doi.org/10.1016/j.tem.2014.07.002.
8. Levine et al., "Low Protein Intake Is Associated with a Major Reduction in IGF-1, Cancer, and Overall Mortality."
9. Chunxue Yang et al., "Persistent Organic Pollutants as Risk Factors for Obesity and Diabetes," *Current Diabetes Reports* 17, no. 12 (2017): 132, https://doi.org/10.1007/s11892-017-0966-0.
10. Farideh Shishehbor, Anahita Mansoori, and Fatemeh Shirani, "Vinegar Consumption Can Attenuate Postprandial Glucose and Insulin Responses; a Systematic Review and Meta-Analysis of Clinical Trials," *Diabetes Research and Clinical Practice* 127 (2017): 1–9, https://doi.org/10.1016/j.diabres.2017.01.021.
11. Michael Boschmann et al., "Water Drinking Induces Thermogenesis Through Osmosensitive Mechanisms," *Journal of Clinical Endocrinology and Metabolism* 92, no. 8 (2007): 3334–7, https://doi.org/10.1210/jc.2006-1438.
12. Hao Wu et al., "Metformin Alters the Gut Microbiome of Individuals with Treatment-Naive Type 2 Diabetes, Contributing to the Therapeutic Effects of the Drug," *Nature Medicine* 23, no. 7 (2017): 850–8, https://doi.org/10.1038/nm.4345.
13. Jotham Suez et al., "Artificial Sweeteners Induce Glucose Intolerance by Altering the Gut Microbiota," *Nature* 514, no. 7521 (2014): 181–6, https://doi.org/10.1038/nature13793.

14. Xiaofa Qin, "The Effect of Splenda on Gut Microbiota of Humans Could Be Much More Detrimental Than in Animals and Deserves More Extensive Research," *Inflammatory Bowel Diseases* 25, no. 2 (2019): e7, https://doi.org/10.1093/ibd/izy181.

15. Romo-Romo et al., "Sucralose Decreases Insulin Sensitivity in Healthy Subjects."

16. Shishehbor, Mansoori, and Shirani, "Vinegar Consumption Can Attenuate Postprandial Glucose and Insulin Responses."

17. David J. A. Jenkins et al., "Effect of a Very-High-Fiber Vegetable, Fruit, and Nut Diet on Serum Lipids and Colonic Function," *Metabolism* 50, no. 4 (2001): 494–503, https://doi.org/10.1053/meta.2001.21037.

18. Annika S. Axelsson et al., "Sulforaphane Reduces Hepatic Glucose Production and Improves Glucose Control in Patients with Type 2 Diabetes," *Science Translational Medicine* 9, no. 394 (2017): eaah4477, https://doi.org/10.1126/scitranslmed.aah4477.

19. Axelsson et al., "Sulforaphane Reduces Hepatic Glucose Production."

20. F. Javier Basterra-Gortari et al., "Effects of a Mediterranean Eating Plan on the Need for Glucose-Lowering Medications in Participants with Type 2 Diabetes: A Subgroup Analysis of the PREDIMED Trial," *Diabetes Care* 42, no. 8 (2019): 1390–7, https://doi.org/10.2337/dc18-2475.

21. J. Salas-Salvadó et al., "Reduction in the Incidence of Type 2 Diabetes with the Mediterranean Diet: Results of the PREDIMED-Reus Nutrition Intervention Randomized Trial," *Diabetes Care* 34, no. 1 (2011): 14–9, https://doi.org/10.2337/dc10-1288.

22. Agathi Ntzouvani, Smaragdi Antonopoulou, and Tzortzis Nomikos, "Effects of Nut and Seed Consumption on Markers of Glucose Metabolism in Adults with Prediabetes: A Systematic Review of Randomised Controlled Trials," *British Journal of Nutrition* 122, no. 4 (2019): 361–75, https://doi.org/10.1017/s0007114519001338.

23. Vita Dikariyanto et al., "Snacking on Whole Almonds for 6 Weeks Improves Endothelial Function and Lowers LDL Cholesterol but Does Not Affect Liver Fat and Other Cardiometabolic Risk Factors in Healthy Adults: The ATTIS Study, a Randomized Controlled Trial," *American Journal of Clinical Nutrition* 111, no. 6 (2020): 1178–89, https://doi.org/10.1093/ajcn/nqaa100.

24. Vahideh Ebrahimzadeh Attari et al., "A Systematic Review of the Anti-Obesity and Weight Lowering Effect of Ginger (Zingiber Officinale Roscoe) and Its Mechanisms of Action," *Phytotherapy Research* 32, no. 4 (2017): 577–85, https://doi.org/10.1002/ptr.5986.

25. Shen et al., "Effect of Oat β-Glucan Intake on Glycaemic Control and Insulin Sensitivity of Diabetic Patients."

26. Amir Hadi et al., "Effect of Flaxseed Supplementation on Lipid Profile: An Updated Systematic Review and Dose-Response Meta-Analysis of Sixty-Two Randomized Controlled Trials," *Pharmacological Research* 152 (2020): 104622, https://doi.org/10.1016/j.phrs.2019.104622.

27. Dan Ramdath, Simone Renwick, and Alison M. Duncan, "The Role of Pulses in the Dietary Management of Diabetes," *Canadian Journal of Diabetes* 40, no. 4 (2016): 355–63, https://doi.org/10.1016/j.jcjd.2016.05.015.

28. Heitor O. Santos and Guilherme A. R. da Silva, "To What Extent Does Cinnamon Administration Improve the Glycemic and Lipid Profiles?" *Clinical Nutrition ESPEN* 27 (2018): 1–9, https://doi.org/10.1016/j.clnesp.2018.07.011.

29. Alexander Kokkinos et al., "Eating Slowly Increases the Postprandial Response of the Anorexigenic Gut Hormones, Peptide YY and Glucagon-Like Peptide-1," *Journal of Clinical Endocrinology and Metabolism* 95, no. 1 (2010): 333–7, https://doi.org/10.1210/jc.2009-1018.

30. Drinda et al., "Effects of Periodic Fasting on Fatty Liver Index."

31. Toledo et al., "Safety, Health Improvement and Well-Being During a 4 to 21-Day Fasting Period."

32. Li et al., "Effects of a One-Week Fasting Therapy in Patients with Type-2 Diabetes Mellitus."

33. Nicholas J. Schork, "Personalized Medicine: Time for One-Person Trials," *Nature* 520, no. 7549 (2015): 609–11, https://doi.org/10.1038/520609a.

34. C. B. Esselstyn, "A Plant-Based Diet and Coronary Artery Disease: A Mandate for Effective Therapy," *Journal of Geriatric Cardiology* 14, no. 5 (2017): 317–20, https://doi.org/10.11909/j.issn.1671-5411.2017.05.004.

35. "Dean Ornish, MD: A Conversation with the Editor. Interview by William Clifford Roberts, MD," *American Journal of Cardiology* 90, no. 3 (2002): 271–98, https://doi.org/10.1016/s0002-9149(02)02486-4.

36. Hadi et al., "Effect of Flaxseed Supplementation on Lipid Profile."

37. Arpita Basu, Michael Rhone, and Timothy J. Lyons, "Berries: Emerging Impact on Cardiovascular Health," *Nutrition Reviews* 68, no. 3 (2010): 168–77, https://doi.org/10.1111/j.1753-4887.2010.00273.x.

38. De Lorgeril, "Mediterranean Diet and Cardiovascular Disease: Historical Perspective and Latest Evidence."

39. Ganiyu Oboh et al., "Inhibitory Effect of Garlic, Purple Onion, and White Onion on Key Enzymes Linked with Type 2 Diabetes and Hypertension," *Journal of Dietary Supplements* 16, no. 1 (2019): 105–18, https://doi.org/10.1080/19390211.2018.1438553.

40. Marian Grman et al., "The Aqueous Garlic, Onion and Leek Extracts Release Nitric Oxide from S-Nitrosoglutathione and Prolong Relaxation of Aortic Rings," *General Physiology and Biophysics* 30, no. 4 (2011): 396–402, https://doi.org /10.4149/gpb_2011_04_396.

41. Sawsan G. Mohammed and M. Walid Qoronfleh, "Nuts," *Advances in Neurobiology: Personalized Food Intervention and Therapy for Autism Spectrum Disorder Management* (2020): 395–419, https://doi.org/10.1007/978-3-030-30402-7_12.

42. Natalia Dos Santos Tramontin et al., "Ginger and Avocado as Nutraceuticals for Obesity and Its Comorbidities," *Phytotherapy Research* 34, no. 6 (2020): 1282–90, https://doi.org/10.1002/ptr.6619.

43. Si Qin et al., "Efficacy and Safety of Turmeric and Curcumin in Lowering Blood Lipid Levels in Patients with Cardiovascular Risk Factors: A Meta-Analysis of Randomized Controlled Trials," *Nutrition Journal* 16, no. 1 (2017): 68, https://doi.org/10.1186/s12937-017-0293-y.

44. Malika Bouchenak and Myriem Lamri-Senhadji, "Nutritional Quality of Legumes, and Their Role in Cardiometabolic Risk Prevention: A Review," *Journal of Medicinal Food* 16, no. 3 (2013): 185–98, https://doi.org/10.1089/jmf.2011.0238.

45. David Khalaf et al., "The Effects of Oral l-Arginine and l-Citrulline Supplementation on Blood Pressure," *Nutrients* 11, no. 7 (2019): 1679, https://doi.org/10.3390/nu11071679.

46. Jibran Khatri et al., "It Is Rocket Science—Why Dietary Nitrate Is Hard to 'Beet'! Part I: Twists and Turns in the Realization of the Nitrate-Nitrite-NO Pathway," *British Journal of Clinical Pharmacology* 83, no. 1 (2017): 129–39, https://doi.org/10.1111/bcp.12913.

47. Michael D. Sumner et al., "Effects of Pomegranate Juice Consumption on Myocardial Perfusion in Patients with Coronary Heart Disease," *American Journal of Cardiology* 96, no. 6 (2005): 810–4, https://doi.org/10.1016/j.amjcard.2005.05.026.

48. Hiroshi Nakamura et al., "Effects of Acute Protein Loads of Different Sources on Renal Function of Patients with Diabetic Nephropathy," *Tohoku Journal of Experimental Medicine* 159, no. 2 (1989): 153–62, https://doi.org/10.1620/tjem.159.153.

49. A. Simon, "Renal Haemodynamic Responses to a Chicken or Beef Meal in Normal Individuals," *Nephrology Dialysis Transplantation* 13, no. 9 (1998): 2261–4, https://doi.org/10.1093/ndt/13.9.2261.

50. María M. Adeva and Gema Souto, "Diet-Induced Metabolic Acidosis," *Clinical Nutrition* 30, no. 4 (2011): 416–21, https://doi.org/10.1016/j.clnu.2011.03.008.

51. Peter Deriemaeker et al., "Nutrient Based Estimation of Acid-Base Balance in Vegetarians and Non-Vegetarians," *Plant Foods for Human Nutrition* 65, no. 1 (2010): 77–82, https://doi.org/10.1007/s11130-009-0149-5.

52. William F. Clark et al., "Effect of Coaching to Increase Water Intake on Kidney Function Decline in Adults with Chronic Kidney Disease," *Journal of the American Medical Association* 319, no. 18 (2018): 1870–9, https://doi.org/10.1001/jama.2018.4930.

53. Y. Liu et al., "Gut Microbiota and Obesity-Associated Osteoarthritis," *Osteoarthritis and Cartilage* 27, no. 9 (2019): 1257–65, https://doi.org/10.1016/j.joca.2019.05.009.

54. Michalsen and Li, "Fasting Therapy for Treating and Preventing Disease."

55. Michalsen and Li, "Fasting Therapy for Treating and Preventing Disease."

56. Olaf Adam et al., "Anti-Inflammatory Effects of a Low Arachidonic Acid Diet and Fish Oil in Patients with Rheumatoid Arthritis," *Rheumatology International* 23, no. 1 (2003): 27–36, https://doi.org/10.1007/s00296-002-0234-7.

57. Hedi Harizi, Jean-Benoît Corcuff, and Norbert Gualde, "Arachidonic-Acid-Derived Eicosanoids: Roles in Biology and Immunopathology," *Trends in Molecular Medicine* 14, no. 10 (2008): 461–9, https://doi.org/10.1016/j.molmed.2008.08.005.

58. Clara M. Yates, Philip C. Calder, and G. Ed Rainger, "Pharmacology and Therapeutics of Omega-3 Polyunsaturated Fatty Acids in Chronic Inflammatory Disease," *Pharmacology and Therapeutics* 141, no. 3 (2014): 272–82, https://doi.org/10.1016/j.pharmthera.2013.10.010.

59. T. Buclin et al., "Diet Acids and Alkalis Influence Calcium Retention in Bone," *Osteoporosis International* 12, no. 6 (2001): 493–9, https://doi.org/10.1007/s001980170095.

60. Rahul Bodkhe, Baskar Balakrishnan, and Veena Taneja, "The Role of Microbiome in Rheumatoid Arthritis Treatment," *Therapeutic Advances in Musculoskeletal Disease* 11 (2019), https://doi.org/10.1177/1759720x19844632.

61. Kevin D. Deane et al., "Genetic and Environmental Risk Factors for Rheumatoid Arthritis," *Best Practice and Research Clinical Rheumatology* 31, no. 1 (2017): 3–18, https://doi.org/10.1016/j.berh.2017.08.003.

62. Harizi, Corcuff, and Gualde, "Arachidonic-Acid-Derived Eicosanoids."

63. Anne Baron and Eric Lingueglia, "Pharmacology of Acid-Sensing Ion Channels—Physiological and Therapeutical Perspectives," *Neuropharmacology* 94 (2015): 19–35, https://doi.org/10.1016/j.neuropharm.2015.01.005.

64. Olov Lindahl, "Metabolic Treatment in Diffuse Pain (Varialgia)," *Acta Rheumatologica Scandinavica* 12, no. 1–4 (1966): 153–60, https://doi.org/10.3109/rhe1.1966.12.issue-1-4.18.

65. Nicola Wilck et al., "Salt-Responsive Gut Commensal Modulates TH17 Axis and Disease," *Nature* 551, no. 7682 (2017): 585–9, https://doi.org/10.1038/nature24628.

66. Buchinger, *Das Heilfasten und Seine Hilfsmethoden Als Biologischer Weg.*

67. Kjeldsen-Kragh et al., "Controlled Trial of Fasting and One-Year Vegetarian Diet in Rheumatoid Arthritis."

68. Müller, De Toledo, and Resch, "Fasting Followed by Vegetarian Diet in Patients with Rheumatoid Arthritis."

69. Lars Sköldstam, "Preliminary Reports: Fasting and Vegan Diet in Rheumatoid Arthritis," *Scandinavian Journal of Rheumatology* 15, no. 2 (1986): 219–21, https://doi.org/10.3109/03009748609102091.

70. Rebecca M. Lovell and Alexander C. Ford, "Global Prevalence of and Risk Factors for Irritable Bowel Syndrome: A Meta-Analysis," *Clinical Gastroenterology and Hepatology* 10, no. 7 (2012): 712–21, https://doi.org/10.1016/j.cgh.2012.02.029.

71. Paul Enck et al., "Irritable Bowel Syndrome," *Nature Reviews Disease Primers* 2 (2016): 16014, https://doi.org/10.1038/nrdp.2016.14.

72. Enck et al., "Irritable Bowel Syndrome."

73. Gerald J. Holtmann, Alexander C. Ford, and Nicholas J. Talley, "Pathophysiology of Irritable Bowel Syndrome," *Lancet Gastroenterology and Hepatology* 1, no. 2 (2016): 133–46, https://doi.org/10.1016/s2468-1253(16)30023-1.

74. William D. Chey, Jacob Kurlander, and Shanti Eswaran, "Irritable Bowel Syndrome: A Clinical Review," *Journal of the American Medical Association* 313, no. 9 (2015): 949–58, https://doi.org/10.1001/jama.2015.0954.

75. Sophie Leclercq et al., "Intestinal Permeability, Gut-Bacterial Dysbiosis, and Behavioral Markers of Alcohol-Dependence Severity," *Proceedings of the National Academy of Sciences* 111, no. 42 (2014): E4485–93, https://doi.org/10.1073/pnas.1415174111.

76. Ingvar Bjarnason, Kevin Ward, and Timothy J. Peters, "The Leaky Gut of Alcoholism: Possible Route of Entry for Toxic Compounds," *Lancet* 323, no. 8370 (1984): 179–82, https://doi.org/10.1016/s0140-6736(84)92109-3.

77. Lyn Guenther and Wayne Gulliver, "Psoriasis Comorbidities," *Journal of Cutaneous Medicine and Surgery* 13, no. 5_suppl (2009), https://doi.org/10.2310/7750 .2009.00024.

78. Emilia Rusu et al., "Prebiotics and Probiotics in Atopic Dermatitis (Review)," *Experimental and Therapeutic Medicine* 18, no. 2 (2019): 926–31, https://doi.org /10.3892/etm.2019.7678.

79. M. Andreassi et al., "Efficacy of γ-Linolenic Acid in the Treatment of Patients with Atopic Dermatitis," *Journal of International Medical Research* 25, no. 5 (1997): 266–74, https://doi.org/10.1177/030006059702500504.

80. Negar Foolad et al., "Effect of Nutrient Supplementation on Atopic Dermatitis in Children," *JAMA Dermatology* 149, no. 3 (2013): 350–5, https://doi.org/10.1001 /jamadermatol.2013.1495.

81. Bo Lundbäck et al., "Is Asthma Prevalence Still Increasing?" *Expert Review of Respiratory Medicine* 10, no. 1 (2016): 39–51, https://doi.org/10.1586/17476348 .2016.1114417.

82. Cheng S. Wang et al., "Is the Consumption of Fast Foods Associated with Asthma or Other Allergic Diseases?" *Respirology* 23, no. 10 (2018): 901–13, https://doi .org/10.1111/resp.13339.

83. Alfonso Mario Cepeda et al., "Diet and Respiratory Health in Children from 11 Latin American Countries: Evidence from ISAAC Phase III," *Lung* 195, no. 6 (2017): 683–92, https://doi.org/10.1007/s00408-017-0044-z.

84. L. Garcia-Marcos et al., "Influence of Mediterranean Diet on Asthma in Children: A Systematic Review and Meta-Analysis," *Pediatric Allergy and Immunology* 24, no. 4 (2013): 330–8, https://doi.org/10.1111/pai.12071.

85. Hsin-Jen Tsai and Alan C. Tsai, "The Association of Diet with Respiratory Symptoms and Asthma in Schoolchildren in Taipei, Taiwan," *Journal of Asthma* 44, no. 8 (2007): 599–603, https://doi.org/10.1080/02770900701539509.

86. Craig McKenzie et al., "The Nutrition-Gut Microbiome-Physiology Axis and Allergic Diseases," *Immunological Reviews* 278, no. 1 (2017): 277–95, https://doi .org/10.1111/imr.12556.

87. Heike Stier, Veronika Ebbeskotte, and Joerg Gruenwald, "Immune-Modulatory Effects of Dietary Yeast Beta-1,3/1,6-D-Glucan," *Nutrition Journal* 13 (2014): 38, https://doi.org/10.1186/1475-2891-13-38.

88. C. Kirmaz et al., "Effects of Glucan Treatment on the Th1/Th2 Balance in Patients with Allergic Rhinitis: A Double-Blind Placebo-Controlled Study," *European Cytokine Network* 16, no. 2 (2005): 128–34.

89. G. Mortuaire et al., "Specific Immunotherapy in Allergic Rhinitis," *European Annals of Otorhinolaryngology, Head and Neck Diseases* 134, no. 4 (2017): 253–8, https://doi.org/10.1016/j.anorl.2017.06.005.

90. Hans-Christoph Diener et al., "Medication-Overuse Headache: Risk Factors, Pathophysiology and Management," *Nature Reviews Neurology* 12, no. 10 (2016): 575–83, https://doi.org/10.1038/nrneurol.2016.124.

91. "Antidepressant Use Among Persons Aged 12 and Over: United States, 2011–2014," Centers for Disease Control and Prevention, https://www.cdc.gov/nchs/products /databriefs/db283.htm.

92. Vikram Patel et al., "Addressing the Burden of Mental, Neurological, and Substance Use Disorders: Key Messages from Disease Control Priorities, 3rd Edition," *Lancet* 387, no. 10028 (2016): 1672–85, https://doi.org/10.1016/s0140 -6736(15)00390-6.

93. Klaus Munkholm, Asger Sand Paludan-Müller, and Kim Boesen, "Considering the Methodological Limitations in the Evidence Base of Antidepressants for Depression: A Reanalysis of a Network Meta-Analysis," *BMJ Open* 9, no. 6 (2019): e024886, https://doi.org/10.1136/bmjopen-2018-024886.

94. Felice N. Jacka et al., "A Randomised Controlled Trial of Dietary Improvement for Adults with Major Depression (the 'SMILES' Trial)," *BMC Medicine* 15, no. 1 (2017): 23, https://doi.org/10.1186/s12916-017-0791-y.

95. Kaijun Niu et al., "A Tomato-Rich Diet Is Related to Depressive Symptoms Among an Elderly Population Aged 70 Years and Over: A Population-Based, Cross-Sectional Analysis," *Journal of Affective Disorders* 144, no. 1–2 (2013): 165–70, https://doi.org/10.1016/j.jad.2012.04.040.

96. Mojtaba Shafiee et al., "Saffron in the Treatment of Depression, Anxiety and Other Mental Disorders: Current Evidence and Potential Mechanisms of Action," *Journal of Affective Disorders* 227 (2018): 330–7, https://doi.org/10.1016/j.jad .2017.11.020.

97. Sarah E. Dixon Clarke and Rona R. Ramsay, "Dietary Inhibitors of Monoamine Oxidase A," *Journal of Neural Transmission* 118, no. 7 (2010): 1031–41, https:// doi.org/10.1007/s00702-010-0537-x.

98. Andreas Nievergelt et al., "Identification of Serotonin 5-HT1A Receptor Partial Agonists in Ginger," *Bioorganic and Medicinal Chemistry* 18, no. 9 (2010): 3345–51, https://doi.org/10.1016/j.bmc.2010.02.062.

99. Laura R. LaChance and Drew Ramsey, "Antidepressant Foods: An Evidence-Based Nutrient Profiling System for Depression," *World Journal of Psychiatry* 8, no. 3 (2018): 97–104, https://doi.org/10.5498/wjp.v8.i3.97.

100. Dixon Clarke and Ramsay, "Dietary Inhibitors of Monoamine Oxidase A."

101. Sushrut Jangi et al., "Alterations of the Human Gut Microbiome in Multiple Sclerosis," *Nature Communications* 7 (2016): 12015, https://doi.org/10.1038/ncomms12015.

102. Dean M. Wingerchuk and Brian G. Weinshenker, "Disease Modifying Therapies for Relapsing Multiple Sclerosis," *BMJ* 354 (2016): i3518, https://doi.org/10.1136 /bmj.i3518.

103. Ilana Katz Sand, "The Role of Diet in Multiple Sclerosis: Mechanistic Connections and Current Evidence," *Current Nutrition Reports* 7, no. 3 (2018): 150–60, https://doi.org/10.1007/s13668-018-0236-z.

104. Choi et al., "A Diet Mimicking Fasting Promotes Regeneration."

105. Kassandra L. Munger et al., "Dietary Intake of Vitamin D During Adolescence and Risk of Multiple Sclerosis," *Journal of Neurology* 258, no. 3 (2011): 479–85, https://doi.org/10.1007/s00415-010-5783-1.

106. Johannes Guggenmos et al., "Antibody Cross-Reactivity Between Myelin Oligodendrocyte Glycoprotein and the Milk Protein Butyrophilin in Multiple Sclerosis," *Journal of Immunology* 172, no. 1 (2004): 661–8, https://doi.org/10.4049 /jimmunol.172.1.661.

107. Stefanie Haase et al., "Sodium Chloride Triggers Th17 Mediated Autoimmunity," *Journal of Neuroimmunology* 329 (2019): 9–13, https://doi.org/10.1016/j.jneuroim.2018.06.016.

108. Fatemeh Ayoobi et al., "Achillea Millefolium Is Beneficial as an Add-on Therapy in Patients with Multiple Sclerosis: A Randomized Placebo-Controlled Clinical Trial," *Phytomedicine* 52 (2019): 89–97, https://doi.org/10.1016/j.phymed.2018.06.017.

109. Klarissa Hanja Stürner et al., "A Standardised Frankincense Extract Reduces Disease Activity in Relapsing-Remitting Multiple Sclerosis (the SABA Phase IIa Trial)," *Journal of Neurology, Neurosurgery and Psychiatry* 89, no. 4 (2018): 330–8, https://doi.org/10.1136/jnnp-2017-317101.

110. Camandola and Mattson, "Brain Metabolism in Health, Aging, and Neurodegeneration."

111. Choi et al., "A Diet Mimicking Fasting Promotes Regeneration."

112. Lina Samira Bahr et al., "Ketogenic Diet and Fasting Diet as Nutritional Approaches in Multiple Sclerosis (NAMS): Protocol of a Randomized Controlled Study," *Trials* 21 (2020): 3, https://doi.org/10.1186/s13063-019-3928-9.

113. James Parkinson, "An Essay on the Shaking Palsy," *Journal of Neuropsychiatry and Clinical Neurosciences* 14, no. 2 (2002): 223–36, https://doi.org/10.1176/jnp.14.2.223.

114. Anouck Becker et al., "A Punch in the Gut—Intestinal Inflammation Links Environmental Factors to Neurodegeneration in Parkinson's Disease," *Parkinsonism and Related Disorders* 60 (2019): 43–5, https://doi.org/10.1016/j.parkreldis.2018.09.032.

115. Susanne Fonseca Santos et al., "The Gut and Parkinson's Disease—A Bidirectional Pathway," *Frontiers in Neurology* 10 (2019): 574, https://doi.org/10.3389/fneur.2019.00574.

116. Bryan A. Killinger et al., "The Vermiform Appendix Impacts the Risk of Developing Parkinson's Disease," *Science Translational Medicine* 10, no. 465 (2018): eaar5280, https://doi.org/10.1126/scitranslmed.aar5280.

117. Agata Mulak and Bruno Bonaz, "Brain-Gut-Microbiota Axis in Parkinson's Disease," *World Journal of Gastroenterology* 21, no. 37 (2015): 10609–20, https://doi.org/10.3748/wjg.v21.i37.10609.

118. Katherine C. Hughes et al., "Intake of Dairy Foods and Risk of Parkinson Disease," *Neurology* 89, no. 1 (2017): 46–52, https://doi.org/10.1212/wnl.0000000000004057.

119. Alastair J. Noyce et al., "Meta-Analysis of Early Nonmotor Features and Risk Factors for Parkinson Disease," *Annals of Neurology* 72, no. 6 (2012): 893–901, https://doi.org/10.1002/ana.23687.

120. Susan Searles Nielsen et al., "Nicotine from Edible Solanaceae and Risk of Parkinson Disease," *Annals of Neurology* 74, no. 3 (2013): 472–7, https://doi.org/10.1002/ana.23884.

121. X. Gao et al., "Habitual Intake of Dietary Flavonoids and Risk of Parkinson Disease," *Neurology* 78, no. 15 (2012): 1138–45, https://doi.org/10.1212/wnl.0b013e31824f7fc4.

122. V. Chandra et al., "Incidence of Alzheimer's Disease in a Rural Community in India: The Indo-US Study," *Neurology* 57, no. 6 (2001): 985–9, https://doi.org/10.1212/wnl.57.6.985.

123. Topiwala et al., "Moderate Alcohol Consumption as Risk Factor for Adverse Brain Outcomes."

124. Annelien C. van den Brink et al., "The Mediterranean, Dietary Approaches to Stop Hypertension (DASH), and Mediterranean-DASH Intervention for Neuro-degenerative Delay (MIND) Diets Are Associated with Less Cognitive Decline and a Lower Risk of Alzheimer's Disease—A Review," *Advances in Nutrition* 10, no. 6 (2019): 1040–65, https://doi.org/10.1093/advances/nmz054.

125. Martha Clare Morris et al., "MIND Diet Slows Cognitive Decline with Aging," *Alzheimer's and Dementia* 11, no. 9 (2015): 1015–22, https://doi.org/10.1016/j .jalz.2015.04.011.

126. Elizabeth E. Devore et al., "Dietary Intakes of Berries and Flavonoids in Relation to Cognitive Decline," *Annals of Neurology* 72, no. 1 (2012): 135–43, https://doi .org/10.1002/ana.23594.

127. Qi Dai et al., "Fruit and Vegetable Juices and Alzheimer's Disease: The Kame Project," *American Journal of Medicine* 119, no. 9 (2006): 751–9, https://doi.org /10.1016/j.amjmed.2006.03.045.

128. Haroon Khan et al., "Neuroprotective Effects of Quercetin in Alzheimer's Dis-ease," *Biomolecules* 10, no. 1 (2020): 59, https://doi.org/10.3390/biom10010059.

129. Daniela Mastroiacovo et al., "Cocoa Flavanol Consumption Improves Cognitive Function, Blood Pressure Control, and Metabolic Profile in Elderly Subjects: The Cocoa, Cognition, and Aging (CoCoA) Study—A Randomized Controlled Trial," *American Journal of Clinical Nutrition* 101, no. 3 (2015): 538–48, https:// doi.org/10.3945/ajcn.114.092189.

130. Marco Cascella et al., "The Efficacy of Epigallocatechin-3-Gallate (Green Tea) in the Treatment of Alzheimer's Disease: An Overview of Pre-Clinical Studies and Translational Perspectives in Clinical Practice," *Infectious Agents and Cancer* 12 (2017): 36, https://doi.org/10.1186/s13027-017-0145-6.

131. Balu Muthaiyah et al., "Dietary Supplementation of Walnuts Improves Memory Deficits and Learning Skills in Transgenic Mouse Model of Alzheimer's Disease," *Journal of Alzheimer's Disease* 42, no. 4 (2014): 1397–405, https://doi.org/10.3233 /jad-140675.

132. Abha Chauhan and Ved Chauhan, "Beneficial Effects of Walnuts on Cognition and Brain Health," *Nutrients* 12, no. 2 (2020): 550, https://doi.org/10.3390/nu12020550.

133. Long Tan et al., "Investigation on the Role of BDNF in the Benefits of Blueberry Extracts for the Improvement of Learning and Memory in Alzheimer's Disease Mouse Model," *Journal of Alzheimer's Disease* 56, no. 2 (2017): 629–40, https:// doi.org/10.3233/jad-151108.

134. Devore et al., "Dietary Intakes of Berries and Flavonoids in Relation to Cognitive Decline."

135. Ting-Ting Hou et al., "Sulforaphane Inhibits the Generation of Amyloid-β Oligomer and Promotes Spatial Learning and Memory in Alzheimer's Disease (PS1V97L) Transgenic Mice," *Journal of Alzheimer's Disease* 62, no. 4 (2018): 1803–13, https://doi.org/10.3233/jad-171110.

136. Shahin Akhondzadeh et al., "A 22-Week, Multicenter, Randomized, Double-Blind Controlled Trial of Crocus Sativus in the Treatment of Mild-to-Moderate

Alzheimer's Disease," *Psychopharmacology* 207, no. 4 (2010): 637–43, https://doi
.org/10.1007/s00213-009-1706-1.

137. K. Prehn et al., "Caloric Restriction in Older Adults—Differential Effects of
Weight Loss and Reduced Weight on Brain Structure and Function," *Cerebral
Cortex* 27, no. 3 (2017): 1765–78, https://doi.org/10.1093/cercor/bhw008.

138. M. Mattson and R. Wan, "Beneficial Effects of Intermittent Fasting and Caloric
Restriction on the Cardiovascular and Cerebrovascular Systems," *Journal of Nutritional Biochemistry* 16, no. 3 (2005): 129–37, https://doi.org/10.1016/j.jnutbio
.2004.12.007.

139. Susan T. Mayne, Mary C. Playdon, and Cheryl L. Rock, "Diet, Nutrition, and
Cancer: Past, Present and Future," *Nature Reviews Clinical Oncology* 13, no. 8
(2016): 504–15, https://doi.org/10.1038/nrclinonc.2016.24.

140. Estefanía Toledo et al., "Mediterranean Diet and Invasive Breast Cancer Risk Among
Women at High Cardiovascular Risk in the PREDIMED Trial," *JAMA Internal
Medicine* 175, no. 11 (2015): 1752–60, https://doi.org/10.1001/jamainternmed
.2015.4838.

141. Michel de Lorgeril et al., "Mediterranean Dietary Pattern in a Randomized Trial,"
Archives of Internal Medicine 158, no. 11 (1998): 1181–7, https://doi.org/10.1001
/archinte.158.11.1181.

142. Mingyang Song et al., "Association of Animal and Plant Protein Intake with All-
Cause and Cause-Specific Mortality."

143. Levine et al., "Low Protein Intake Is Associated with a Major Reduction in IGF-
1, Cancer, and Overall Mortality."

144. Li Jiao et al., "Dietary Consumption of Advanced Glycation End Products and
Pancreatic Cancer in the Prospective NIH-AARP Diet and Health Study," *American Journal of Clinical Nutrition* 101, no. 1 (2015): 126–34, https://doi.org/10.3945
/ajcn.114.098061.

145. Willett and Ludwig, "Milk and Health."

146. Mayne, Playdon, and Rock, "Diet, Nutrition, and Cancer."

147. Rowan T. Chlebowski et al., "Low-Fat Dietary Pattern and Breast Cancer Mortality in the Women's Health Initiative Randomized Controlled Trial," *Journal of
Clinical Oncology* 35, no. 25 (2017): 2919–26, https://doi.org/10.1200/jco.2016
.72.0326.

148. Kyle B. Zuniga et al., "Diet and Lifestyle Considerations for Patients with Prostate
Cancer," *Urologic Oncology* 38, no. 3 (2020): 105–17, https://doi.org/10.1016
/j.urolonc.2019.06.018.

149. Temidayo Fadelu et al., "Nut Consumption and Survival in Patients With Stage
III Colon Cancer: Results From CALGB 89803 (Alliance)," *Journal of Clinical
Oncology* 36, no. 11 (2018): 1112–20, https://doi.org/10.1200/jco.2017.75.5413.

150. Yu Ma et al., "Dietary Fiber Intake and Risks of Proximal and Distal Colon
Cancers," *Medicine* 97, no. 36 (2018): e11678, https://doi.org/10.1097/md
.0000000000011678.

151. Erin L. Richman et al., "Intakes of Meat, Fish, Poultry, and Eggs and Risk of
Prostate Cancer Progression," *American Journal of Clinical Nutrition* 91, no. 3
(2010): 712–21, https://doi.org/10.3945/ajcn.2009.28474.

152. Griswold et al., "Alcohol Use and Burden for 195 Countries and Territories, 1990–2016."

153. Griswold et al., "Alcohol Use."

154. Richard Béliveau, Denis Gingras, and Barbara Sandilands, *Foods That Fight Cancer: Preventing Cancer Through Diet* (Buffalo, NY: Firefly Books, 2016).

155. Valter D. Longo, Michael R. Lieber, and Jan Vijg, "Turning Anti-Ageing Genes Against Cancer," *Nature Reviews Molecular Cell Biology* 9, no. 11 (2008): 903–10, https://doi.org/10.1038/nrm2526.

156. Longo, Lieber, and Vijg, "Turning Anti-Ageing Genes Against Cancer."

157. Lizzia Raffaghello et al., "Fasting and Differential Chemotherapy Protection in Patients," *Cell Cycle* 9, no. 22 (2010): 4474–6, https://doi.org/10.4161/cc.9.22.13954.

158. Bauersfeld et al., "The Effects of Short-Term Fasting on Quality of Life and Tolerance to Chemotherapy."

159. Nencioni et al., "Fasting and Cancer."

160. Wei et al., "Fasting-Mimicking Diet and Markers/Risk Factors for Aging."

161. Catherine R. Marinac et al., "Prolonged Nightly Fasting and Breast Cancer Prognosis," *JAMA Oncology* 2, no. 8 (2016): 1049–55, https://doi.org/10.1001/jamaoncol.2016.0164.

162. Bauersfeld et al., "The Effects of Short-Term Fasting on Quality of Life and Tolerance to Chemotherapy."

163. Madeo et al., "Spermidine in Health and Disease."

164. Madeo et al., "Spermidine Delays Aging in Humans."

165. Kiechl et al., "Higher Spermidine Intake Is Linked to Lower Mortality."

166. Miranka Wirth et al., "The Effect of Spermidine on Memory Performance in Older Adults at Risk for Dementia: A Randomized Controlled Trial," *Cortex* 109 (2018): 181–8, https://doi.org/10.1016/j.cortex.2018.09.014.

167. Chisato Nagata et al., "Association of Dietary Fat, Vegetables and Antioxidant Micronutrients with Skin Ageing in Japanese Women," *British Journal of Nutrition* 103, no. 10 (2010): 1493–8, https://doi.org/10.1017/s0007114509993461.

168. Katherine M. Appleton et al., "The Value of Facial Attractiveness for Encouraging Fruit and Vegetable Consumption: Analyses from a Randomized Controlled Trial," *BMC Public Health* 18 (2018): 298, https://doi.org/10.1186/s12889-018-5202-6.

169. Yuhi Saito et al., "Effects of Intake of Lactobacillus Casei Subsp. Casei 327 on Skin Conditions: A Randomized, Double-Blind, Placebo-Controlled, Parallel-Group Study in Women," *Bioscience of Microbiota, Food and Health* 36, no. 3 (2017): 111–20, https://doi.org/10.12938/bmfh.16-031.

170. K. Miyazaki et al., "Bifidobacterium Fermented Milk and Galacto-Oligosaccharides Lead to Improved Skin Health by Decreasing Phenols Production by Gut Microbiota," *Beneficial Microbes* 5, no. 2 (2014): 121–8, https://doi.org/10.3920/bm2012.0066.

171. Talita Pizza Anunciato Pedro Alves da Rocha Filho, "Carotenoids and Polyphenols in Nutricosmetics, Nutraceuticals, and Cosmeceuticals," *Journal of Cosmetic Dermatology* 11, no. 1 (2012): 51–4, https://doi.org/10.1111/j.1473-2165.2011.00600.x.

172. Wioleta Grabowska, Ewa Sikora, and Anna Bielak-Zmijewska, "Sirtuins, a Promising Target in Slowing Down the Ageing Process," *Biogerontology* 18, no. 4 (2017): 447–76, https://doi.org/10.1007/s10522-017-9685-9.

173. Yong-Ru Chen et al., "Calorie Restriction on Insulin Resistance and Expression of SIRT1 and SIRT4 in Rats," *Biochemistry and Cell Biology* 88, no. 4 (2010): 715–22, https://doi.org/10.1139/o10-010.

174. Frank Madeo et al., "Caloric Restriction Mimetics Against Age-Associated Disease: Targets, Mechanisms, and Therapeutic Potential," *Cell Metabolism* 29, no. 3 (2019): 592–610, https://doi.org/10.1016/j.cmet.2019.01.018.

COVID-19

175. Stephen S. Morse et al., "Prediction and Prevention of the Next Pandemic Zoonosis," *Lancet* 380, no. 9857 (2012): 1956–65, https://doi.org/10.1016/s0140-6736(12)61684-5.

176. Felicia Keesing et al., "Impacts of Biodiversity on the Emergence and Transmission of Infectious Diseases," *Nature* 468, no. 7324 (2010): 647–52, https://doi.org/10.1038/nature09575.

177. Toph Allen et al., "Global Hotspots and Correlates of Emerging Zoonotic Diseases," *Nature Communications* 8, no. 1 (2017): 1124, https://doi.org/10.1038/s41467-017-00923-8.

178. Kate E. Jones et al., "Global Trends in Emerging Infectious Diseases," *Nature* 451, no. 7181 (2008): 990–3, https://doi.org/10.1038/nature06536.

179. Annemarie B. Docherty et al., "Features of 16,749 Hospitalised UK Patients with COVID-19 Using the ISARIC WHO Clinical Characterisation Protocol" (2020), https://doi.org/10.1101/2020.04.23.20076042.

180. Jennifer Lighter et al., "Obesity in Patients Younger Than 60 Years Is a Risk Factor for COVID-19 Hospital Admission," *Clinical Infectious Diseases* (2020): ciaa415, https://doi.org/10.1093/cid/ciaa415.

181. Qingxian Cai et al., "Obesity and COVID-19 Severity in a Designated Hospital in Shenzhen, China" *Diabetes Care* 43, no. 7 (2020): 1392–8, https://doi.org/10.2337/dc20-0576.

182. F. Eichelmann et al., "Effect of Plant-Based Diets on Obesity-Related Inflammatory Profiles: A Systematic Review and Meta-Analysis of Intervention Trials," *Obesity Reviews* 17, no. 11 (2016): 1067–79, https://doi.org/10.1111/obr.12439.

183. Naveed Sattar, Iain B. McInnes, and John J. V. McMurray, "Obesity a Risk Factor for Severe COVID-19 Infection: Multiple Potential Mechanisms," *Circulation* (2020), https://doi.org/10.1161/circulationaha.120.047659.

184. Choi, Lee, and Longo, "Nutrition and Fasting Mimicking Diets."

185. Daniela Martini, "Health Benefits of Mediterranean Diet," *Nutrients* 11, no. 8 (2019): 1802, https://doi.org/10.3390/nu11081802.

186. Fontana and Partridge, "Promoting Health and Longevity Through Diet."

187. Sameera A. Talegawkar et al., "A Higher Adherence to a Mediterranean-Style Diet Is Inversely Associated with the Development of Frailty in Community-Dwelling

Elderly Men and Women," *Journal of Nutrition* 142, no. 12 (2012): 2161–6, https://doi.org/10.3945/jn.112.165498.

188. Henry Redel and Bruce Polsky, "Nutrition, Immunity and Infection," in Mandell, Douglas, and Bennett, *Principles and Practice of Infectious Diseases*, vol. 2, 9th ed., ed. John Bennett, Raphael Dolin, and Martin J. Blaser (Philadelphia: Elsevier, 2019), 4328.

189. Andrew Gibson et al., "Effect of Fruit and Vegetable Consumption on Immune Function in Older People: A Randomized Controlled Trial," *American Journal of Clinical Nutrition* 96, no. 6 (2012): 1429–36, https://doi.org/10.3945/ajcn.112 .039057.

190. Jürgen Reichling et al., "Essential Oils of Aromatic Plants with Antibacterial, Antifungal, Antiviral, and Cytotoxic Properties—An Overview," *Forschende Komplementärmedizin/Research in Complementary Medicine* 16, no. 2 (2009): 79– 90, https://doi.org/10.1159/000207196.

191. M. E. Gershwin, J. B. German, and C. L. Keen, *Nutrition and Immunology: Principles and Practice* (Berlin: Springer Science & Business Media, 1999).

192. Reichling et al., "Essential Oils of Aromatic Plants."

193. Chih-Chun Wen et al., "Specific Plant Terpenoids and Lignoids Possess Potent Antiviral Activities Against Severe Acute Respiratory Syndrome Coronavirus," *Journal of Medicinal Chemistry* 50, no. 17 (2007): 4087–95, https://doi.org/10.1021 /jm070295s.

194. H. Hemilä and E. Chalker, "Vitamin C as a Possible Therapy for COVID-19," *Infection and Chemotherapy* 52, no. 2 (2020): e22, https://icjournal.org/Synapse /Data/PDFData/0086IC/ic-52-c22.pdf.

195. Kazuke Ide et al., "Anti-Influenza Virus Effects of Catechins: A Molecular and Clinical Review," *Current Medicinal Chemistry* 23, no. 42 (2016): 4773–83, https://doi.org/10.2174/0929867324666161123091010.

196. Muhareva Raekiansyah et al., "Inhibitory Effect of the Green Tea Molecule EGCG Against Dengue Virus Infection," *Archives of Virology* 163, no. 6 (2018): 1649–55, https://doi.org/10.1007/s00705-018-3769-y.

197. Daisuke Furushima, Kazuki Ide, and Hiroshi Yamada, "Effect of Tea Catechins on Influenza Infection and the Common Cold with a Focus on Epidemiological /Clinical Studies," *Molecules* 23, no. 7 (2018): 1795, https://doi.org/10.3390 /molecules23071795.

198. Elisa Fanunza et al., "Quercetin Blocks Ebola Virus Infection by Counteracting the VP24 Interferon Inhibitory Function," *Antimicrobial Agents and Chemotherapy* 64, no. 7 (2020): e00530-20, https://doi.org/10.1128/aac.00530-20.

199. Gaber El-Saber Batiha et al., "The Pharmacological Activity, Biochemical Properties, and Pharmacokinetics of the Major Natural Polyphenolic Flavonoid: Quercetin," *Foods* 9, no. 3 (2020): 374, https://doi.org/10.3390/foods9030374.

200. Scott A. Read et al., "The Role of Zinc in Antiviral Immunity," *Advances in Nutrition* 10, no. 4 (2019): 696–710, https://doi.org/10.1093/advances/nmz013.

201. Kazuo Yamagata et al., "Dietary Apigenin Reduces Induction of LOX-1 and NLRP3 Expression, Leukocyte Adhesion, and Acetylated Low-Density Lipoprotein Uptake in Human Endothelial Cells Exposed to Trimethylamine-N-Oxide,"

Journal of Cardiovascular Pharmacology 74, no. 6 (2019): 558–65, https://doi.org /10.1097/fjc.0000000000000747.

202. Venkidasamy Baskar, Se Won Park, and Shivraj Hariram Nile, "An Update on Potential Perspectives of Glucosinolates on Protection Against Microbial Pathogens and Endocrine Dysfunctions in Humans," *Critical Reviews in Food Science and Nutrition* 56, no. 13 (2016): 2231–49, https://doi.org/10.1080/10408398 .2014.910748.

203. Siti Khaerunnisa et al., "Potential Inhibitor of COVID-19 Main Protease (Mpro) from Several Medicinal Plant Compounds by Molecular Docking Study," (2020), https://doi.org/10.20944/preprints202003.0226.v1.

204. Bui Thi Phuong Thuy et al., "Investigation into SARS-CoV-2 Resistance of Compounds in Garlic Essential Oil," *ACS Omega* 5, no. 14 (2020): 8312–20, https:// doi.org/10.1021/acsomega.0c00772.

205. Ranil Jayawardena et al., "Enhancing Immunity in Viral Infections, with Special Emphasis on COVID-19: A Review," *Diabetes and Metabolic Syndrome* 14, no. 4 (2020): 367–82, https://doi.org/10.1016/j.dsx.2020.04.015.

206. Jessie Hawkins et al., "Black Elderberry (Sambucus Nigra) Supplementation Effectively Treats Upper Respiratory Symptoms: A Meta-Analysis of Randomized, Controlled Clinical Trials," *Complementary Therapies in Medicine* 42 (2019): 361–5, https://doi.org/10.1016/j.ctim.2018.12.004.

207. Z. Zakay-Rones et al., "Randomized Study of the Efficacy and Safety of Oral Elderberry Extract in the Treatment of Influenza A and B Virus Infections," *Journal of International Medical Research* 32, no. 2 (2004): 132–40, https://doi.org /10.1177/147323000403200205.

208. Evelin Tiralongo, Shirley Wee, and Rodney Lea, "Elderberry Supplementation Reduces Cold Duration and Symptoms in Air-Travellers: A Randomized, Double-Blind Placebo-Controlled Clinical Trial," *Nutrients* 8, no. 4 (2016): 182, https:// doi.org/10.3390/nu8040182.

209. Jing-Ru Weng et al., "Antiviral Activity of Sambucus FormosanaNakai Ethanol Extract and Related Phenolic Acid Constituents Against Human Coronavirus NL63," *Virus Research* 273 (2019): 197767, https://doi.org/10.1016/j.virusres.2019 .197767.

210. Brandhorst et al., "A Periodic Diet That Mimics Fasting Promotes Multi-System Regeneration."

211. Cheng et al., "Prolonged Fasting Reduces IGF-1/PKA."

212. Beth Newcomb, "What and When We Eat Affects Our Immune System. Here's How," USC Leonard Davis School of Gerontology, https://gero.usc.edu/2020/04 /22/fasting-mimicking-diet-immune-system-function.

213. Newcomb, "What and When We Eat Affects Our Immune System."

214. Andrew Wang et al., "Opposing Effects of Fasting Metabolism on Tissue Tolerance in Bacterial and Viral Inflammation," *Cell* 166, no. 6 (2016): 1512–25.e12, https://doi.org/10.1016/j.cell.2016.07.026.

215. Emily L. Goldberg et al., "Ketogenic Diet Activates Protective $\Gamma\delta$ T Cell Responses Against Influenza Virus Infection," *Science Immunology* 4, no. 41 (2019):eaav2026, https://doi.org/10.1126/sciimmunol.aav2026.

216. Nathalie Le Floc'h et al., "Effect of Feed Restriction on Performance and Post-prandial Nutrient Metabolism in Pigs Co-Infected with Mycoplasma Hyopneu-moniae and Swine Influenza Virus," *PLoS One* 9, no. 8 (2014): e104605, https://doi.org/10.1371/journal.pone.0104605.

217. Nils C. Gassen et al., "SKP2 Attenuates Autophagy Through Beclin1-Ubiquitination and Its Inhibition Reduces MERS-Coronavirus Infection," *Nature Communications* 10, no. 1 (2019): 5770, https://doi.org/10.1038/s41467-019-13659-4.

218. Nils C. Gassen et al., "Analysis of SARS-CoV-2-Controlled Autophagy Reveals Spermidine, MK-2206, and Niclosamide as Putative Antiviral Therapeutics" (2020), https://doi.org/10.1101/2020.04.15.997254.

219. Michela Silvestri and Giovanni A. Rossi, "Melatonin: Its Possible Role in the Management of Viral Infections—A Brief Review," *Italian Journal of Pediatrics* 39 (2013): 61, https://doi.org/10.1186/1824-7288-39-61.

220. Rüdiger Hardeland, "Aging, Melatonin, and the Pro- and Anti-Inflammatory Networks," *International Journal of Molecular Sciences* 20, no. 5 (2019): 1223, https://doi.org/10.3390/ijms20051223.

Index